EDUCATION AND HIV/AIDS

A Sourcebook of HIV/AIDS Prevention Programs

Contents

Acronyms

ACESS	Alliance for Children's Entitlement to Social Security
ACI	Africa Consultants International
AIC	AIDS Information Centre
AIDS	acquired immunodeficiency syndrome
AIDSCAP	AIDS Control and Prevention Project
AIDSCOM	AIDS Technical Support: Public Health Communication Component
AMREF	African Medical and Research Foundation
AMODEFA	*Associacão Mozambican para Defesa da Familia*
ANC	antenatal clinic
ARVs	antiretrovirals
ASRH	adolescent sexual and reproductive health
BBC	British Broadcasting Corporation
BP	British Petroleum
CAA	Community AIDS Abroad
CBD	community-based distributor
CBO	community-based organization
CBoH	Central Board of Health
CEO	chief executive officer
CEFOREP	*Centre de Formation et de Recherche en Santé de la Reproduction*
CHEP	Copperbelt Health Education Project
CIDA/SAT	Southern African Training Program
CINDI	Children in Distress (project)
COIN	*Centre d'Orientation et d'Information des Jeunes* (Youth Corner)
CPDs	condom promoters and distributors
CRDI	*Centre de Recherche pour le Développement International*
CRETF	*Centre Régional d'Enseignement Technique Féminin*
CTA	chief technical adviser
DAAC	District AIDS Action Committee
DAC	development assistance committee
DANIDA	Danish International Development Agency
DEO	District Education Officer
DFID	Department for International Development (United Kingdom)
DHMT	district health management team
DoE	Department of Education
DoH	Department of Health

DPE	disease prevention education
DSW	German Foundation for World Population
EDF	European Development Fund
EFS	*économie familiale et sociale* (social and family economics)
EJAF	Elton John AIDS Foundation
EMP	*éducation en matière de population* (population education)
EU	European Union
EVF	*éducation à la vie familiale* (family life education)
EPS	*éducation pour la santé* (health education)
FHT	Family Health Trust
FLE	family life education
FLMZ	Family Life Movement of Zambia
FNUAP	*Fonds des Nations Unies pour la Population* (United Nations Population Fund)
FRESH	Focusing Resources on Effective School and Health
GEEP	*Groupe pour l'Etude et l'Enseignement de la Population* (Group for the Study and Teaching of Population Issues)
GPA	Global Programme on AIDS
GTZ	*Deutsche Gesellschaft für Technische Zusammenarbeit* (German Agency for Technical Cooperation)
HALIRA	Health and Lifestyle Research
HIV	human immunodeficiency virus
HST	Health Systems Trust
IATT	Inter-Agency Task Team
IBE	International Bureau of Education
ICT	information communication technology
IDRC	International Development Research Centre
IEC	information, education, and communication
IIED	International Institute for Environment and Development
IIEP	International Institute for Educational Planning
INDE	*Institute Nacional de Desenvolvimento Educacional* (National Institute of Educational Development)
IPPF	International Planned Parenthood Foundation
IT	information technology
KAB	knowledge, attitudes, and behavior
KABP	knowledge, attitudes, behavior, and practices
KAP	knowledge, attitudes, and practice
KAPB	knowledge, attitudes, practices, and beliefs
KARHP	Kafue Adolescent Reproductive Health Project
KASH	knowledge, attitudes, skills, and habits
LSE	life skills education
LSHTM	London School of Hygiene and Tropical Medicine
MASO	Midlands AIDS Service Organisation
MBOD	Medical Bureau for Occupational Diseases
MFD	Media for Development
MoE	Ministry of Education
MoEC	Ministry of Education and Culture
MoH	Ministry of Health

MoYS	Ministry of Youth and Sport
MPH	Master's Degree in Public Health (degree)
MTCT	mother-to-child transmission
MTN	Mobile Telephone Network
NACP	National AIDS Control Program
NAFCI	National Adolescent Friendly Clinic Initiative
NASHI	National Adolescent Sexual Health Initiative
NCRC	National Children's Rights Committee
NGO	nongovernmental organization
NIMR	National Institute for Medical Research
NORAD	Norwegian Agency for Development Cooperation
NPA	National Plan of Action
NSHP	National School Health Program
PDIS	*Programme de Développement Intégré de la Santé* (Integrated Health Development Program)
PEEP	Parent Elder Education Program
PHC	primary health care
PNLS	*Programme Nationale de Lutte contre le SIDA* (National Program for the Fight Against AIDS)
PNPF	National Family Planning Programme
PPASA	Planned Parenthood Association of South Africa
PPAZ	Planned Parenthood Association of Zambia
PPP	peer, parent, and provider
PSG	project support group
PSI/CMS	Population Services International
PTA	Parent-Teacher Association
PTC	Prevention Training Centres
PWAs	persons living with AIDS
RFSU	Swedish Association for Sexuality Education
RHRU	Reproductive Health Research Unit
SABC	South Africa Broadcasting Corporation
SAFAIDS	Southern Africa AIDS Information Dissemination Service
SANASO	Southern Africa AIDS Network
SCF	Save the Children Fund
SCI	Sara Communication Initiative
SDC	Swiss Agency for Development and Cooperation
SHEP	School Health Education Program
SIDA	Swedish International Development Authority
SPW	Students Partnership Worldwide
SRH	sexual and reproductive health
STD	sexually transmitted disease
STF	Straight Talk Foundation
STI	sexually transmitted infection
SYFA	Safeguard Youth from AIDS
TA	technical adviser
TAMWA	The Tanzania Media Women's Association
TANESA	Tanzania Netherlands Support for AIDS

TASO	The AIDS Support Organisation
TOP	trainer of peers
TOT	trainer of trainers
TSh	Tanzanian shilling(s)
UMATI	National Family Planning Association
UNAIDS	Joint United Nations Programme on HIV/AIDS
UNDP	United Nations Development Programme
UNESCO	United Nations Educational, Scientific, and Cultural Organization
UNFPA	United Nations Population Fund
UNICEF	United Nations Children's Fund
UNIFEM	United Nations Development Fund for Women
USAID	United States Agency for International Development
US	Ugandan shilling(s)
VCT	voluntary counseling and testing
WHO	World Health Organization
YCDG	youth community development group
YDC	Youth Development Centre
YFHS	youth-friendly health service
YFM	Youth FM
YWCA	Young Women's Christian Association
ZD	Zimbabwean dollar(s)
ZECAB	Zambia Educational Capacity Building Program
ZIHP	Zambia Integrated Health Program

Acknowledgments

This document was prepared by members of the World Bank's education team led by Alexandria Valerio and Don Bundy, with technical support from Helen Baños Smith, Katie Tripp, and Lesley Drake (Partnership for Child Development, Department of Infectious Disease Epidemiology, Imperial College, United Kingdom), and Seung-Hee F. Lee (World Bank). We appreciated the leadership and overall support of Birger Fredriksen, Ruth Kagia, Debrework Zewdie, Oey Meesook, Keith Hansen, and Dzingai Mutumbuka (World Bank). Production of the *Sourcebook* was supported by Development Cooperation Ireland.

We are grateful to El Hadji Habib Camara, Glynis Clacherty, David Kaweesa, Esther Kazilimani-Pale, Adeline Kimambo, Anne Salmi, and Evelyn Serima for collecting the data and writing drafts of the program reports. We also thank Carolien Albers, Nicola Brennan, Ebrahim Jassat, Kevin Kelly, Michael Kelly, Dr. Kiwara, Nicole McHugh, Pronch Murray, Warren Naamara, Justin Nguma, and Malick Semebene for providing their expert advice and guidance in the participating countries.

Many other people have contributed to discussions of the issues considered here and made contributions to the reviewing process: David Clarke (Department for International Development, United Kingdom), Delia Barcelona (UNFPA), Amaya Gillespie (UNICEF), Michael Kelly (University of Zambia), Brad Strickland (United States Agency for International Development), Jack Jones (World Health Organization), Inon Schenker (UNESCO), and Carol Coombe (University of Pretoria, South Africa), and from the World Bank, Sheila Dutta, Hope Phillips, Elizabeth Lule, and Mercy Tembon.

We appreciated input from our partner agencies. Special thanks go to Christine Abbo (Straight Talk Foundation), Terry Allsop (Department for International Development, United Kingdom), Rita Badiani (Pathfinder International, Mozambique), Tara Bukow (UNESCO International Institute for Education Planning), Kevin Byrne (Save the Children, South Africa), Isabel Byron (UNESCO International Bureau of Education), Jim Cogan (Students Partnership Worldwide, United Kingdom), Mary Crewe (University of Pretoria, South Africa), Amy Cunningham (United States Agency for International Development), Babacar Fall (GEEP, Senegal), Craig Ferla (Students Partnership Worldwide, Tanzania), Laura Ferguson (AMREF, United Kingdom), Alexander Heroys (AMREF, United Kingdom), Anna-Marie Hoffman (UNESCO), Aida Girma (UNAIDS, Mozambique), Sue Goldstein (Soul City, South Africa), Simon Gregson (Imperial College, United Kingdom), Liz Higgins (Ireland Aid), Clement Jumbe (Ministry of Education, Sport and Culture, Zimbabwe), Virgilio Juvane (Ministry of Education, Mozambique), Gloria Kodzwa (UNICEF, Mozambique), Irene Malambo (Ministry of Education, Zambia), Peter Masika (Youth Aware, Tanzania), Kirsten Mitchell (GOAL, Uganda), Alick Nyirenda (CHEP, Zambia), Vera Pieroth (AMREF, Tanzania), Faye Richardson and David

Ross (London School of Hygiene and Tropical Medicine, United Kingdom), Berit Rylander (Swedish International Development Authority), Alfredo Santos (Action Aid, Mozambique), Bobby Soobrayan (Ministry of Education, South Africa), Angela Stewart-Buchanan (loveLife, South Africa), Kenau Swaru (Ministry of Health, South Africa), George Tembo (UNAIDS, Zimbabwe), Miriam Temin (Department for International Development, United Kingdom), Alan Whiteside (University of Natal, South Africa), and John Williamson (United States Agency for International Development), and from the World Bank, Jaap Bregman, Donald Hamilton, Cathal Higgins, Wacuka Ikua, Bruce Jones, Noel Kulemeka, Rest Lasway, Emmanuel Malangalila, Mmamtsetsa Marope, Paud Murphy, Khama Rogo, and Clement Siamatowe.

We thank Jess Lipson for technical input; the staff of Grammarians, Inc., for editing, design, and layout of the book; and Gillian Lonsdale and Bakary Diaby for their translation of the French into English.

Section 1:
About the *Sourcebook*

About the *Sourcebook*

The education sectors of affected countries are playing an increasingly important role in the fight against HIV/AIDS. In part this is a response to the dramatic impact of HIV/AIDS on education themselves, an impact that affects education supply, demand, and quality, which for many countries poses a major threat to the achievement of Education for All and of the Millennium Development Goals.

But the increasing role of education sectors is also a recognition that a good education is one of the most effective ways of helping young people to avoid HIV/AIDS. Children of school age have the lowest prevalence of infection, and even in the worst affected countries, the vast majority of schoolchildren are uninfected. For these children, there is a window of hope, a chance of a life free from AIDS if they can acquire the knowledge, skills, and values to help them protect themselves as they grow up. Providing young people with the "social vaccine" of education offers them a real chance of productive life (see *Education and HIV/AIDS: A Window of Hope* [World Bank 2002]).

This *Sourcebook* aims to support efforts by countries to strengthen the role of the education sector in the prevention of HIV/AIDS. It was developed in response to numerous requests for a simple forum to help countries share their practical experiences of designing and implementing programs that are targeted at school-age children. The *Sourcebook* seeks to fulfill this role by providing concise summaries of programs, using a standard format that highlights the main elements of the programs and makes it easier to compare the programs with each other.

For many countries, HIV/AIDS is a newly recognized challenge to the education sector, and as a result, very few programs have been in place long enough to be formally evaluated. Rather than delaying access to program information until success was confirmed, the *Sourcebook* combines two approaches to offer some assurance of program quality. First, the programs were selected by national experts because they show promise where they have been implemented. Second, all the programs were benchmarked against criteria that the Joint United Nations Programme on HIV/AIDS (UNAIDS) Inter-Agency Task Team (IATT) for Education considers to be sound programming practice. This provides a framework for exploring the strengths and weaknesses of the program design, pending more conclusive evaluation.

The *Sourcebook* has been developed rapidly to fill an important gap in information on programming within the education sector. It is a work in progress, and the content will be expanded and refined in use.

Objectives of the *Sourcebook*

The *Sourcebook* aims to document a variety of promising programs for school-age children in a user-friendly format. It will begin to build a database, which will be updated periodically, to offer some insight into what kinds of programs are running and what appears to be working.

The *Sourcebook* will provide an opportunity to share ideas on how programs may be re-contextualized to fit a variety of local circumstances; readers will be able to apply what they have learned from the reports.

Target Audience

The *Sourcebook* is intended to be relevant to anyone who is seeking to launch or improve an HIV/AIDS prevention program targeted at school-age children. By sharing practical experiences of HIV/AIDS prevention programs options, the *Sourcebook* can serve as the foundation for decisions to be made by education policymakers, planners, managers, and practitioners in government and in civil society.

The Format of the *Sourcebook*

All the programs are summarized in section 2, which allows those seeking advice on program design to browse through the various options and identify those that might reward further study. The full program reports for each country are given in section 3. Each program report follows the same format, so the reader can more easily find those aspects of the program that are of specific interest. The consistent design also allows for ease of comparison between programs.

There are four main sections within each full program report.

Part A: Description of the Program

This section gives an overview of the program, describing the rationale, the aims and objectives, the target audience, the components, and the main approaches.

Part B: Implementing the Program

This section describes the process from the initial needs assessment, through the development of materials and training, to the practical details of implementation. There is an attempt made to estimate unit costs, but these should be seen only as indicative, because the number of beneficiaries is often uncertain and because costs in newly implemented programs may be artificially high.

Part C: Assessment and Lessons Learned

This section begins with comments from implementers on the challenges faced and the lessons learned, followed in a few cases by a description of any formal evaluation of the program. The final part explores the extent to which the program complies with a set of benchmarks that, on the basis of expert opinion, contribute to an effective program. The benchmarks were adapted by the UNAIDS IATT from a United Nations Children's Fund (UNICEF) analysis, "Lessons Learned About School Based Approaches to Reducing HIV/AIDS Related Risk" (see Appendix 1).

Part D: Additional Information

This gives details of the organization(s) involved with the program, including their contact information. It lists all the materials that are available to the reader, along with an order code number. Please use the materials ordering form to obtain copies of these materials.

Country	Program Name	Program Type
Mozambique	Action Aid	Community based "stepping stones" approach
	UNFPA/Pathfinder International	Voluntary counseling and testing, peer education
Senegal	*Group pour l'Etude et l'Enseignement de la Population*	College- and secondary-school-level peer education, counseling
South Africa	loveLife	Mass media campaign
	Soul Buddyz	Television show, mass media campaign
Tanzania	Mema kwa Vijana	Primary-school-level peer education
	Student Partnership Worldwide	Secondary-school-level peer education
Uganda	GOAL: Baaba Project	Outreach program for street children
	Straight Talk	Newsletters, radio show
Zambia	Copperbelt Health Education Program	School clubs, community, behavior change through fun activities
	Kafue Adolescent Reproductive Health	School clubs, health clinics, peer education
Zimbabwe	Africare	Secondary-school clubs, income generation, peer education
	Midlands AIDS Service Organisation	Secondary-school clubs, counseling, peer education

Developing the *Sourcebook*

These steps were taken in each country to develop the *Sourcebook*:

- The *Sourcebook* concept was shared with government, civil society, donors, and other stakeholders.
- A focal point was identified to coordinate expert advice and identify which programs should be included in the *Sourcebook*.
- The candidate programs were visited, and one or two selected for each country, with the aim of including a diversity of approaches, activities, and target groups.
- Using a standardized questionnaire, a consultant interviewed program managers, implementers, and target groups and prepared a draft report.
- A review of available research, including "gray" literature, was undertaken and used to enrich the draft report.

- The draft report was edited into a standard format and sent to the program head for comments, and the final version of the report was added to the *Sourcebook*.

Availability of the *Sourcebook*

The *Sourcebook* is available electronically at http://www.schoolsandhealth.org or http://www.unesco.org/education/ibe/ichae.

Reports in French and Portuguese and in CD format are planned for the *Sourcebook*.

For further information or to order printed copies of the *Sourcebook* or CDs, contact the World Bank Education Advisory Service on the Web at http://www.worldbank.org/education.

By e-mail:
eservice@worldbank.org

By mail:
Education Advisory Service
The World Bank
1818 H Street, NW
Washington, DC 20433
USA

Section 2:
Program Summaries

Mozambique

Action Aid: Stepping Stones Program

Action Aid uses "Stepping Stones" methodology to target communities at risk of HIV/AIDS. This helps give communities skills and information so that they can respond to their own needs. It is based on the following principles:

- The best solutions are those developed by people themselves.
- Men and women each need private time and space with their peers to explore their own needs and concerns about relationships and sexual health.
- Behavior change is much more likely to be effective and sustained if the whole community is involved.

Therefore, the overall aim of the program is to enable individuals, their peers, and the community as a whole to change behavior individually and collectively.

In Maputo province, members of the community who have chosen to participate in the program meet once a week for Stepping Stones workshops. They are divided into four groups: young women, older women, young men, and older men. Trained facilitators use the *Stepping Stones Manual* as a guide to discuss topics of concern to the community, such as cultural and gender issues, relationships, and HIV/AIDS. Through drama, song, dance, and other participatory activities, issues are brought to the attention of the community and can then be discussed. Problems are identified, and the group members come up with realistic solutions, which are shared with the other groups. At the end of the workshops, a pledge is made to the community outlining changes that they promise to implement.

This year, if the trickle-down effect of the program is taken into consideration, an estimated 500,000 people have benefited from the program. The estimated cost of the program is US$0.30 per person per year. Of the 16 UNAIDS benchmarks for effective programs, the program was found to have successfully met 10 and partially met 4.

Mozambique

UNFPA and Pathfinder International: *Geração Biz*, Youth-Friendly Health Clinics

Geração Biz is the youth-friendly health service (YFHS) component of an integrated United Nations Population Fund (UNFPA)–Pathfinder International–government program that includes school- and community-based interventions. The overall aim of the program is to increase in- and out-of-school 15- to 24-year–olds' awareness of sexual and reproductive health issues and to encourage the adoption of safe, responsible, and gender-sensitive sexual and reproductive behavior. This report discusses the clinic-based component of the program (*Geração Biz*) that began in Maputo City, the capital of Mozambique, in 1999.

The overall aim of *Geração Biz* is to improve adolescents' access to sexual and reproductive health services through the development of specialized, youth-friendly clinical and counseling services. Youth are counseled on sexually transmitted diseases (STDs), contraception, condom use, and relationships. Nurses and doctors are trained in counseling skills that are accepting of youth. Peer educators visit the clinics to talk to young people about adopting safer sexual practices, as well as to give them information concerning HIV/AIDS.

In Maputo City, there are six YFHSs, with the biggest at the central hospital. The YFHSs are overseen by a UNFPA-Pathfinder International technical adviser who works closely with the Ministry of Health (MoH) counterpart and the clinic coordinators of the health centers.

In 2001, the program underwent an evaluation, resulting in 2002 in the program being expanded to the provinces of Maputo, Gaza, and Tete.

In the first year of the program, 1,173 youth used these services. In 2002, more than 11,000 young people used them. More than 91,550 condoms have been distributed. The estimated cost per person served is US$80.76. Of the 16 UNAIDS benchmarks for effective programs, the program has met 12 and partially met 3, and 1 was not applicable.

Senegal

The Group for the Study and Teaching of Population Issues (GEEP): An Experiment to Prevent the Spread of HIV/AIDS among Schoolchildren

The Group for the Study and Teaching of Population Issues (*Groupe pour l'Etude et l'Enseignement de la Population* [GEEP]) is a multidisciplinary, nonprofit, nongovernmental organization (NGO) created in May 1989. GEEP's initial strategy concentrated on two main areas: population education and family life education (FLE) clubs designed to bring population issues, notably sexual and reproductive health of adolescents, prevention of sexually transmitted diseases (STDs), and understanding of HIV/AIDS, into the classroom and to situate them within the framework of socioeducational and extracurricular activities.

In November 1994, GEEP launched a program entitled "Promotion of Family Life Education (FLE)" in middle and secondary schools in Senegal. The program targets teachers and 12- to 19-year-old pupils and aims to promote responsible sexual behavior through training activities, peer education, social mobilization, and provision of support materials and equipment (audiovisual and information technology).

After this, in response to a demand for information unmet by previous mass awareness campaigns, Youth Information and Advice Centers (*Centres d'Information et d'Orientation des Jeunes* [COIN-Jeunes]) were set up in some schools and at Cheikh University. These centers deal with reproductive health issues, STDs, and HIV/AIDS.

GEEP has benefited from the institutional, technical, and financial support of temporary and permanent partners, including government institutions (Ministries of Education, Health, Prevention, Economy, and Finance), foreign government agencies (United States Agency for International Development [USAID]), *Centre de Recherche pour le Développement International* [CRDI]), United Nations agencies (UNFPA, UNESCO, United Nations Development Fund for Women [UNIFEM]), and NGOs (Population Council, Rainbo, Club 2/3 Canada, Schools Online).

Of the 16 UNAIDS benchmarks for effective programs, the program has met 12 and partially met 3, and 1 was not applicable.

South Africa

loveLife: Promoting Sexual Health and Healthy Lifestyles for Young People in South Africa

Launched in September 1999, loveLife is one of the largest and most ambitious HIV prevention efforts in the world today. The program aims to reduce the incidence of HIV among 15- to 20-year-olds in South Africa by at least 50 percent over the next five years and is a brand-driven, comprehensive national program targeting 12- to 17-year-olds. It focuses on reducing the negative consequences of premature and adolescent sex by promoting sexual health and healthy lifestyles for young people.

The loveLife program is informed by the following imperatives:

- Education must deal with the broader context of sexual behavior.
- Condom use must become a normal part of youth culture.
- Education and prevention must be sustained over many years at a sufficient level of intensity to hold public attention.

Its program consists of three main components:

1. a media campaign that includes television, radio, and print advertising,
2. a social response that includes the establishment of youth centers and adolescent-friendly clinics, and
3. a research component that informs the development of the program and undertakes evaluation and monitoring.

All the activities emphasize that young people can make choices for a healthy lifestyle. In addition, the values of shared responsibility and positive sexuality are promoted. The behavioral goals of "delay, reduce, and protect" are also embedded in the media and other activities.

Evaluations of the first few years of implementation show that the program has been successful in raising sexual and reproductive health awareness among young people in South Africa. Youth are more aware of the risks of unprotected sex, and young people report that they have delayed having sexual relations or abstained from sex. In addition, they say that the program has created opportunities for them to talk about HIV/AIDS with their parents.

Of the 16 UNAIDS benchmarks for effective programs, the program was found to have successfully met 14 and partially met 1, and 1 was not applicable.

South Africa

Soul *Buddyz*: A Multimedia Edutainment Project for Children in South Africa

South Africa has one of the most extensive AIDS epidemics in the world, with 4.7 million people infected with HIV. It is the major cause of death in South Africa and is *the* national public health priority.

Soul *Buddyz* is a mass media edutainment vehicle for South African children aged 8 to 12, based on the successful Soul City adult vehicle. It is used to reach children with important messages about AIDS, youth sexuality, and gender.

The Soul *Buddyz* series was developed through an interactive process involving children; it consists of a 26-part television drama, a 26-part radio magazine program in three local languages, and a life skills book distributed to 1 million 12-year-olds. The series was accompanied by an advocacy campaign to reach policymakers and enrich NGOs' ability to act as child rights activists.

The evaluation of the series shows that 67 percent of South African children accessed Soul *Buddyz*. These children had increased knowledge, showed improved attitudes, and discussed the issues more than those who did not access the materials. Further, the materials improved parents' understanding and willingness to interact with children about such difficult issues as sex, AIDS, and gender.

The program costs approximately US$0.38 per child. It was found to have successfully met 14 and partially met 2 of the 16 UNAIDS benchmarks for effective programs.

Tanzania

AMREF, LSHTM, and NIMR: MEMA Kwa Vijana Program

The African Medical and Research Foundation (AMREF), in collaboration with the London School of Hygiene and Tropical Medicine (LSHTM) and the (Tanzanian) National Institute for Medical Research (NIMR), initiated a program in 62 primary schools and 18 health facilities in Mwanza region of Tanzania in January 1999.

Its main objective was to improve reproductive health knowledge among 12- to 19-year-olds and decrease the rate of sexually transmitted infections (STIs) and HIV infection as well as the number of unwanted pregnancies. To do this, teacher-led peer educators use informal and participatory techniques to teach young people about reproductive health. Health workers are also trained to make health services more youth friendly, and the community is mobilized to participate in Youth Health Weeks, which are held once a year.

The program reaches approximately 2,850 new adolescent participants a year, at an estimated cost of US$1.37 per child per year. Of the 16 UNAIDS benchmarks for effective programs, the program was found to have successfully met 13 and partially met 2, and 1 was not applicable.

Tanzania

Students Partnership Worldwide: School Health Education Program (SHEP)

Students Partnership Worldwide (SPW) is a nonprofit NGO whose aim is to make young people central to the development process. Working under the Tanzanian Ministry of Education and Culture, SPW Tanzania advocates that young people have much to offer, and their age can be an advantage when discussing sensitive issues.

Currently, SPW Tanzania has just completed its third year of implementing a Demonstration Model of School Health Education in 35 secondary schools in all seven districts of Iringa region. The program trains and deploys 18- to 25-year-old Tanzanians and Europeans as peer educators in the frontline of a schools-based campaign to mobilize young people against HIV/AIDS. The peer educators use participatory activities in both the classroom and extracurricular activities to educate students in adolescent sexual and reproductive health (ASRH). They also work toward facilitating easier access to youth-friendly services, both within and outside the school.

These appropriately trained, committed, and well-educated young peer educators are proving very effective in challenging the culture of stigma and denial among the older generation and also in effecting the necessary behavior change through exerting a positive influence among their younger peers. The students exposed to the School Health Education Program (SHEP) can also educate their own peers, both in and out of school, as well as older generations.

So far, approximately 16,250 students have benefited from the program at an estimated cost of US$24.12 per student per year. However, it should be noted that 15,000 adults have also benefited, along with a huge number of other school-aged children and adults in the community. The program was found to have successfully met 11 and partially met 5 of the 16 UNAIDS benchmarks for effective programs.

Uganda

GOAL: The Baaba Project

The Baaba project aims to promote the sexual and reproductive health of street children by providing training, resources, and ongoing technical and financial support to NGOs working with these children.

Established in January 2001, the project builds partnerships with NGOs catering for the immediate and longer-term needs of street children. The project adopts a nonjudgmental and life skills approach in tackling HIV/AIDS prevention and other issues such as growing up, sexual relationships, drug abuse, and rape.

In the local Luganda language, *baaba* is the term for a respected older sibling. Baabas are peer educators who teach fellow street children about HIV/AIDS. The Baaba project seeks to empower youth from the streets and other disadvantaged youth with confidence, knowledge, and skills to prevent the spread of HIV. This is done in collaboration with existing NGOS that serve youth and street children in the towns of Kampala, Jinja, Malaba, Masaka, and Mbale. The project is currently working with 12 NGOs.

Project activities include peer education, outreach, NGO staff support, improving access to sexual and reproductive health clinics, and advocacy within the community.

The total cost of the project per year is US$92,703, with an approximate cost of US$18.50 per child per year. Of the 16 UNAIDS benchmarks for effective programs, the program was found to have successfully met 13 and partially met 1, and 2 were not applicable.

Uganda

Straight Talk Foundation

The Straight Talk Foundation has a print media and outreach campaign that began in 1993 with the *Straight Talk* newspaper. The overall aim of the program is to increase adolescents' (and adults') understanding of adolescent sexuality and reproductive health. It also aims to promote safer sex and the development of life skills, as well as to raise awareness of child and adolescent rights.

The program targets 10- to 14-year-olds with the *Young Talk* newspaper and 15- to 19-year-olds with the *Straight Talk* newspaper. Both newspapers are delivered to schools and appear as supplements in a national Sunday newspaper. *Young Talk* and *Straight Talk* are published monthly and discuss topics suggested by the readers themselves. They provide accurate and frank information and guidance on issues related to adolescent sexual and reproductive health (ASRH). *Straight Talk* also encourages young people (15- to 24-year–olds) and teachers to set up Straight Talk Clubs in schools to further advance the messages given in the newspapers. There is also a radio show targeted at 15- to 24–year-olds, which follows the themes of the newspapers, that broadcasts once a week in English and local languages.

The Straight Talk Foundation also carries out school visits by a team of health experts and counselors to help teachers and pupils devise a plan to make sure the adolescents remain healthy. They also conduct sensitization workshops with primary school teachers (and parents) to raise awareness of ASRH needs and services and to encourage them to discuss issues with young people.

An evaluation of the program has shown that the majority of adolescents have access to and read the newspapers and listen to the radio shows, and this is raising awareness of important ASRH issues. The Straight Talk program has directly responded to the information needs of adolescents, and its work is increasingly recognized and appreciated by the government.

The program was found to have succesfully met 14 of the 16 UNAIDS benchmarks for effective programs, and 2 were not applicable.

Zambia

Copperbelt Health Education Project (CHEP): The In-School Program

The Copperbelt Health Education Project (CHEP) focuses on health education and HIV/AIDS prevention in the Copperbelt province of Zambia. The project started in January 1988. The main focus during the first year was information dissemination to members of the general public on the dangers of HIV/AIDS, how it is transmitted and how to protect yourself and others against it.

CHEP's mission statement notes that the project collaborates with all sectors of the community to help develop knowledge, values, and life skills that enable creativity, responsibility, and healthy lifestyles. CHEP has focused its efforts by working under three specific target program units: Child and Youth-, Community-, and Occupation-Focused Units.

The Child and Youth-Focused Unit has three programs targeting children and youth in urban and rural areas: an in-school youth program, an out-of-school youth program, and a program for vulnerable children and other youths in the community.

The in-school program is CHEP's largest program in terms of reach and resources and, together with the out-of-school youth program, represents the core of CHEP's work. The in-school youth program comprises children and youth aged 3 to 35 years in preschools, basic schools, secondary/high schools, colleges, universities, as well as children with special needs. The main goal for the in-school program is to ensure that children and youth form and maintain behaviors that will not put them at risk of contracting STDs and HIV. The main components of the in-school program include Anti-AIDS Clubs, the Sara Communication Initiative, Education Through Entertainment, Games for Life, and youth-friendly health services.

Since its inception in 1988, CHEP has been funded mainly by the Norwegian Agency for Development Cooperation (NORAD). The estimated yearly cost of running this program is US$350,000. Of the 16 UNAIDS benchmarks for effective programs, the program was found to have successfully met 12 and partially met 2, and 2 were not aplicable.

Zambia

Planned Parenthood Association of Zambia (PPAZ), Family Life Movement of Zambia (FLMZ), and Swedish Association for Sexuality Education (RFSU): Kafue Adolescent Reproductive Health Project (KARHP), Peer Education through Family Life Education Clubs

KARHP is a multifaceted school-, community-, and clinic-based intervention that began in 1997 in the Kafue district of Zambia. The overall aim of the program is to develop strategies for the delivery of sexual and reproductive health (SRH) and family life education (FLE) information and services to in-school youth between 10 and 24 years of age. To achieve this, the program adopted an approach called "triple Ps": peers, parents, and providers. Trained peer educators, parent-elder educators, and health providers act as channels to deliver SRH and FLE information and services to in-school youth, as well as to mobilize and sensitize the wider community.

The main program component for in-school youth is the peer education program through FLE Clubs in the schools. FLE Clubs are extracurricular activities. The club activities are facilitated by trained peer educators and supervised by trained teachers (called matrons and patrons). Several topics related to sexual health are discussed, such as abstinence, decisionmaking, and communication skills. Abstinence is promoted as the preferred sexual health decision for young people in the schools, but for those young people who are already sexually active, effective condom use is encouraged and taught.

Initially, the program targeted 10,700 in-school adolescents. In 2000, an evaluation led to a subsequent expansion, to cover most of Kafue district. The estimated total number of adolescent beneficiaries (both in and out of school) over the duration of the program is 53,000, at an average cost of US$2.26 per youth per year. NGO involvement came to an end in 2002, and the program is now under the control of the District Offices of the Zambian Ministry of Health, Ministry of Education, and Ministry of Community and Social Development.

Of the 16 UNAIDS benchmarks for effective programs, the program fulfills 10 and partially fulfills 4, and 2 were not applicable.

Zimbabwe

Africare: Adolescent Reproductive Health Project; AIDS Action Clubs In Schools

Africare, a Zimbabwean NGO, established its AIDS Action Clubs Program in collaboration with the District Education Office in 2000. The clubs target youth aged 10 to 24 years in both primary and secondary schools. The program started in 26 schools in the Bindura and Mount Darwin districts (Mashonaland Central Province) and has since expanded to work in 61 schools: 16 in Bindura, 10 in Mount Darwin, 10 in Makoni South, 10 in Makoni North, and 15 in urban Harare.

The goal of the program is to contribute toward a reduction in the transmission of HIV/AIDS through effectively reaching adolescents with reproductive health information and promoting positive attitudes and behavior. The project has two main components: AIDS Action Clubs, which involve peer education, life skills training, and awareness of child abuse, and income generation activities to promote self-sufficiency.

So far, the program has reached 25,200 in-school and 10,000 out-of-school youth at an estimated cost of US$8.89 per youth per year. Of the 16 UNAIDS benchmarks for effective programs, the program was found to have successfully met 9 and partially met 5, and 2 were not applicable.

Zimbabwe

Midlands AIDS Service Organisation (MASO): Youth Alive Initiatives Project

The Midlands Aids Service Organisation (MASO), a Zimbabwean NGO, started the Youth Alive Initiative Project in 1996. The program targets 10- to 24-year-old, in- and out-of-school youth in urban and rural areas of the Midlands province of Zimbabwe. It aims to encourage safer sexual practices among youth, reduce the prevalence of HIV/AIDS in the general population, and promote positive living among people who haved been infected and affected.

To achieve these aims, volunteer teachers are trained to lead youth clubs. Young people become members of the clubs voluntarily, and those who attend are trained by the teachers in peer education and adolescent sexual and reproductive health issues. These youth then disseminate information among their peers to encourage life skills development, communication, and behavior change. This dissemination takes place either on a one-to-one counseling basis or during outreach activities. These activities involve performances for youth and other community members. The main focus of the clubs and outreach activities is on abstinence.

The teachers and peer educators are also trained in counseling about child abuse to equip them with skills to respond to children's needs and problems.

The program has put together a number of manuals and materials that can be obtained from the MASO offices (see MASO report, Part D).

To date, more than 10,000 youth and 1,000 adults have benefited from the program at an estimated cost of US$71 per youth per year. Of the 16 UNAIDS benchmarks for effective programs, the program was found to have successfully met 11 and partially met 3, and 2 were not applicable.

Section 3:
The Programs

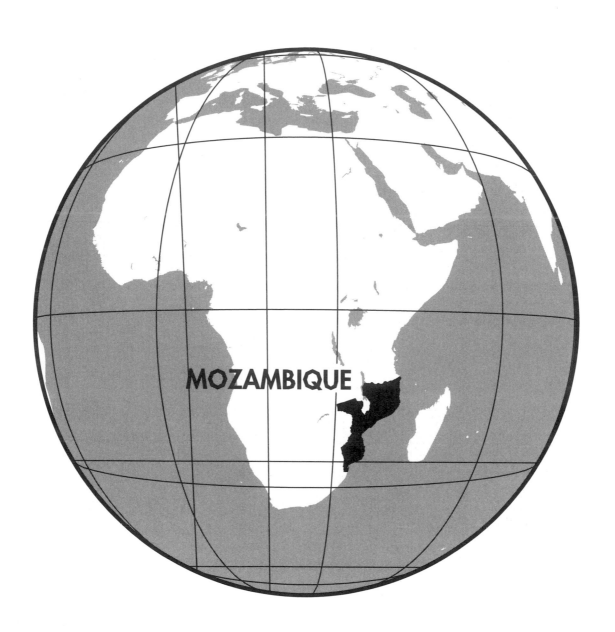

MOZAMBIQUE

Action Aid:
Stepping Stones Program

PART A: DESCRIPTION OF THE PROGRAM

Program Rationale and History

Action Aid began work in Mozambique in 1988, during the civil war. They were asked by the government of Mozambique to carry out emergency work in Zambezia province because few NGOs were active there. By 1994, the impact of HIV/AIDS had become more noticeable, so Action Aid began to introduce prevention programs in Zambezia.

In 1997, Action Aid expanded this work to the Manhica and Marracuene districts in Maputo province. Again, they did this largely because very few NGOs and donor agencies were working there, and little work was being conducted on HIV/AIDS prevention in that province.

At first, Action Aid trained activists and worked with cultural groups to disseminate preventive messages about sexually transmitted diseases (STDs) to communities through dance, song, and drama activities.

In 1999, Action Aid introduced the "Stepping Stones" methodology into its existing program in Zambezia to increase the profile and effectiveness of HIV/AIDS activities. The Stepping Stones method was pioneered by Alice Welbourne of Action Aid Uganda. It arose in recognition of the drawbacks of the "ABC" (abstain, be faithful, and use condoms) and "information = behavior change" approaches that had previously been used. Stepping Stones had proved successful in other African countries, therefore it was selected and adapted to make it more appropriate for Mozambique.

> In order to provide the necessary time and skills for the community to tackle its problems, it is necessary to work through a progression of themes. The community needs to start by identifying and talking about its problems. Next, they have to analyse them. Lastly, they have to come up with workable solutions.
>
> *Program manager*

The main aim of the program was to teach communities about the risk of HIV infection and increase their capacity to respond to this risk. Community facilitators were identified and trained for two weeks in Stepping Stones methods. For their first three months of work, Action Aid supervised them and assessed their capabilities.

27

After the 2000 flood, Action Aid started using the Stepping Stones methods in the Manhica and Marracuene districts in Maputo province. It was thought that the Stepping Stones methods would help bring together people who had been displaced from their areas by the floods.

Intensive advocacy was conducted, particularly with local government officials and community leaders because their full participation in the program was necessary. The program was evaluated in 2001 by an external consultant, and the limitations identified were used to make the current phase of the program more relevant to its target communities.

From 1998 to 2001, the program was financed principally by the British government (Department for International Development [DFID]), the Elton John AIDS Foundation, and UNICEF. The program plans on running at least until 2006, when current funding ends. An external evaluation will be conducted with the aim of assessing the impact of the Stepping Stones program and finding areas for improvement.

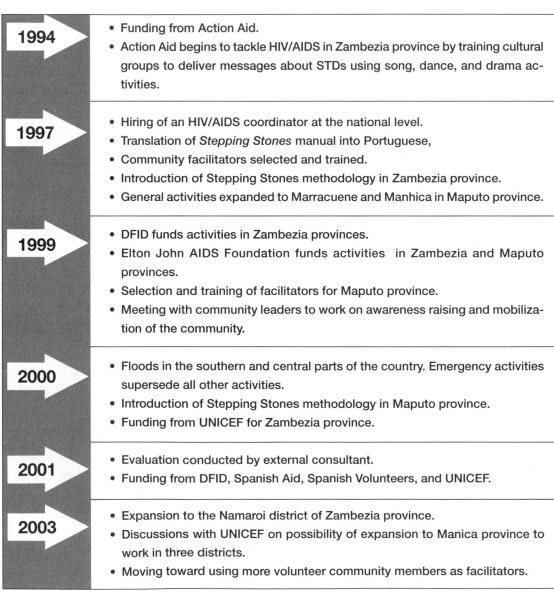

1994
- Funding from Action Aid.
- Action Aid begins to tackle HIV/AIDS in Zambezia province by training cultural groups to deliver messages about STDs using song, dance, and drama activities.

1997
- Hiring of an HIV/AIDS coordinator at the national level.
- Translation of *Stepping Stones* manual into Portuguese,
- Community facilitators selected and trained.
- Introduction of Stepping Stones methodology in Zambezia province.
- General activities expanded to Marracuene and Manhica in Maputo province.

1999
- DFID funds activities in Zambezia provinces.
- Elton John AIDS Foundation funds activities in Zambezia and Maputo provinces.
- Selection and training of facilitators for Maputo province.
- Meeting with community leaders to work on awareness raising and mobilization of the community.

2000
- Floods in the southern and central parts of the country. Emergency activities supersede all other activities.
- Introduction of Stepping Stones methodology in Maputo province.
- Funding from UNICEF for Zambezia province.

2001
- Evaluation conducted by external consultant.
- Funding from DFID, Spanish Aid, Spanish Volunteers, and UNICEF.

2003
- Expansion to the Namaroi district of Zambezia province.
- Discussions with UNICEF on possibility of expansion to Manica province to work in three districts.
- Moving toward using more volunteer community members as facilitators.

Figure 1. Time Line of Major Program Events

Program Overview

Aim

The program aims to help individuals and the community as a whole combat the problems they face, including that of HIV/AIDS. It teaches them about how to make informed decisions, as well as how to act responsibly and change behavior, both individually and together as a community.

Objectives

According to the program coordinator, the program objectives are

- to contribute to the reduction of individual and group vulnerability to infection by HIV,
- to reduce the impact of AIDS through increasing the community's understanding of the risk of infection and increasing their capacity to respond effectively,
- to contribute to the creation of a positive environment to support people living with HIV/AIDS and their families, and
- to encourage people living with HIV/AIDS to get involved in the development and implementation of preventive and care programs for HIV/AIDS.

Target Groups

Primary Target Group

The Stepping Stones Program primarily targets people in the community who attend the specialized program workshops. Ideally, this would be all the women and men of the community, but in practice, about 40 women and 40 men attend the workshops.

Secondary Target Group

The secondary target group includes people in the community who do not participate in the workshops but hear about the issues from their neighbors and friends who attend the workshops. The Stepping Stones program attempts to reach the whole community.

Site

The Stepping Stones workshops take place at community meeting points. These are often in the center of the community, underneath trees.

> We will talk about HIV/AIDS prevention, but we will not tell the community to use condoms. Instead, we present and discuss the advantages and disadvantages of condom use and then leave the community to decide what is right for them.
>
> ***Program manager***

Program Length

In Maputo province, workshops are run once a week for a period of four months. (In Zambezia province, workshops are run every day for a month in each community.) About 40 men and 40 women attend the workshops, and each workshop lasts approximately two hours. Three to six months after the end of the workshops, Action Aid conducts feedback sessions (discussions with community members who attended the workshops) to see how the community is responding. If there are problems, they talk with the community to try to find solutions.

Program Goals

Figure 2 shows how the program coordinator ranked the program goals. Program implementers were in agreement with the objectives and stated that the main focus of the program was behavior change through group discussions.

Program Approaches

Because the program has a holistic approach to the prevention and mitigation of HIV/AIDS, it is impossible to rank the approaches in order of importance. The underlying concept of Stepping Stones is to enable communities to explore their problems and negotiate solutions; these skills are seen as essential for sustained behavior change. People are encouraged to learn from their experiences and examine their needs and priorities. An important feature of the Stepping Stones program is that it works in groups of peers of the same sex and age drawn from the community rather than concentrating on individual or segregated risk groups. The community is encouraged to take responsibility for itself, and the program attempts to equip them with the necessary skills and information to be able to do this.

Activities

Different activities are used depending on the workshop's theme and the guidelines drawn from a detailed manual of activities (see "Program Materials" in Part B).

The facilitators often use activities that involve the participation of the whole group because these seem to be more enjoyable and empowering to community members. For example, role plays have the advantage of attracting people who are not usually involved in the workshops and are effective in getting discussions going. A role play in which someone has sex and is later in pain may spark a discussion of STDs and their symptoms. Often, this may lead to discussions on how to avoid STDs.

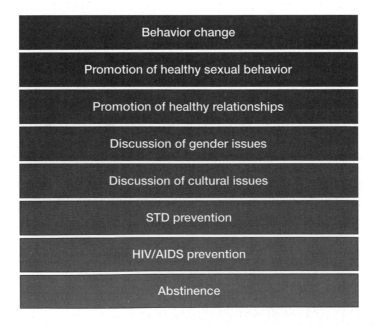

Figure 2. Program Goals Ranked in Increasing Importance by Program Manager

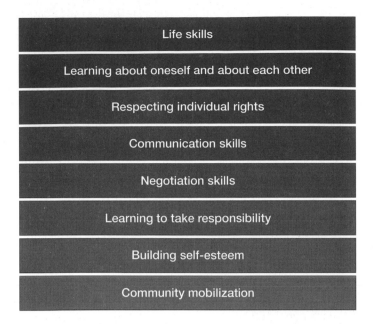

Figure 3. Program Approaches Unranked

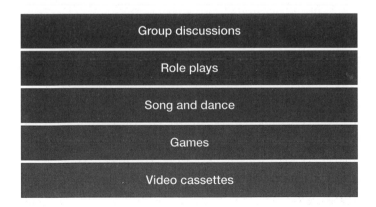

Figure 4. Program Activities Unranked

Components

The program consists of one main component, the community workshops, which are discussed below.

At a time and place agreed between the community members and the facilitators, each community holds a workshop once a week. When the facilitators arrive, they begin each session with brief greetings. If there are visitors, the participants welcome them with a song and dance. The community then breaks into four groups:

- younger women,
- older women,
- younger men,
- older men.

One or two facilitators are assigned to each of the four groups. It is important to note that facilitators are of a similar age and of the same sex as the group they are working with. They begin the session by reviewing the work that was conducted the week before. The group is then given a chance to reflect and ask questions. After making sure there are no more questions or misunderstandings, the current week's topic, taken from the Stepping Stones manual, is introduced. Various approaches (described above) are used to reflect on the weekly topic, which is then discussed by the group. All groups discuss the same topics. The topics include

- Gender
- Cultural issues
- Relationships
- Sexuality/HIV-AIDS education
- Abstinence
- Contraceptive education
- Moral behavior and social values
- Respecting individual rights
- Self-efficacy and self-esteem
- Behavioral and life skills development
- Sexual reproductive health services/information access
- Condom access

The groups work separately much of the time to ensure they have a safe, supportive space for talking about intimate issues. However, the four groups meet as one group every four to six weeks to share insights. The facilitators also meet with each other once a week to discuss any problems or difficulties with their respective groups and plan for the activities of the next week.

We like the group discussions as questions are answered on the spot.

Program implementers and participants

After four months, the weekly workshops come to an end. In the final workshop, each group presents a special request and an action plan to the whole community. The community discusses the requests and decides whether they will be accepted or dismissed. For those accepted, a committee is elected to implement the action plan and follow up on its progress.

Facilitators then return to the communities at intervals of three to six months to conduct feedback sessions, evaluate whether the requests are being implemented, and assess informally whether behavior change has taken place. When requests are not honored, Action Aid holds a meeting with the selected community representatives to find out the main problem and discuss ways of resolving the problem.

Case Study of a Manhica Workshop

After greeting each other, workshop members moved into their four groups. In the older women's group, the facilitator began the session by discussing the previous week's workshop on the consequences of one's behavior. They then turned to this week's topic and begin with a role play.

In the role play, two young women decide not to go to school, but to have fun in another part of town instead. They go to a bar, where they drink alcohol and where one of them tries to rob someone. The police are called. They chase the young women, and one of them falls and hurts herself.

When the young women get home, their mother asks why one of them is hurt. They lie and say she fell at school. The mother says someone told her they were seen being chased by the police, so the young women confess and tell their mother that they had been drinking.

After the role play, the participants discussed why the young women had behaved in that way. The older women said they find it hard to talk to or control their children. They thought that teachers should inform them about truancy. With guidance from the facilitator, they also talked about how to communicate with adolescents and be involved in their lives in and out of school. The session closed by asking the participants to think about ways to improve communication within the family to discuss next week.

PART B: IMPLEMENTING THE PROGRAM

Needs Assessment

A Participatory Rural Appraisal was conducted by Action Aid in 1997 to look at issues affecting the community, such as knowledge of HIV/AIDS, educational level, and everyday chores and activities.

They found that people knew very little about HIV/AIDS and how to avoid it, and that community perceptions of gender and relationships could increase the likelihood of HIV infection. However, because of staffing changes and office relocation, no further information was available.

> Role plays are effective because they involve a wide variety of the audience.
>
> *Program manager*

Program Materials

The Stepping Stones program relies on the manual and video prepared by Alice Welbourne of Action Aid Uganda. It took three months to translate the manual into Portuguese and one month to print and distribute it. The manual is currently undergoing further adaptation: Names of people, places, and stories are being changed to reflect the Mozambican context. The community and workshop members are actively involved in this process, explaining which parts of the book are less suitable in Mozambique and suggesting alternatives.

The Stepping Stones manual is a training package on HIV/AIDS communication and relationship skills. Although the manual does not offer solutions, it helps communities to develop their own solutions to their own problems and concerns.

Copies of the manual and the video are available. Please see "Available Materials" at the end of this chapter.

> The whole community is asked to participate in the workshops. They are split into four groups so that they can feel more free to talk to one another. This helps each peer group to bond together and creates a safe, friendly atmosphere in which to explore sensitive issues. Ideally facilitators come from the same community as the participants.
>
> **Program manager**

Target Group Materials

The facilitator uses the Stepping Stones manual during workshops. This manual focuses on social issues such as gender, culture, and relationships and relates them to sexual and reproductive health. The manual can be divided into three sections.

Section One

The first section focuses on exercises to develop group cooperation and communication that help participants to recognize their own perspectives and needs. The participants explore facts and feelings about relationships, HIV infection prevention, and safer sex. The men's and women's groups each have a chance to assess their priorities in sexual health and family life, in the context of a greater understanding of their potential vulnerability to HIV.

Section Two

The second section aims to help participants analyze individual behavior and attitudes and identify the influences that shape them. Society's expectations of men and women (gender roles), which are often closely tied up with cultural traditions, are examined. Other influences, such as the economic pressures to make a living (the need for money), the use and abuse of alcohol or drugs, and people's personalities, are also considered in some depth.

Involving men in this reflection is key to transforming gender relations and harmful practices. Participants — both male and female — evaluate for themselves the advantages and disadvantages of current relations and practices, as well as the factors influencing them. For example, cultural traditions such as wife inheritance, polygamy, initiation, and cleansing rites are used for reflection. Community members are encouraged to question for themselves the benefits of these practices, the risks involved, and the alternatives that can be devised.

> The old women asked if they could remain in the village after their husbands had died, rather than being sent back to their home villages. The young women asked the men to stop chasing after them and asking for sex, so that they could finish school.
>
> **Young and older women's groups**

Section Three

The final section helps participants to think and practice ways in which they can change behavior in a manner that allows them to become more assertive and to take responsibility for personal and community-wide actions. How to sustain more assertive behavior is also discussed.

The process culminates in a special request from each peer group to the whole community, presented in the form of a role play, to illustrate the change each group sees as its top priority. Because these requests are collectively made, in a community forum, they are more effective than a request made by an individual.

Staff Training Materials

The Stepping Stones manual is also used for instructing trainers and facilitators because it is the primary tool for conducting workshops.

Staff Selection and Training

All staff receive training. Staff selection methods may change over time; however, the training program the staff receives remains constant. Training is performed using a cascade approach.

> I would like to see pictures of the diseases we talk about, like HIV/AIDS and other STDs, so that I can know what they look like.
>
> *Program participant*

Trainers' Instruction

Two people from the Institute of Social Communication, based in Maputo, received training in the Stepping Stones methodology in Zimbabwe. This training was conducted by SANASO (Southern Africa AIDS Network), an HIV/AIDS network for Southern Africa based in Harare, Zimbabwe.

Trainers of Facilitators

- These are two consultants, one male and one female.
- They are trained in Stepping Stones methodology by the trainers' instructor. During training, the participants are sometimes separated by gender.
- Training takes two weeks.
- Training involves familiarization with the Stepping Stones manual and strategies to use in a variety of situations presented. They are also trained in interpersonal communication and how to be sensitive to community environment.

Facilitators

- There are usually eight facilitators (four female, four male) per four communities. They have to belong to one of these communities.
- The facilitators are chosen by the village leaders.
- The facilitators are selected to participate in the program based on their ability to read and write Portuguese and the local language, knowledge of reproductive health, open attitude, ability to listen and communicate openly in the community environment, ability to speak openly about issues of relationships and sexuality, ability to work as a team, and willingness to change their own behavior and act as role models.

> It would make our work easier if we had picture books, so that when we talk about sexuality, we can point to the male and female reproductive organs to show the changes that are taking place.
>
> *Program implementers*

- The facilitators are trained for two weeks by the trainers of facilitators.
- Training involves familiarization with the Stepping Stones manual. They are also trained on how to help people communicate so that they can discuss their problems and identify solutions.
- Facilitators receive refresher training once a year.

Setting Up the Program

Before the program was set up, a meeting was held with the provincial and district health officials to obtain government approval and find out if there was a particular district or community that the government would like the organization to focus on. Meetings were also held with community leaders to explain the program and to gain their support.

Setting Up a Workshop

- Participatory Rural Appraisals are used to decide which communities are most in need. Usually Action Aid starts with one community and then expands the number of communities covered as the facilitators become more familiar with the work.
- Facilitators are selected and trained and the first workshops established.
- The workshops are publicized to the whole community through community meetings, talking to people at community gatherings, and word of mouth.
- Those members of the community who choose to participate are divided into groups according to age and gender.
- Facilitators meet with each other once a week to discuss workshop curriculum and activities. They meet with the Action Aid program assistant once a month.

Program Resources

In addition to the Stepping Stones manual, materials used in the workshops include pens, paper, and markers. These are sent from the head office to Action Aid offices in the provinces. The facilitators take the materials to the workshop venues. In practice, too often the reference materials are kept in the head office, making them hard to obtain. The project has no resource center where facilitators can obtain materials for their work. Thus, facilitators use the Stepping Stones manual as the main resource.

One of the program's biggest weakness is the training. It is difficult to implement and sustain for two principal reasons. Firstly, few rural people speak Portuguese, and facilitators are rarely able to speak or write the local language. Secondly, literacy levels are very low in rural areas, so it is difficult to use the manual effectively.

Former HIV/AIDS coordinator

Advocacy

The provincial Ministries of Education and Health are informed of Action Aid's program in the community through discussions and presentation of action plans and proposals. At the district level, the administrator is informed about the program through monthly or quarterly meetings in his or her office, and sometimes the district-level administrator is invited to attend meetings.

In Zambezia province, the Ministries of Health and Education participated in a training of trainers workshop. This was done to encourage them to supervise the Stepping Stones facilitators at the community level. However, as a result of the workload of ministry staff and the lack of funds to support this supervision, this did not occur.

The Stepping Stones program is advocacy based in that it aims for change in the community through discussions. The support of community leaders is seen as crucial. Action Aid discusses the program with them so that they can ensure their support. Community leaders call the first meeting and introduce the organization to the community. They are also encouraged to attend the workshops to urge others to go.

Program Finances

Funding has been received from Action Aid (1997, 1999), DFID (1999, 2001), the Elton John Foundation (2000), Spanish Aid (2001), Spanish Volunteers (2001), and Unicef (2001). Table 1 summarizes how the funding has been used.

There have been approximately 500,000 adult beneficiaries over the past year. If we assume that there will be the same number of beneficiaries each year, the average cost per person per year is approximately US$0.30 (597,000/[500,000*4]).

Table 1. Program Costs

Spent on	Cost in US$*
Manual (production and adaptation)	33,000
Training of trainers	22,000
Refresher training	7,000
Training of facilitators	90,000
Community workshops	60,000
Supervision at provincial and national level	15,000
Networking and provincial meetings	8,000
Salary and support costs	
Stepping Stone coordinators	160,000
Two vehicles (Maputo and Zambezia)	60,000
Two motorbikes (Maputo and Zambezia)	16,000
Administrative and logistical support	30,000
Computer and office equipment	6,000
Monitoring and evaluation	20,000
Total	597,000

*Costs are over a four-year period.

PART C: ASSESSMENT AND LESSONS LEARNED

Challenges and Solutions

At one time, work on HIV/AIDS was the responsibility of a separate department, but now there is recognition that it needs to be streamlined into Action Aid's other departments. The challenge is how this is going to be implemented.

Program Manager

- The greatest challenge is to obtain the necessary level of facilitator training in order for the program to be effective. At present, most facilitators are not highly educated; thus they require training to
    - change their own behaviors and internalize the Stepping Stones message and
    - learn to be flexible and know how to change the approach according to what works best for the community.
- The facilitators also require continuous updates in training to develop the skills to maintain good-quality program implementation.
- Ideally then, a permanent team of trainers is required.

- Monitoring and evaluation is weak. There is a need for a system to follow up on the issues that are put forward by the community during the sessions. Action Aid does not have the time or resources to do this frequently. One possible solution would be for other partners, such as NGOs and governments, to get involved.

- Children should be included in the Stepping Stones program because they are also affected by what happens in the family and community. For the first time Action Aid has recently begun to pilot the use of Stepping Stones in schools.

> It would be good to have a resource center where we could go and consult books on topics we are not familiar with, since sometimes people ask us things we do not know about. When this happens, we sometimes resort to seeking out nurses at the health post or someone else, depending on the topic.
>
> **Program facilitator**

Facilitators

- Facilitators need access to expertise and up-to-date information in areas that they have not been trained in. This could be either
  - a resource center that has books, videos, and posters, that the facilitators can refer to, or;
  - access to local experts (e.g., nurses, doctors, and counselors) that can help them with the technical components of certain workshops.
- For some topics, the Stepping Stones manual and video are not enough. There is a need for posters or picture books that show the different types of disease at their various stages. Posters showing reproductive organs should also be made available. In general, other simple educational materials are needed to reinforce the manual and video.

Report Author

- Links with other organizations working in this area are weak and can be strengthened. There is currently an effort to collaborate with Population Services International (PSI) to distribute condoms.
- If a high percentage of community members participate in the workshops, there is a high probability of change. However, where few members participate, it is likely that further workshops will be needed if any real change is to occur.

> For any organization to work at community level, the political structure needs to be informed.
>
> **Program manager**

- Where participation is low, interested participants should be trained as facilitators to encourage continuity and internalization of the Stepping Stones methodology.
- There should be more supervision of the facilitators to ensure that they are doing a good job.
- People from the community should be trained so they can follow up on whether changes are being implemented, rather than relying on underresourced Action Aid staff.
- In areas where there is no electricity, efforts should be made to have a portable car battery, generator, or other appropriate technology to enable participants to see the Stepping Stones video or at least some aspects of it.
- There should be systematic monitoring of progress after the final workshop.
- Observations showed that certain group members appeared to be participating more than others in the workshops. It is very important to think of ways to make sure everybody is participating and learning equally.

Evaluation

Facilitators return to the communities at intervals of three to six months after the final workshop has taken place. They check to see whether the changes the community promised to make are actually being implemented through discussions with community members who participated in the workshop.

Changes are noticeable in many communities. For example, in one community, women had asked that men give them more money for household expenditures. This now happened. Furthermore, changes are sometimes noticed in those who did not attend workshops — they saw their neighbors changing and they followed suit.

However, there is no systematic evaluation of the program.

UNAIDS Benchmarks

	Benchmark	Attainment	Comments
1	Recognizes the child/youth as a learner who already knows, feels, and can do in relation to healthy development and HIV/AIDS-related prevention.	Partially fulfilled	Sometimes children participate when the workshops are conducted outside school hours.
2	Focuses on risks that are most common to the learning group and that responses are appropriate and targeted to the age group.	✓	Participants discuss their problems and are encouraged to learn from their own experiences.
3	Includes not only knowledge but also attitudes and skills needed for prevention.	✓	Participants reflect on their attitudes and come up with behavioral change solutions to their problems.
4	Understands the impact of relationships on behavior change and reinforces positive social values.	✓	In trying to understand the impact of relationships on behavior change, this program strives for positive social values.
5	Is based on analysis of learners' needs and a broader situation assessment.	✓	Participatory Rural Appraisal is conducted to assess the needs of the community.
6	Has training and continuous support of teachers and other service providers.	Partially fulfilled	Facilitators are trained. Little backup training or resources provided.
7	Uses multiple and participatory learning activities and strategies.	✓	Activities such as group discussions and role plays are participatory.
8	Involves the wider community.	✓	The foundation of this program is the community and the collective and individual life experiences.
9	Ensures sequence, progression, and continuity of messages.	✓	Through following the manual and the exercises, there is sequence, progression, and continuity of messages.

	Benchmark	Attainment	Comments
10	Is placed in an appropriate context in the school curriculum.	Not applicable	
11	Lasts a sufficient time to meet program goals and objectives.	✓	There is enough time in each workshop to be able to discuss a topic fully. The whole manual can be covered in the four allocated months.
12	Is coordinated with a wider school health promotion program.	Not applicable	There is no school program.
13	Contains factually correct and consistent messages.	✓	The organization of the manual goes from what the community knows to building on their knowledge and giving information on different issues in sequence.
14	Has established political support through intense advocacy to overcome barriers and go to scale.	✓	Stepping Stones has the support of the government and the local communities. The program is expanding, not only through Action Aid but also through other international and national NGOs.
15	Portrays human sexuality as a healthy and normal part of life, and is not derogatory against gender, race, ethnicity, or sexual orientation.	Partially fulfilled	Portrays human sexuality as a healthy and normal part of life. The program does not talk about homosexuality.
16	Includes monitoring and evaluation.	Partially fulfilled	Action Aid goes back to the communities to see whether changes have taken place. There is no scientific or systematic monitoring or evaluation of program impact.

PART D: ADDITIONAL INFORMATION

Organizations and Contacts
Action Aid Mozambique
Alfredo Santos, National AIDS Coordinator
Rua Comandante Augusto Cardoso 327/9
C.P. 2608
Maputo, Mozambique
E-mail: admin@actionaidmozambique.org
or
aamozhiv@teledata.mz
Website: www.actionaid.org

Contributors to the Report
Program report prepared by Esther Kaziliman-Pale.

Edited by Helen Baños Smith.

We appreciate the help of the following people at Action Aid in providing much of the information in this report:

Alfredo Santos — HIV/AIDS coordinator
Antonio Banze — Project officer
Janet Duffield — Former HIV/AIDS coordinator
Simao Hilario Ferreira Tima — Facilitator
Joaquim Alberto Chau — Facilitator
Gabriel Jacob Mimbirri — Facilitator
Raimundo Valente Dzimba — Facilitator
Celia Maria Marques — Facilitator
Sandra Macho Bonzela — Facilitator
Adelaide Filipe Machaua — Facilitator
Ricardina Valente Chapo — Facilitator

Available Materials
To obtain these materials, please contact ibeaids@ibe.unesco.org or Education for HIV/AIDS Prevention, International Bureau of Education, C.P. 199, 1211 Geneva 20, Switzerland.

Stepping Stones: A Training Package on HIV/AIDS, Communication and Relationship Skills
(order number: ActionAid01)

Stepping Stones Summary
(order number: ActionAid02)

"Final evaluation: Adolescent RH in Maputo City and Zambezia, July 2001"
(order number: ActionAid03)

"Report of the Evaluation of the HIV/AIDS Programme 1998–2001"
(order number: ActionAid04)

Gender, Sex, and HIV: How to Address Issues that No One Wants to HearAbout
(order number: ActionAid05)

Video
(order number: ActionAid06)

APPENDIX 1. MAIN STAFF ROLES, ACTION AID PROGRAM

Country Directors, Action Aid

The directors are in charge of the whole country program. They allocate funds and approve changes to program activities.

HIV/AIDS Coordinator

The coordinator reports directly to the country director and is in charge of the day-to-day administrative and technical running of the program. He is assisted by the administration and human resources departments. The provincial HIV/AIDS coordinators, the HIV/AIDS assistants, and the facilitators report to him. At the district level, he is assisted by the district area coordinators. With the assistance of the program officer, he is responsible for selection of trainers for the facilitators.

HIV/AIDS Program Officer (Maputo Province)

The program officer is responsible for supervision of the HIV/AIDS program in Maputo province. He or she reports directly to the HIV/AIDS coordinator and assists in the selection and training of facilitators.

Provincial Coordinator (Zambezia Province)

The provincial coordinator oversees the whole provincial program and supervises the HIV/AIDS program.

District Area Coordinator (DAC)

The DAC is in charge of the whole Action Aid program at the district level and is responsible for seeing to it that the facilitators are working and planning for their community visits. If there are problems, DACs act as the link between the facilitators and the HIV/AIDS assistant.

HIV/AIDS Assistant

The HIV/AIDS assistants are responsible for assisting the provincial coordinator in overseeing the HIV/AIDS program. They have direct supervisory responsibility over the facilitators, and they also conduct facilitator training when needed.

Facilitators

Facilitators are responsible for conducting the workshops within the communities. Their training and supervision are important because they are the people who can make or break the Stepping Stones program.

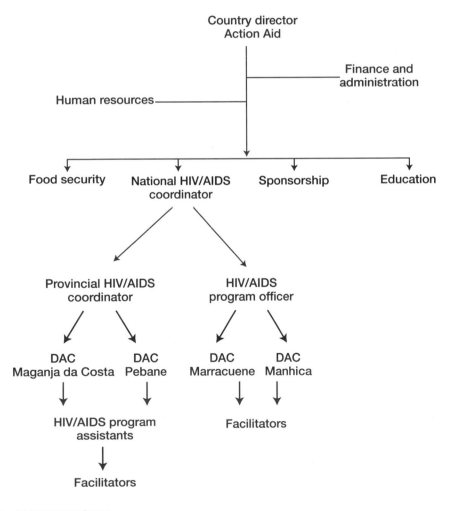

Note: DAC = district area coordinator

Figure A.1. Staff Structure

APPENDIX 2. STAFF DATA

	Number of staff	Position/title	Gender
Full-time and paid	1	National coordinator	Male
	1	HIV/AIDS program officer	Male
	1	Provincial coordinator	Female
	2	HIV/AIDS program assistant	1 male, 1 female
	1	Program assistant	Male
Part-time and paid	1	District coordinator, Manhica	Female
	1	District coordinator, Marracuene	Female
	1	District coordinator, Pebane	Male
	1	District coordinator, Manja de Costa	Male
Volunteer peer educators (not receiving allowances/ incentives)	32	Facilitators	16 female, 16 male
	3	Supervisors	All male

UNFPA and Pathfinder International: *Geração Biz*, Youth-Friendly Health Clinics

PART A: DESCRIPTION OF THE PROGRAM

Program Rationale and History

Since 1999, three Ministries (Youth and Sports, Education, and Health) have coordinated a multisectoral program in collaboration with selected NGOs, associations, and youth networks. This program aims to address Mozambican youths' lack of knowledge, skills, and access to youth-friendly sexual and reproductive health services. It is called *Geração Biz*, a name chosen by the young people themselves to represent a busy generation and to stress that they want to play a major role in protecting their own reproductive health.

The program began at the central level and implemented activities in Maputo City and Zambezia province. By 2002, activities had also started in Gaza, Maputo, and Tete provinces. Program expansion throughout these provinces and to new provinces is expected in the coming years.

In the school-based component, which is implemented in collaboration with the Ministry of Education, students are trained to advise and empower their in- and out-of-school peers on topics such as sexuality, teen pregnancy, abortion, and STDs/HIV/AIDS. To do this, they use counseling, drama, film shows, group debates, and youth discussion corners. The community-based component works with the Ministry of Youth and Sport and youth associations. Youth centers are established where young people can go to receive counseling, condoms, and referral service to youth-friendly health services (YFHSs). Youth also help in preparing and airing community radio programs. This helps to set up links between the school and the community and maximizes resources and the impact of efforts.

In this report, only the Maputo City clinic-based component of the overall program in Maputo City is discussed.

In 1999, a needs assessment was carried out by the Ministry of Health in Maputo City to evaluate the situation of the health centers and their services to youth. The assessors found that most of the health centers needed renovation and equipment to serve the needs of youth. Furthermore, the head of the Gynaecology and Obstetrics Department at Maputo Central Hospital had noticed a large number of adolescents coming in for abortion-related complications. At the same time, the United Nations Population Fund (UNFPA) was developing an adolescent sexual and reproductive health (ASRH) program. The two organizations decided to collaborate by incorporating youth-friendly services into government health facilities. Funding for this was received from UNFPA and the German Agency for Technical Cooperation (*Gesellschaft für Technische Zusammenarbeit;* GTZ), which is the German government's development agency.

Five youth-friendly clinics, located in existing health centers, were opened in October 1999 in Maputo City. In November 1999, another clinic was opened in Maputo Central Hospital and two more have opened since. These clinics provide separate private spaces for youth where they can receive confidential, youth-friendly clinical and counseling services from trained staff. When the youth-friendly clinics first opened, about 150 young people visited per month. This figure has since increased to about 700 per month.

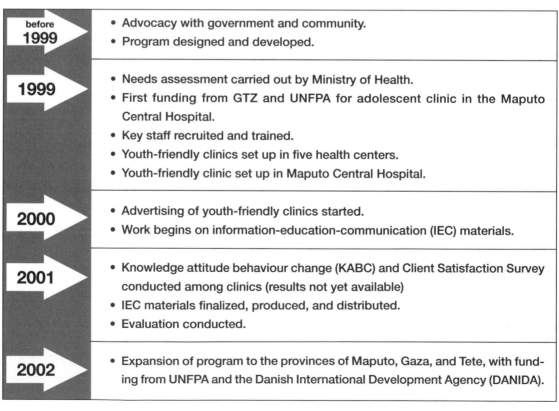

Figure 1. Time Line of Major Program Events

Program Overview

Aim
The aim of the multisectoral program is to improve the sexual and reproductive health of adolescents, including reducing early or unwanted pregnancies, as well as STDs and HIV infection. The specific aim of the youth-friendly clinics it to provide 15- to 24-year-olds with youth-friendly reproductive health services and counseling through government health facilities.

Objectives
According to the program coordinator, the program objectives are
- to offer improved accessibility to ASRH services (including information, education, and counseling) to in- and out-of-school youth through the development of specialized, youth-friendly clinical and counseling services in reproductive health;
- to achieve increased awareness and adoption of safe, responsible, and gender-sensitive sexual and reproductive behavior;
- to increase the use of reproductive health services by in- and out-of-school young people;
- to strengthen the mechanisms for involving youth of both sexes in all aspects of the program as well as to foster gender awareness and equity as a fundamental component of ASRH activities; and
- to build technical and institutional capacity of government ministries, their partners, and civil society to plan, implement, and monitor sectoral activities.

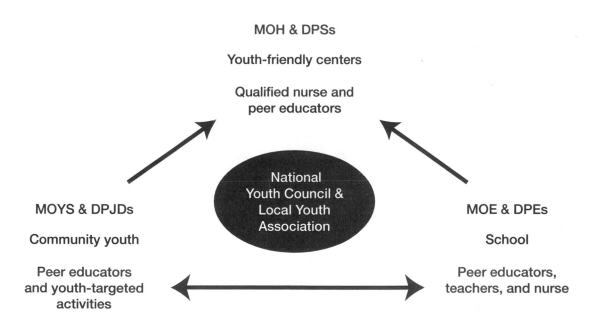

Note: MOH — Ministry of Health; DPSs — Provincial Directorate of Health; MOE — Ministry of Education; DPEs — Provincial Directorate of Education; MOYS — Ministry of Youth and Sports; DPJDs — Provincial Directorate of Youth and Sports.

Figure 2. Program Overview

Target Groups

Primary Target Group

The primary target group is youth between the ages of 15 and 24 who are living in Maputo City. However, children younger than this age are also welcome to attend the clinics.

Secondary Target Group

The program also targets health providers who are trained in counseling and adolescent communication techniques and in the clinical care of youth.

Site

The program takes place in five health centers and the Maputo Central Hospital. Only the hospital has full-time YFHSs; the health centers are open only on specific afternoons. In the beginning, it was opened twice a week; currently it is opened three to four times per week.

Program Length

This program has been running for three years. Young people attend the clinics whenever they want or need to.

The list in figure 3 shows how the chief technical adviser ranked the program goals. The goal of the YFHS is to provide services and counseling to the youth. However, it should be remem-

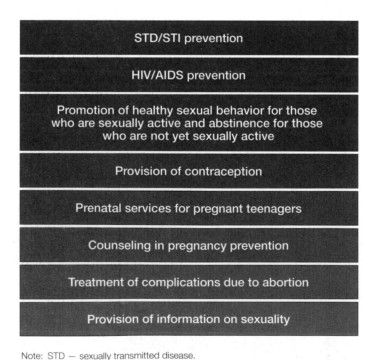

Note: STD — sexually transmitted disease.
STI — sexually transmitted infection.

Figure 3. Program Goals Ranked in Increasing Importance

bered that this is part of a bigger program that is targeting youth in the schools and in the communities. These other components deal with the broader issues of sexuality and gender.

Program Approaches
The main focus of the clinics is to encourage healthy sexuality among youth. All approaches are considered effective but are used to differing degrees, depending on what the patient wants. The nurses thought that counseling was the most important approach because it allows them to introduce a wide range of topics that are not necessarily what the child/youth had attended the clinic to discuss. For example, the nurses can give advice about not confusing sex with love.

Abstinence is considered the least important approach, although children who come to the clinic who are not yet sexually active are encouraged to delay sexual initiation. The school and community components of the program deal more with abstinence, peer education, individual rights, and so forth.

Activities
The nurses felt that one-to-one counseling was effective because they were able to talk to young people and give them advice that helps the youth make decisions on sexual and reproductive health. For example, if a girl comes in with an STD, they counsel her on the benefits of using a condom (dual protection), even though she may already be using some other form of contraception.

Components
The program consists of one main component, the YFHSs. In the five health centers, one or two trained nurses dedicate three or four afternoons a week (from noon to 3:30 pm) to seeing youth. In the mornings, they attend to adult patients. At Maputo Central Hospital, there are three trained

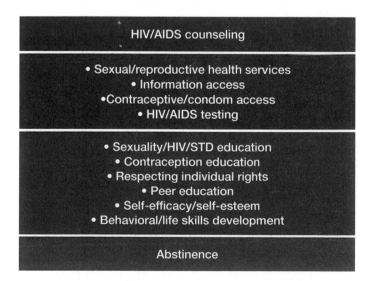

Figure 4. Program Approaches Ranked in Increasing Importance

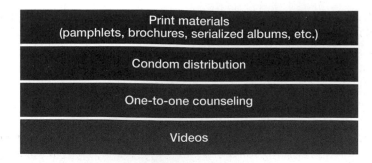

Figure 5. Program Activities Unranked

nurses who work full time at the YFHS. Every day, a physician attends the clinic for at least two hours. Voluntary counseling and testing (VCT) is available at the Maputo Central Hospital but not at the health centers.

The exact nature of what occurs in the clinics will vary from case to case. However, a typical example of the steps followed during a clinic visit are described below.

- When a youth comes in for the first time, she or he is greeted and asked to fill out a card so that she or he can be put in the system.
- While waiting for the nurse, patients can either watch videos on adolescent sexuality and HIV/AIDS/STD prevention or talk to peer educators who are on duty.
- The nurse counsels the young people on whatever they have come in for. For example, if youths come in because they think they have an STD, they are treated and told how they can prevent themselves from contracting STDs in the future. A youth being treated for an STD is also asked to bring his or her partner to the clinic as soon as possible.
- The nurse then talks to the youth about contraception, and the advantages and disadvantages of different methods. This includes teaching them how to use a condom (through the use of a wooden penis) even if the girl/woman is taking birth control pills or is using the calendar method of contraception. The aim of this component of clinic visits is to reduce STD/HIV infection.
- The nurses also conduct face-to-face counseling to try and change behavior. For example, they may discuss self-esteem and techniques for saying no to sex, relationships with parents and family, and so forth.
- Each day, *activistas* (peer educators) from surrounding schools come and talk to youth visiting the YFHSclinics on various topics related to ASRH, including attitude and behavior change.

Counseling usually involves one-to-one discussions, with the use of brochures and serialized albums. If a problem arises that the nurses at the health clinics are not qualified to attend to, the patient is referred to a hospital-based doctor at the youth clinic.

Once a month, the nurses from Maputo Central Hospital meet with the nurses from the health centers and the UNFPA-Pathfinder International technical adviser and manager. These meetings are used to discuss cases and experiences of the past month.

Case Study of Maputo Central Hospital Adolescent Clinic

Almost all patients are female, and they come in with friends. The patients first register at the reception desk. The receptionist is very friendly and takes down the patient's name and looks for her file. Patients are then asked to have a seat in either the television room or in the corridor and await their turn. In the television room, there are videos showing programs on reproductive health, human sexuality, and STDs. Some patients sit and wait in the corridor. After about 10 to 20 minutes, the patient is called by the nurse, with whom she spends about 20 to 30 minutes. Some patients leave carrying contraceptives; others do not. They join up with their friends in the corridor or the waiting room and leave.

PART B: IMPLEMENTING THE PROGRAM

Needs Assessment

A needs assessment was carried out in 1999 by the Ministry of Health. An assessment guide called *Assessment of Friendly Services for Adolescents and Youth,* adapted from the *Reproductive Health Services for Adolescents* manual produced by Pathfinder International was used. This guide looks at and assesses

- the types of service provided by the clinic, including whether:
  - there is a specific package for adolescents,
  - counseling is provided,
  - there are any educational activities, and
  - there is educational material in sufficient quantities;
- the working hours of the health clinic;
- the environment of the health unit (Does it have a comfortable place for adolescents? Does it have a private waiting area?)
- the location of the health clinic — if there is public transport, whether it is near schools or places where adolescents spend most of their free time;
- the capacity of the health clinic (number and types of wards, number of beds, number of patients seen per month, and so forth);
- are staff trained in adolescent health, youth-friendly service provision, and so forth; and
- questions on youth involvement, political support, administrative procedures, recruitment, publicity, and costs for services.

Unfortunately, data on the numbers of health centers visited and people interviewed were not available. However, it is known that data were collected using interviews and observations.

In addition to the above study, a survey was conducted among in- and out-of-school youth using focus group discussions to find out what they liked and did not like about YFHS clinics and what would encourage them to visit clinics. The results showed that:

- Most of the clinics needed renovating to create a space for adolescents.
- The clinics needed better equipment, including materials such as curtains, bed linen, and furniture as well as basic gynecologic/obstetric instruments.
- Staff needed to be trained in adolescent health issues.

The results of the needs assessment were used to set up YFHSs in health centers that were able to provide space for privacy, that were easily accessible to adolescents, and that offered a range of services.

Program Materials

The program materials, which are in Portuguese, were developed and pretested by technical advisers, national counterparts, and the youth with the support of external consultants. The materials took about one year to design, test, produce, and distribute.

Target Group Materials

There are five brochures covering these topics: "Adolescence — So Much Change at the Same Time" (includes a list of YFHSs), "Pregnancy — So Easy to Avoid," "HIV/AIDS — A Lot of Talk but Little Knowledge," "STDs — Protected if You Use Condoms," and "Boys and Girls – Different but the Same." These brochures focus on urban children and adolescents, and they are well written and easy to understand. They are available at the health centers, Maputo Central Hospital, and in schools. A soap opera called *Jaime and Maria* is available to out-of-school and rural youth.

Additional Materials

Stickers and posters with the same branding as the brochures are available at the clinics and at schools. They contain messages about the program and cover topics such as health and pleasure, where to find condoms and how to use them, how to change behavior, and how to communicate with a partner. Video tapes about adolescence, pregnancy, STDs, and other issues relating to ASRH are also available at the clinics.

Staff Training Materials

A manual for health care providers is used to train nurses and doctors in counseling and how to deliver clinical services such as contraception and STD treatment in a youth-friendly way. The manual has been adapted from Pathfinder International's *Health Providers Manual*. The manual has sections where brainstorming, group discussions, and drama take place in which everyone in a group participates and thus contributes their experiences to the training. The manual is divided up into nine units as follows:

Unit One: The Nature of Adolescence
- Why Health Workers Should be Trained in Sexual Reproductive Health for Adolescents
- Adolescents' Rights
- The Different Stages of Adolescent Development
- The Possible Health Problems Found in Adolescence

Unit Two: Risky Behavior and the Vulnerability of Adolescents

- What Makes Adolescents Vulnerable
- Physical, Emotional, and Socioeconomic Vulnerability
- Health Problems
- Why Adolescents Adopt Risky Behaviors

Unit Three: Attending to Adolescents

- Taking Their Clinical History
- Taking Their Family and Personal History
- Taking Their Psychological and Social History
- Taking Their Sexual History
- The Difference Between Taking Male and Female Histories

Unit Four: Contraceptive Options for the Adolescent

- Rumors and Misconceptions Regarding Contraception
- Health Risks in Early Pregnancy
- Consequences of Adolescent Pregnancy
- Different Types of Contraception and Their Advantages and Disadvantages
- Counseling on Contraceptive Methods
- Common Secondary Effects of Contraception and Misconceptions About Contraceptives

Unit Five: Prevention Management of STDs and Prevention of HIV/AIDS

- Clinical History and Manifestation
- Transmission and Clinical Symptoms
- Syndromatic management of STDs
- HIV/AIDS and Our Defense System/Transmission
- Strategies for Successful Prevention of STDs in Adolescents
- Barriers in Services and Information

Unit Six: Safe Sex and Protection for Adolescents

- Techniques for Safe Sex
- Negotiating Safe Sex
- Why Adolescents Do Not Have Safe Sex

Unit Seven: Other Topics in Reproductive Health

- Sexual Abuse and Why Sexual Abuse Is a Reproductive Health Problem
- Physical and Behavioral Indicators of Sexual Abuse
- How to Get Sexual Abuse History
- Barriers to Getting Sexual Abuse History
- Definition and Identification of Sexual Orientation

Unit Eight: Pregnancy, Birth, and Postnatal Care in Adolescents

- Physical Care of a Pregnancy Adolescent
- Physical Examination of a Pregnant Adolescent
- Counseling Adolescents in the Prenatal Period
- Birth Preparations During Prenatal Visits

- Birth
- Support to Adolescents During Birth
- Postpartum Care
- What Adolescent Parents Feel/Need

Unit Nine: Abortion and Postabortion Attention in Adolescence
- Classifications
- Differential Diagnosis
- Unsafe Abortion and Most Frequent Complications
- Adolescents and Abortion
- Counseling
- Emergency Treatment for Incomplete Abortions

In addition to these units, a training of trainers counseling module prepared in 2000 with the support of a UNFPA regional technical team is available for use in training providers.

Staff Selection and Training

One or two mother-child health nurses from the gynecology and obstetrics unit of each health center were trained. At the adolescent health clinic at Maputo Central Hospital, three nurses were trained. Because this was the first selection of nurses and doctors for the program, the criteria for selection were flexible. Health care providers were chosen (by their supervisors) if they were willing to work with adolescents, willing to learn, friendly, open, able to communicate, and treated people with respect.

Nurses and doctors were trained in counseling and as adolescent services providers, using the manual discussed in the section above on staff training materials. Training was provided by the UNFPA-Pathfinder International technical adviser and their counterpart from the Ministry of Health, who have postgraduate training in adolescent health. The training in counseling and adolescent clinical services lasted for about 10 days; consisted of group discussions, brainstorming, and drama by the participants; and included topics such as effective communication.

All staff training covered these core components:
- The concept of an adolescent health clinic.
- The aims and objectives of the program.
- Building on staff clinical knowledge. The emphasis was on how to deal with diagnosis and treatment of STDs, prevention of HIV/AIDS, and contraception for adolescents.
- Skills needed to work with young people (e.g., listening skills, openness, friendliness).

There has been no training since the first in 1999. Rather, there have been monthly technical meetings where nurses can be updated on technical issues. Further training is planned for pharmacists and auxiliary workers, such as receptionists and cleaners, to make the youths' entire experience of the health centers youth friendly.

Setting Up the Program

Before setting up the program, representatives from the department of obstetrics and gynecology at Maputo Central Hospital and the Ministry of Health had discussions with UNFPA and Pathfinder International about how youth-friendly services could be integrated into government health facilities.

As a follow-up to the sexuality and reproductive health curriculum change in schools (which was undertaken by the *Institute Nacional de Desenvolvimento Educacional* (National Institute of Educational Development [INDE]), which is part of the Ministry of Education, meetings were conducted with the communities and schools to let them know that youth-friendly clinics were to be set up and why.

How to Set Up a Youth-Friendly Health Clinic

- Five health centers were selected after a needs assessment conducted by the Ministry of Health and UNFPA. The Maputo Central Hospital was also chosen, although no assessment was done here.
- Senior management were asked if they would like help to provide YFHSs in their health centers and the hospital.
- Advocacy work was done in the community to explain the need for YFHSs.
- Nurses and doctors were selected and trained (see the section on staff selection and training above).
- Health units and the Maputo Central Hospital YFHS clinics were rehabilitated and given equipment and educational materials.
- The YFHS clinics were publicized on the radio and billboards and in schools.
- Nurses meet once a month to discuss the clinics.

Program Resources

A conference room in the adolescent health clinic at Maputo Central Hospital is used for meetings and is currently being established as a library for the nurses and also as a room for group counseling by peer educators. Posters, brochures, and videos are kept there. Condom supplies are kept in the consultation rooms, the waiting room, and the pharmacy.

Advocacy

Meetings are held every month with the program partners — the Ministries of Health, Education, and Youth and Sport — on program progress. Through this collaboration, the program has assisted in obtaining approval of a youth policy by Parliament. The policy emphasizes healthy lifestyles among youth by promoting and implementing programs that asssure youth of access to information and integrated, high-quality sexual and reproductive health services. At the political level, the government is encouraging that YFHSs be made available in all provinces.

Meetings were arranged with the community (through sending letters to parents from schools and through community leaders) to raise awareness of the need for such clinics. The INDE had also raised public awareness through its research into how to include sexuality in the school curriculum. Hence, the public's reaction to the clinics was generally one of acceptance.

Program Finances

The total funding for the YFHS component in Maputo City is US$215,147. (For a breakdown, please see Mozambique UNFPA-Pathfinder International Appendix 3.)

In 2001, 11,726 youth were seen at an estimated cost of approximately US$18.40 (215,147/11,726) per youth.

Table 1. Total Funding Received From UNFPA and DANIDA (US$)

Component	1999	2000	2001	Total
Personnel	190,962	291,939	344,556	827,457
Subcontracting	2,854	20,423	104,185	127,462
Training	81,820	96,850	104,185	282,855
Equipment	163,754	52,232	155,549	371,535
Miscellaneous	17,436	42,853	151,433	211,722
Administration and operational support	0	29,639	87,112	116,751
Total	456,826	533,936	947,020	1,937,782

PART C: ASSESSMENT AND LESSONS LEARNED

Challenges and Solutions

Program Coordinator

Access

ASRH services must be provided in a comprehensive and integrated manner. They must cover both in- and out-of-school adolescents. One way of doing this is institutionalization of youth-friendly services.

Involving the Young

Young people must be engaged in finding solutions to their problems. They should be actively involved in the planning, managing, and implementing of their health services. To begin this process, youth need to be listened to and research needs to be conducted with them to discover their needs.

Condoms

Condoms must be introduced from the starting point of a program, and access to them should be simple and continuous.

Staff Commitment

Personnel working with youth programs must be committed to helping young people deal with sexual and reproductive health concerns.

Targeting Men

Ways of attracting male youth should be developed. There should be more specific targeting of young men and boys in publicity encouraging them to attend the health centers. Services should be provided in an environment that is comfortable for them, and they should be encouraged to assume a responsible role toward their partners.

Sustainability

In fostering sustainability, the overall challenge will be to effectively transfer the high-quality planning and implementation more fully to the government.

Report Author

- Although there are brochures and pamphlets displayed along corridor walls in the health centers, there is also a need for such materials that youth can take away with them.
- At present, clinics are open from 8:00 a.m. to 3:00 p.m., which is during school hours. Clients come in during break times or when they have no lessons. Clinic hours should be extended; maybe clinics should be open in the early morning and in the evening as well.
- Nurses expressed the need to have more continuous training, especially in the area of HIV/AIDS.
- Although nurses from different centers and the hospital are supposed to have monthly meetings, when questioned about this they provided only limited information about what occurred at these meetings. This suggests that these meetings could be better structured to discuss the important issues.
- Focus group discussions should be conducted among youth (particularly male youth) to find out why they do not come to the YFHS and what should be done to encourage them to attend.

Evaluation

In 2001, external consultants and UNFPA regional technical advisers conducted an evaluation of the program. Unstructured interviews were conducted with nurses, students, and youth who were at the clinics when the evaluation team was there. The aim was to discover what they thought of the program.

The evaluation concluded that the clinics were functioning well and provided a useful service for adolescents and youth: Staff were well informed, motivated, respectful, and friendly, and youth and adolescents were well received. The quality of the clinical and counseling services was high. Over the three years the services have been running, youth attendance at clinics has increased by 70 percent and condom use has increased by 28 percent.

The majority of adolescents attending clinics are students, which results in the demand for services increasing during the school holidays. The majority of adolescents and youth attending the clinics are girls. There may be several reasons for this:

- Girls come for prenatal care or contraceptives. (very few boys come for contraceptives.)
- Traditionally, contraception is the responsibility of girls.
- Clinical and counseling services are provided by female nurses.
- Girls find it easier than boys to discuss their problems with people they do not know well.

UNAIDS Benchmarks

	Benchmark	Attainment	Comments
1	Recognizes the child/youth as a learner who already knows, feels, and can do in relation to healthy development and HIV/AIDS-related prevention.	✓	Youth are involved in the design and development of program materials.
2	Focuses on risks that are most common to the learning group and that responses are appropriate and targeted to the age group.	Partially fulfilled	Focuses on youth who are either sexually active or thinking of becoming sexually active. A KAB (knowledge, attitudes behavior) study has been conducted that will help determine whether the approach is relevant and appropriate. The results will be out soon.
3	Includes not only knowledge but also attitudes and skills needed for prevention.	✓	Through counseling, the program tries to give skills and knowledge to youth as well as imparting information.
4	Understands the impact of relationships on behavior change and reinforces positive social values.	✓	*Geração biz* teaches youth to treat disease on time.
5	Is based on analysis of learners' needs and a broader situation assessment.	✓	The youth are counseled on problems that they face and that they bring to the clinic.
6	Has training and continuous support of teachers and other service providers.	Partially fulfilled	Service providers are trained and meet monthly to discuss their problems. At present, no refresher training is available.
7	Uses multiple and participatory learning activities and strategies.	✓	Uses mainly counseling. Uses videos, brochures, etc. Other components of the program use other techniques, such as peer education.
8	Involves the wider community.	Partially fulfilled	The wider community is not involved in this aspect of the program. However, they are involved in other components. For example, they give feedback in the radio shows.

	Benchmark	Attainment	Comments
9	Ensures sequence, progression, and continuity of messages.	✓	Different youth need different messages. As they come in for consultations after their first visit, nurses build on their knowledge of individual participants.
10	Is placed in an appropriate context in the school curriculum.	Not applicable	
11	Lasts a sufficient time to meet program goals and objectives.	✓	Counseling lasts about 20 to 30 minutes, with the opportunity for further sessions if required or desired.
12	Is coordinated with a wider school health promotion program.	✓	The clinic program is part of a wider program that involves school- and community-based interventions.
13	Contains factually correct and consistent messages.	✓	UNFPA is considered an expert in reproductive health, and they helped devise the materials.
14	Has established political support through intense advocacy to overcome barriers and go to scale.	✓	The government has been involved from the very beginning, and the hope is that these YFHSs will be provided in all government health facilities.
15	Portrays human sexuality as a healthy and normal part of life, and is not derogatory against gender, race, ethnicity, or sexual orientation.	✓	Nurses will counsel anyone who comes to them, regardless of gender, race, or sexual orientation.
16	Includes monitoring and evaluation.	✓	Two evaluations have been conducted.

PART D: ADDITIONAL INFORMATION

Organizations and Contacts

UNFPA/Pathfinder International: Mozambique
CTA Rita Badiani
Av. Do Zimbabwe 830
C.P. 1590
Maputo, Mozambique
E-mail- Odete@unfpa.uem.mz
or
RBadiani@pathfind.org
or
Izilhao@pathfind.org

Contributors to the Report

Program report prepared by Esther Kaziliman-Pale.

Edited by Helen Baños Smith.

We appreciate the help of the following people in providing much of the information in this report:

Rita Badiani — Chief technical adviser
Julio Pacca — Technical adviser, Ministry of Education, INDE
Ivonne Zilhao — Technical adviser, Ministry of Health
Celmira Silva — National counterpart, Ministry of Youth and Sport
Joachim Matavele — INDE
Helena Zerinda — INDE
Dr. Nassifa — Clinical coordinator, Adolescent Health Clinic
Ajamia Ibraimo — Nurse youth counselor
Raquel Jose Daniel — Nurse, youth counselor
Deolinda Aurora — Nurse youth counselor, Maputo

Available Materials

To obtain these materials, please contact ibeaids@ibe.unesco.org or Education for HIV/AIDS Prevention, International Bureau of Education, C.P. 199, 1211 Geneva 20, Switzerland.

Programa de saúde escolar e do adolescente: Linhas de orientação para os serviços amigo dos adolescents e jovens (SAAJ)
(order number: UNFPA01)

Direitos reprodutivos dos adolescents
(order number: UNFPA02)

Curriculum de formação de formadores em saúde reprodutive e planeamento familiar: Módulo 16, serviços de saúde reprodutiva para adolescentes
(order number: UNFPA03)

Manual do participante
(order number: UNFPA04)

Pamphlets:
HIV/SIDA: *Nuito se fala mas pouco se sabe…*
DTS: Está *protegido quem usa preservative*
Gravidez: É tão simples evitar
Meninas e rapazes: Diferentes porém iguais
Adolescência: Quanta mudança ao mesmo tempo!
Prazer com saúde
Small cards with messages written on the back
Stickers (order number: UNFPA05)
Posters (order number: UNFPA06)

APPENDIX 1. STAFF ROLES

Main Program Staff Roles

Chief Technical Adviser
Oversees and coordinates all aspects of the program.

Technical Advisers
Support the chief technical adviser on issues of health, education, and youth. Each adviser has a national counterpart team at the ministerial level. Technical advisers work with their national counterparts on the day-to-day running of the program. They are also responsible for supervision of technical advisers at the provincial level.

Health Technical Adviser
Oversees the running of the YFHSs and is responsible for all technical aspects of the program in Maputo City. She works with the city directorate of health, which is responsible for running the city health units.

Physicians
These are government-employed doctors trained in youth-friendly practice who attend to the needs of the youth referred by the nurses. They also support the management and technical aspects of program activities.

Nurses
Attend to the needs of the youth. They are also employed by the government.

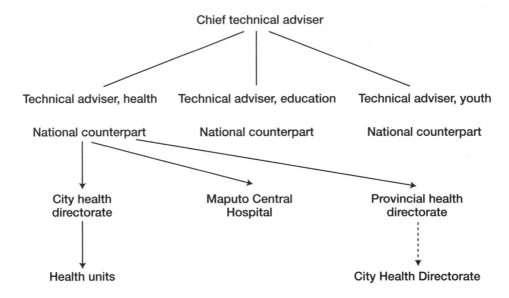

Note: Dotted line indicates occassional contact between provincial health directorate and city health directorate.

Figure A.1. UNFPA/Pathfinder International Program Staff Structure

APPENDIX 2. STAFF DATA

Number of Staff Currently Working on the Clinical Component of the Program in Maputo			
	Number of Staff	Position/title	Gender
Full-time and paid	1	Chief technical advisor	Female
	1	Technical advisor	Female
	1	National counterpart	Female
	1	Clinical coordinator	Female
	15	Nurses	Female
Volunteer peer educators (not receiving allowances/ incentives)	Not constant	Peer educators	

APPENDIX 3. PROGRAM FINANCES (IN US$)

Technical assistant	45,000
International consultant	15,000
Travel/per diem	3,000
National consultant	3,450
Honoraria	4,753
Elaboration of IEC material	10,000
Research knowledge, attitudes, and practices and BCC	8,000
Audiovisual material	8,000
Short external fellowship	3,500
Curricula development workshop	3,957
Training seminar	19,954
Meeting with collaborators	17,628
Study tour	3,243
Management course	996
English and computer courses	355
Expandable equipment	3,270
Rehabilitation costs	48,000
Operations and maintenance	8,988
Printing costs	4,000
Sundry	5,063
Total	**215,147**

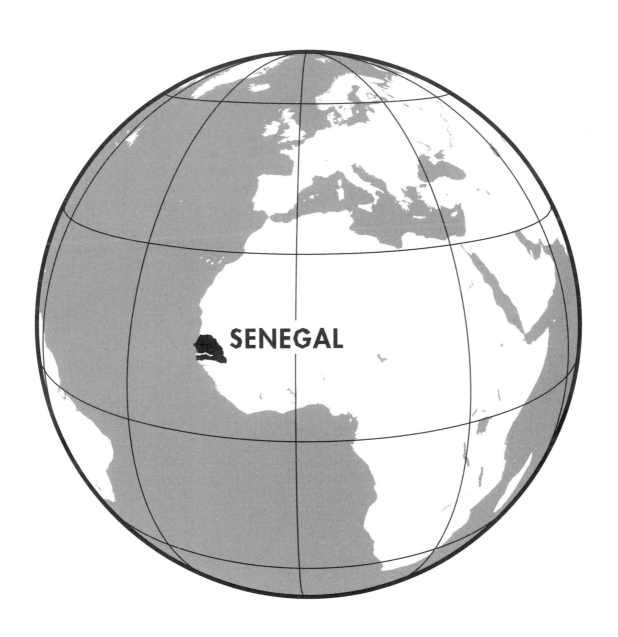

SENEGAL

The Group for the Study and Teaching of Population Issues (GEEP): An Experiment to Prevent the Spread of HIV/AIDS among Schoolchildren

PART A: DESCRIPTION OF THE PROGRAM

Program Rationale and History

In Senegal, as in the majority of African societies, sexuality has long been considered to be a taboo subject for social and religious reasons; the subject is not addressed at home or at school because adults (parents or teachers) are not prepared to talk to young people about sexual and reproductive health (SRH) issues.

Young people have suffered from this lack of discussion about their sexuality, even though a large proportion of them are sexually active (according to a 1990 study by the *Centre de Recherche pour le Développement International* [Research Center for International Development; CRDI]). This sexual activity naturally brings with it the risk of unwanted pregnancies, sexually transmitted diseases (STDs), and HIV/AIDS. It was within this context that the *Groupe pour l'Etude et l'Enseignement de la Population* (Group for the Study and Teaching of Population Issues; GEEP) was created by a group of teachers and health and population professionals.

To better educate young people about their sexuality and their fertility, GEEP, with the support of the Ministry of Health and the Population Council, undertook

- the organization of a series of conferences on adolescent fertility led by health care professionals in the community houses of the *lycées* (upper secondary schools) of Senegal, and

- the creation of information packs on population issues for teachers of geography, life sciences, and social and family economics.

This approach, which focused on specific activities, could not, however, respond satisfactorily to the growing demand from in-school adolescents for information about their sexuality and fertility.

Therefore, based on results from the CRDI study on youth fertility, questions posed by pupils during conferences, and research carried out in 1994 on upper secondary school students in Saint-Louis, GEEP decided in 1994 to implement a program of family life education in the *lycées* and and *collèges* (lower secondary schools) of Senegal. It did this in partnership with the

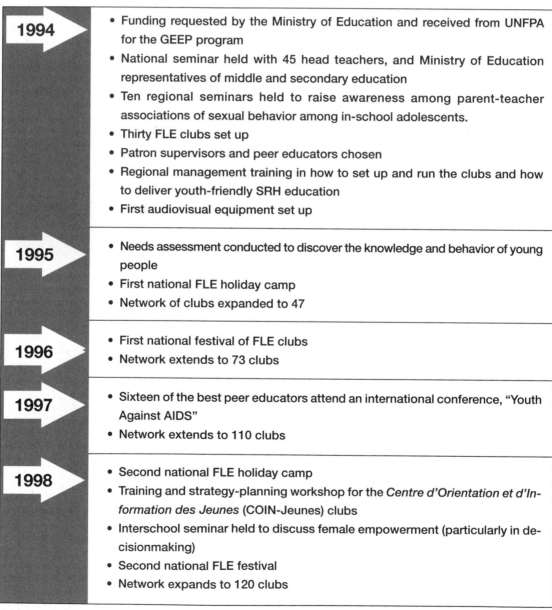

1994
- Funding requested by the Ministry of Education and received from UNFPA for the GEEP program
- National seminar held with 45 head teachers, and Ministry of Education representatives of middle and secondary education
- Ten regional seminars held to raise awareness among parent-teacher associations of sexual behavior among in-school adolescents.
- Thirty FLE clubs set up
- Patron supervisors and peer educators chosen
- Regional management training in how to set up and run the clubs and how to deliver youth-friendly SRH education
- First audiovisual equipment set up

1995
- Needs assessment conducted to discover the knowledge and behavior of young people
- First national FLE holiday camp
- Network of clubs expanded to 47

1996
- First national festival of FLE clubs
- Network extends to 73 clubs

1997
- Sixteen of the best peer educators attend an international conference, "Youth Against AIDS"
- Network extends to 110 clubs

1998
- Second national FLE holiday camp
- Training and strategy-planning workshop for the *Centre d'Orientation et d'Information des Jeunes* (COIN-Jeunes) clubs
- Interschool seminar held to discuss female empowerment (particularly in decisionmaking)
- Second national FLE festival
- Network expands to 120 clubs

Figure 1. Time Line of Major Program Events

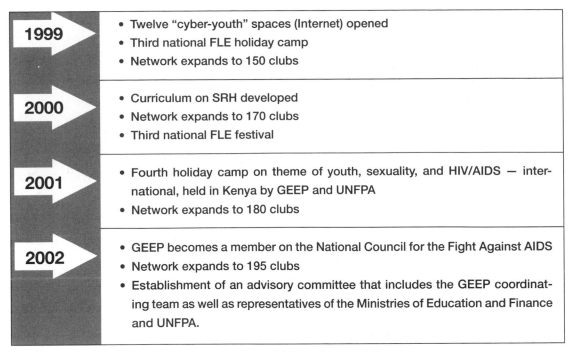

Figure 1. Time Line of Major Program Events

Ministry of Education, with financial support primarily from the United National Population Fund (UNFPA) but also with other backers.

This program aims to respond to the needs of in-school adolescents by establishing family life education (FLE) clubs (activity and communication centers) in schools. There is currently a network of 191 FLE clubs (established in 65 percent of the upper and lower secondary schools of Senegal), of which two out of three are equipped with audiovisual material (television and videotapes) and one out of eight are equipped with computer and Internet access.

At a central level, GEEP has a mobile activity unit, which consists of a vehicle, a video projector, a giant screen, and a public address system, that can present social mobilization activities to schools and sometimes to the wider community.

Program Overview

Aim

Through the FLE program and its participatory approaches, GEEP aims to integrate SRH into the body of knowledge taught at school and encourage responsible sexual behavior among in-school adolescents from the ages of 12 through 19. It also aims to encourage these young people to promote responsible behavior among their peers and in their own communities.

Objectives

The program's objectives are to

- give information and encourage responsible behavior among adolescents in relation to sexual and reproductive health issues, particularly gender issues, STDs, and HIV/AIDS;

- modernize the teaching of SRH issues by training new trainers, producing educational materials, and integrating into the curriculum the need for behavioral changes in matters of adolescent SRH;
- establish participatory information structures in individual schools to advise in-school adolescents on matters of SRH(FLE clubs);
- empower the leaders of these structures (peer educators and patron supervisors) by providing training and support materials and equipment;
- support awareness-raising activities of these structures in both the schools and the wider community;
- train teachers to adopt a global and cross-curricular approach to the teaching of SRH issues; and
- facilitate the integration of SRH issues into the life sciences, family and social economics, and geography curricula.

Target Groups

Primary Target Group
Members of FLE clubs:peer educators, patron supervisors, and 12- to 19-year-old students of public and private secondary schools in Senegal, as well as students at the University of Dakar and the University of Saint-Louis, and their teachers.

Secondary Target Group
Adolescents attending schools that host FLE clubs and members of the community that come in touch with club members.

Site
The program takes place primarily in the school environment, within the framework of classes and extracurricular activities. Some specific activities take place outside schools, particularly in rural areas.

Program Length
Initially planned for two years (1994–96), the FLE program has been renewed two times (1997–2001, 2002–03).

Program Goals
To help school-age children adopt responsible sexual behavior to prevent unwanted pregnancy and sexually transmitted infection (STI)–STD transmission (including HIV) and prepare them to lead responsible adult lives.

Program Approaches
- SRH information access,
- raise awareness of issues related to SRH, and
- listen to school-age children's needs and refer them to appropriate services.

The program's messages take into account the different levels of sexual experience of its audience; abstinence is advocated, but the program also advocates the use of condoms if young people are already sexually active.

Activities

The most effective activities are those in which participants are actively involved. This makes them aware of important SRH issues and their (communal) responsibilities by placing them in specific situations (through such activities as role plays and watching films). Materials production workshops encourage participants to develop their own points of view. Activities that build a rapport between the peer educators and patron supervisors are also important. The least effective training methods are information sessions that lack an interactive dimension.

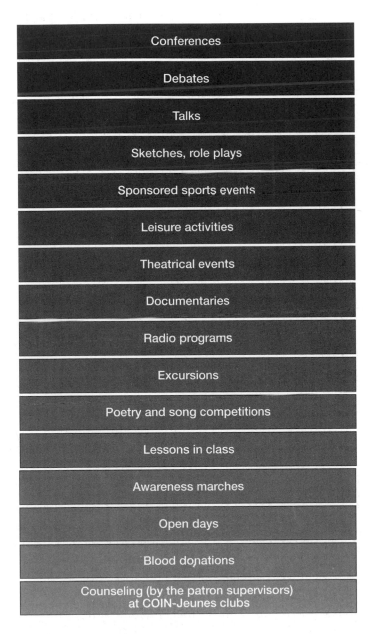

Figure 2. Program Activities Unranked

Components

There are four main components:
1. FLE clubs,
2. COIN-Jeunes clubs,
3. school curricula, and
4. Outreach activities.

FLE Clubs

The clubs are led by 15 peer educators under the supervision of 5 patron supervisors. All pupils are invited to attend voluntarily. Activities generally take place once a week at break times or after school, with each pupil attending for at least one or two half-days each week. In addition to this, the FLE clubs hold extra activities on national and world population days (December 1, March 8, July 11, and so forth). The peer educators provide information and raise awareness on adolescent SRH (sexuality, pregnancy, HIV/AIDS, gender, and so forth) using a variety of activities.

Each FLE club is under the authority of its host school. Working with the peer educators, the school manages all the materials and funds that are given to, or generated by, the club.

Records of activities, feedback, and the use of materials, as well as financial reports prepared by the club's leaders (peer educators and patron supervisors) and the school head are regularly sent to the national head of the FLE clubs to allow him to periodically review the running of the clubs and the state of the program's materials.

The role of the patron-supervisor team is to manage and assist the peer educators in planning and running activities. They also organize and lead conferences and act as a core around which a network of local personnel (doctors, sociologists, psychologists, social workers) gather.

The program also supports and encourages the Generation FLE project. This project has been running for three years, and it aims to reunite former peer educators who are now at a university or working.

COIN-Jeunes Clubs

These are information and advice centers (one at the University of Dakar, as well as at several schools that accommodate regional FLE centers) to meet the special psychological and social needs of certain adolescents who need support beyond that provided by the FLE clubs. Of the 11 COIN-Jeunes clubs that were set up, only 3 are currently functional. Adolescents can go to the centers for confidential and personal advice and counseling on their sexuality and problems at home or at school (often including issues of sexual abuse). Apart from the university COIN-Jeunes, the centers are run by patron supervisors.

School Curricula

In parallel with the FLE and COIN-Jeunes clubs, GEEP has launched another strategy, known as "population education," which aims to bring SRH issues into the classroom by using two linked strategies: a cross-curricular model and a specific curriculum on adolescent SRH. The plan is that matters relating to SRH will permeate all aspects of education.

Outreach Activities

At the school level, each FLE club functions autonomously; on the departmental, regional, and national levels, the clubs work together to organize communal activities planned by the national network of FLE clubs under the supervision of GEEP. These events, which target great numbers of students, are described below.

The community podium event. This is a school-based event, that is also held quarterly in the wider community. It is organized by the regional FLE clubs with support from GEEP's mobile activity unit (see "Program Resources"). This activity targets a large public audience of 200 to 300 people and usually consists of a film on HIV/AIDS and family planning, a talent show on SRH issues, and musical entertainment.

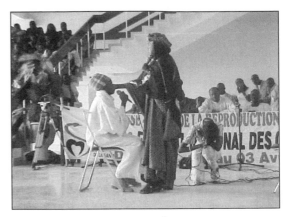

A community podium event

The reproductive health competition. Different FLE clubs compete against each other and test their knowledge of questions relating to SRH and HIV/AIDS. Two teams of four players represent each school. This game is prepared by a large group of students — about 15 to 20 on average — who research the issues. It is from these students that the four team members are chosen. The competition provides an opportunity to evaluate the participants' knowledge and understanding of SRH issues, including HIV/AIDS, and also informs the wider public about the issues. Each game lasts, on average, for 10 to 15 minutes, and the players must combine speed and knowledge to gain the most points. The competition is structured in two phases, an elimination round and a final round.

Regional FLE days. These are organized to encourage the FLE clubs to meet with others in their areas. Patron representatives from different regions meet to discuss program activities and exchange experiences. Sometimes they also carry out regional awareness-raising activities, such as marches and speeches.

The FLE festival. This three-day event brings together representatives from all the FLE clubs in Senegal (four peer educators and one patron supervisor per club). It takes place in Dakar every three years under the patronage of the president of the republic and offers the representatives an opportunity to meet and exchange information and ideas.

The FLE festival agenda is made up of
- intellectual and psychological play activities,
- information panels led by reproductive health specialists,
- workshops for sharing experiences,
- demonstration sessions,
- artistic expression activities,
- evaluation sessions by the national network, and
- launching of new initiatives.

Holiday camps. This is an extension of the national network's activities in rural areas. Camps are organized during the long school holidays. They last seven days and provide the opportunity for peer educators, who often come from urban areas, to become familiar with the realities of rural life and share their experiences with young people from rural areas. The location of these

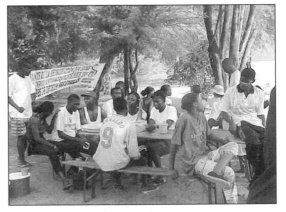

Youth at a camp

camps is chosen by taking into account the extent of the health and environmental problems facing the local population. These events foster social exchange and mobilization in rural environments. They also provide an opportunity for young people to be creative and consequently learn that they are in a position to solve their problems and make changes.

The holiday camps are generally run by about 50 of the most dynamic peer educators, who are chosen by individual FLE clubs. They are structured around the following activities:

- workshops for the production of information and awareness-raising materials;
- multimedia information and sensitization campaigns targeted at the local community dealing with health problems, notably family planning, STDs, HIV/AIDS, and malaria;
- community demonstration activities on sanitary techniques and reforestation;
- cyberspace activities to introduce the rural population to the Internet; and
- research on population and health issues in the area in which the camp is held.

The idea of the FLE holiday camps (which have been held since 1995 in different parts of Senegal) was "exported" in August 2001 to Nakuru, Kenya. On this occasion, young people from 13 different southern African countries adopted an African declaration on HIV/AIDS (see the discussion of the manual *Youth, Sexuality, and HIV/AIDS* in "Program Materials" below).

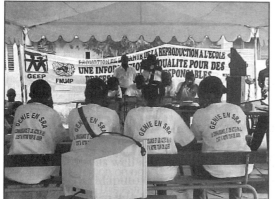

Cyberspace activities

Essay on population and development issues. This is an annual dissertation competition organized by GEEP in collaboration with the Ministry of Education. It is targeted at the best students in the upper secondary schools' premier classes (final level). The competition evaluates their knowledge and understanding of SRH and environmental issues.

A huge sensitization campaign prepares the students in premier classes for this competition, which takes place nationally on the second and third Wednesday of May between 3:00 P.M. and 7:00 P.M., under the supervision of the patron supervisors.

The award ceremony (prizes of grants and school manuals) for the winners takes place on July 11, which is World Population Day. The prizes are given by the Ministry of Education and the Ministry of Finance and Economy.

PART B: IMPLEMENTING THE PROGRAM

Needs Assessment

The program design was based on

- the findings of an analysis of questions posed by secondary school students during GEEP conferences between 1990 and 1994,

- the findings of a 1994 study of the sexual behavior of upper secondary school students in Saint–Louis.
- the findings of a 1990 CRDI study on adolescent fertility in Senegal,
- a national study conducted by GEEP in 1995 of the sexual behavior of upper secondary school students, and
- a study in the town of Mbour, conducted by GEEP in 1996, of the sexual behavior of upper secondary school students.

These studies revealed that young people had certain experiences and held certain beliefs that were putting them at risk in a variety of ways:
- Growing numbers of young people are sexually active.
- Many youth engage in unprotected sex.
- There is a lack of communication within families.
- Some young people question the very existence of HIV/AIDS.
- There is a tendency among some young people to regard HIV/AIDS as a disease that effects only prostitutes and drug addicts.

The findings of these various studies were used to develop the program. Unfortunately, further details of these studies are not available.

Program Materials

To fully equip the young people and the teachers involved in the project, GEEP has produced a range of support materials, listed below. These materials took between six months and one year to develop, produce, and distribute.
- Educational support
  - training modules,
  - information packs, and
  - manuals for peers.
- Sensitization support materials
  - information packs,
  - cassettes,
  - films,
  - posters,
  - cartoons, and
  - T-shirts.

These are described in more detail below.

Target Group Materials

A variety of print materials has been developed for use in the classroom, the FLE clubs, and COIN-Jeunes centers. They are described in detail below.

Manuals

Three manuals on adolescent SRH have been produced by peer educators under the supervision of the patron supervisors and other specialists:
- *Adolescence, sexualité précoce, MST-SIDA pour des comportements responsables (1999) (Adolescence, Early Sexuality, STD-AIDS for Responsible Behavior),*

- *Droits en santé de la reproduction = brisons le silence (2000) (Reproductive Health Rights = Breaking the Silence)*, and
- *Les jeunes, la sexualité et le VIH-SIDA (2001) (Youth, Sexuality, and HIV/AIDS).*

Through these materials, the authors seek to educate themselves and others about SRH issues, notably premature pregnancy, HIV/AIDS, and adolescent SRH rights.

Each manual is structured into training units that consist of a dialogue, a personal narrative, or a cartoon strip, followed by questionnaire that aims to help the user to make his or her evaluation. For example, Youth, Sexuality, and HIV/AIDS is structured into three training units that represent three different stages:

1. "Let's Discover'" presents a personal narrative, a letter, or a brief dialogue designed to inform and catch the user's attention.
2. "Let's Understand" comprises dialogues to encourage the user to reflect on the issues.
3. "'Let's Suggest" consists solely of questions that encourage the user to express his or her point of view and suggest possible solutions to the problems.

The STOP AIDS information pack is a three-part information pack that makes HIV/AIDS information accessible to both in-school and out-of-school adolescents. It is made up of both text and illustrations and contains information on:

- the nature of HIV/AIDS,
- situations in which the HIV/AIDS virus can be caught and transmitted,
- situations in which the virus cannot be caught, and
- preventive methods, including protection against HIV/AIDS.

For further information about materials, see Senegal GEEP Program Appendix 2.

Staff Training Materials

These materials are used to train patron supervisors and peer educators.

The cross-curricular model for teaching SRH issues is presented in a brochure, "Teaching SRH Issues: A Cross-curricular Approach." This model integrates three subjects — geography, life sciences, and social and family economics — into SRH education.

It aims to

- encourage teachers to have a global, multidimensional, and integrated vision of SRH issues, whether they involve world, regional, or local questions; and
- draw on the different training and knowledge of each teacher to encourage new, but scientifically sound, perspectives on SRH issues.

The brochure is structured in four parts:

1. The theoretical framework describes methodology and identifies references.
2. The discussion of SRH issues draws together the four main areas of SRH studies (SRH dynamics, SRH and the environment, health and SRH, SRH and the family).
3. The section on general objectives outlines how the four areas described in the second part of the brochure may be drawn together in a scientific way.
4. The section on delivery of such information shows how SRH issues can be incorporated into the official curriculum and identifies appropriate pedagogical approaches.

The sexual health curriculum, "Managed Evolution," is the work of several specialists (doctors, lawyers, sociologists, psychologists, educational psychologists, and teachers). It provides patron supervisors and peer educators with information they can use to help FLE club members to

- deal with adolescent crisis,
- become informed about their SRH rights,
- prevent the spread of HIV/AIDS,
- make enlightened choices about their own behavior, and
- actively promote positive changes in behavior and become aware of the need to use health services.

The curriculum consists of four parts:
1. references and pedagogical intentions;
2. five training modules on self awareness, human reproduction, STDs and HIV/AIDS, the legal rights of adolescents in relation to SRH, and communication and reproductive health;
3. teaching, training, and evaluation strategies; and
4. scientific advice on the training modules, which draws together all related knowledge from the themes treated in the modules.

This curriculum has been piloted in schools in three regions (Dakar, Saint-Louis, and Thiès), and an evaluation is planned for the end of 2002.

The AIDS-gender module, produced by GEEP's educational team, aims to contribute to the social and emotional development of young people by dealing with the question of HIV/AIDS. Many ideological and sociocultural barriers to understanding HIV/AIDS still exist; these can make it difficult for young people to build new relationships and communicate with others.

The module is delivered in six sessions on different themes:
1. introduction,
2. the notion of gender,
3. HIV/AIDS,
4. the spread of HIV/AIDS (the group or the gender most at risk, responsibilities, etc.),
5. attitudes to adopt toward gender, and
6. planning of FLE and COIN-Jeunes activities regarding young people's approach to gender.

For further information about materials, see Senegal GEEP Program appendix 2.

Staff Selection and Training

Training activities aim to enable the peer educators and patron supervisors to become leaders and promote positive behavioral changes in both the school and the local community. Peer educators and patron supervisors receive the same training, which is described below.

- Patron supervisors are school teachers. The choice of teachers is made by the school head and the GEEP national coordination group. The patrons are volunteers and are chosen for their openness and moral reputation.
- The choice of peer educators is overseen by the patron supervisors in agreement with the school authority and is based on the following criteria:
  - the student's grades in classes,
  - his or her good behavior in school, and
  - his or her open-mindedness and dynamism.
- Peer educators and patron supervisors are usually trained together.
- Training lasts between three and five days.

- Training is led by the GEEP educational team, assisted when necessary by extra personnel (life sciences, geography, and social and family economics teachers; experts from the U.N. Development Fund for Women (UNIFEM); and representatives from the Education Service for Health).
- Training sessions are often in the form of interactive workshops.
- Training content varies, but generally includes the cross-curricular model, strategic planning, activity leadership techniques, message delivery techniques, management, the Population Policy Declaration, the fight against HIV/AIDS, gender and HIV/AIDS, adolescent SRH, family planning, and counseling.
- The most effective training activities are those organized as workshops.

For further information about staff structure, see the GEEP organizational chart in Appendix 1 to this chapter.

For further information about materials, see Senegal GEEP Program Appendix 2.

Setting up the Program

No information was available on how to set up the program.

Program Resources

Each FLE club is provided with its own equipment (a television, a cassette recorder, a filing cabinet, and, in special cases, a computer).

Advocacy

GEEP works with three different ministry departments: The Office for Middle and Secondary Education, the General Inspectorate for National Education, and the Bureau for Educational Planning and Research. It sends them reports as well as the significant educational materials and other brochures that have been produced and asks them to promote the principles behind GEEP. The FLE program is also authorized by the Ministry of Education. Furthermore, in addition to the financial support provided to GEEP through the *Programme de Développement Intégré de la Santé* (PDIS; Integrated Health Sector Development Program), the Ministry of Health has incorporated it into the National Council for the Fight Against AIDS. However, GEEP does not work with any of the other HIV/AIDS prevention associations.

On the local level, the school head authorizes, and sometimes presides over, the FLE club's activities. To overcome resistance from parents and teachers, who often worry that SRH education will encourage promiscuity, GEEP demonstrates their openness by involving parents and teachers in the program's design and inviting them to various activities.

Program Finances

GEEP has received funding from the government (Ministries of Education, Health, Prevention, and Economy and Finance), foreign government agencies (the United States Agency for International Development [USAID], CRDI), United Nations agencies (UNFPA, the United Nations Educational, Scientific, and Cultural Organization [UNESCO], UNIFEM), and NGOs (Population Council, Rainbo, Club 2/3 Canada, Schools Online). Table 1 shows the grants received in 2001.

For the year 2001, the balance was positive, with an amount of US$12,.290, which was included in the planning programs for 2002.

FLE clubs also often raise financial support from their partners (through collections, sponsorship, parent-teacher association grants, and other fund-raising activities). GEEP also supports the clubs by allocating *fonds d'impulsion* (action funds) grants.

Table 1. Funding Received in 2001

Donor	Amount (US$)
UNFPA	62,415
Ministry of Health	41,096
Population Council (CEFOREP)	16,438
Club 2/3	12,637
Rainbo	3,877
Schools Online	20,852
Total	157,316

Table 2. 2001 Spending (US$)

Activities and Programs	UNFPA	IDRC Schools Online	Club 2/3	Ministry of Health	Rainbo	Population Council	Total
Training/ capacity building	35,042	3,000	10,200	6,000		6,500	60,742
Survey/ICT in schools		4,352			3,875	5,255	13,482
Equipment for FLE clubs (e.g., computers, TV)	8,265	13,500		20,547			42,312
Personal salaries (5 people)	10,273			6,947			17,220
Overhead	8,334		2,436				11,270
Total	62,414	20,852	12,636	33,494	3,875	11,755	145,026

PART C: ASSESSMENT AND LESSONS LEARNED

Challenges and Solutions

Program Coordinator

- The implementation of the FLE school program in the early 1990s was not easy. There were parents, certain heads of schools, and even some teachers who were completely against any discussion of sexuality at school because they feared it would encourage students to engage in premature sexual activity.

- Knowledge of the school environment is essential. Schools, with their emphasis on conservatism and routine, are institutions with their own particular cultures; innovations should only be introduced with care. Pedagogical innovations such as the FLE clubs should be implemented only by education professionals, because they are most aware of the complex dynamics that exist within schools. Teachers should manage the program. Their involvement in the program should be seen as an extension of their professional engagement and not as an extra duty for which they are paid.

- It is necessary to run the program as an ongoing research project. This means that the program can consistently identify problems and new needs while seeking the most appropriate responses and solutions.

Report Author

The originality of GEEP's program lies in its main areas:

- emphasis on a cross-curricular approach in class,
- the way it makes young people aware of their own responsibilities and involves them more effectively in socioeducational activities, and
- emphasis on a participatory approach to activities.

GEEP's program is pioneering particularly in its cross-curricular approach, its use of games (role plays, drama) as a training method in class, and the way young people themselves produce its educational and sensitization materials.

Nevertheless, the GEEP program could improve in these areas:

- Educational materials that are developed by the program are not pretested, and there is no formal system in place to record feedback about their use.
- There is a problem concerning the institutional validation of the educational materials that are produced.
- There are no appropriate systems to capitalize on the program's findings in terms of approaches and educational materials.
- There is no consideration in planning school timetables to take advantage of the opportunities presented by a cross-curricular approach.
- There are no groups developing cross-curricular programs at the school level.

A solution to these problems could be found in an agreement between the Ministry of Education and GEEP to introduce the FLE program into the Institute of Teacher Training's curriculum and to have a more centralized, institutional approach to training methods and the validation and use of educational materials.

Evaluation

The clubs' activity reports and annual reports are used to evaluate the program. However, no formal system is in place to evaluate the impact of messages.

In 2000, an evaluative study entitled "*Etats des lieux*" showed an increased knowledge of SRH and more responsible behaviors among adolescents who had attended GEEP's clubs than among those who had not.

To ensure that the program's messages are consistent and effective in the long term, a longitudinal evaluation was planned for 2002.

UNAIDS Benchmarks

	Benchmark	Attainment	Comments
1	Recognizes the child/youth as a learner who already knows, feels, and can do in relation to healthy development and HIV/AIDS-related prevention.	✓	Young people are at the center of a training process that enables them to gain the knowledge and develop the attitudes to change their own behavior and promote positive behavior changes among their peers. They are trained in communication and leadership techniques that enable them to influence their peers most effectively. Many of the printed support materials are produced by young people. Peer educators also run the FLE club activities, both within and outside school.
2	Focuses on risks that are most common to the learning group and that responses are appropriate and targeted to the age group.	✓	Premature pregnancy, STDs, and, in particular, fear of HIV/AIDS are the main concerns of the target group, as revealed by an analysis of questions posed by students during GEEP conferences before 1994 and during a 1994 study of the sexual behavior of upper secondary school pupils in Saint Louis. In response to these concerns, the program has favored peer education; moreover, the program uses communication styles and techniques that young people can best relate to (cartoon strips, sketches, musical productions, drama). Messages are generally formulated by young people who are aware of their peers' needs and concerns. The messages are aimed specifically at their target group; for example, although abstinence is advocated, HIV/AIDS prevention messages always take into account the fact that some young people are already sexually active and so the importance of using a condom is stressed.

	Benchmark	Attainment	Comments
3	Includes not only knowledge but also attitudes and skills needed for prevention.	✓	The gender-AIDS module challenges young people's attitudes.
			The program tries to influence behavior and attitudes in its socialization activities (role plays, use of audiovisual equipment, etc.) and in its activities, which are designed to make young people aware of their responsibilities (initiative, production of support materials, leading activities).
			By favoring peer education, the program is able to develop positive role models for young people from within their own community.
			Interactivity is seen as the key to all the activities, and participant are always encouraged to develop and defend a point of view.
			Activities are designed to help young people become responsible, adult members of society so that they can influence opinion and promote behavioral changes.
4	Understands the impact of relationships on behavior change and reinforces positive social values.	✓	Gender is a key concept in the program, and the GEEP logo underlines this. The program seeks to develop self-esteem in young people, respect for others, and negotiating skills, which will help them deal more effectively with peer pressure.
5	Is based on analysis of learners' needs and a broader situation assessment.	Partially fulfilled	The program design was based on the findings of an analysis of questions posed by students during GEEP conferences between 1990 and 1994, and of a 1994 study of the sexual behavior of upper secondary school pupils in Saint-Louis and of a 1990 CRDI study on adolescent fertility in Senegal.
			GEEP has also carried out two additional studies into the sexual behavior of upper secondary school students (a national study in 1995 and a study in the town of Mbour in 1996).
			As the program's sphere of influence is limited to schools, GEEP has not conducted studies in the wider community. Although it is a member of the National Council for the Fight Against HIV/AIDS, GEEP does not work with any of the other AIDS prevention associations.

	Benchmark	Attainment	Comments
6	Has training and continuous support of teachers and other service providers.	Partially fulfilled	The training of peer educators and patron supervisors on HIV/AIDS and on adolescent SRH issues is delivered by the GEEP educational team in collaboration with professionals from the Service for Health Education or the National Council for the Fight Against AIDS. This consists of initial training; specific, one-time training courses, and training sessions requested by individual FLE clubs. However, there is no systematic refresher training.
7	Uses multiple and participatory learning activities and strategies.	✓	As interactive and participative approach is evident in all the program's activities. Training sessions take the form of workshops, with the leaders making use of a wide range of support materials and techniques (manuals, role plays, films, posters). Activities such as role plays, talent shows, debates, community podium events, drama, and forums all encourage interactivity between the activity leaders and participants. Information activities (specialist conferences, debates, testimony from AIDS sufferers) are always followed by discussions.
8	Involves the wider community.	✓	The program reaches out to the wider community through its various activities (marches, community podium events, FLE holiday camps, sports tournaments, etc). Health workers are involved in the organization of the community podium events; youth clubs help organize the sports tournaments sponsored by the FLE clubs, who provide the musical entertainment and the prizes (including sensitization materials). These specific activities are not, however, supported by follow-up work with the local community.
9	Ensures sequence, progression, and continuity of messages.	✓	The manuals used in the FLE clubs build up knowledge and understanding gradually. They introduce topics and then ask children to reflect on what they have learned and then to come up with solutions to problems they may face.

	Benchmark	Attainment	Comments
10	Is placed in an appropriate context in the school curriculum.	✓	The program is delivered by both class activities (the formal educational section) and socioeducational activities (the FLE clubs). The formal educational section of the program (especially the part relating to HIV/AIDS) is delivered by the following school subjects; life sciences (in class 3 and 4 of lower secondary school) and family and social economics (in class 4 of lower secondary school).
11	Lasts a sufficient time to meet program goals and objectives.	✓	It takes two years to establish about 30 clubs and make them them fully operational, but their effect on behavior can be evaluated only in the longer term.
12	Is coordinated with a wider school health promotion program.	Not applicable	In addition to the prevention of HIV/AIDS, the program aims to reduce premature pregnancies and campaigns against female genital mutilation. The coordination and delivery of school health programs are in principle the responsibility of the School of Medical Inspectorate. However, this has not been evident in schools, where up until now, the fight against HIV/AIDS has been led by the FLE clubs, the anti-AIDS association, and life sciences teachers.
13	Contains factually correct and consistent messages.	✓	Information transmitted by the program through the FLE clubs comes from health specialists (the Health Educator Service, health workers) and life sciences and family and social economics teachers. The involvement of local health workers in community activities ensures that all information on health issues is accurate.

	Benchmark	Attainment	Comments
14	Has established political support through intense advocacy to overcome barriers and go to scale.	✓	The FLE program is authorized by the Ministry of Education. GEEP works with three different ministry departments; the Office for Middle and Secondary Education, the General Inspectorate for National Education, and the Bureau for Educational Planning and Research. It sends them reports as well as the significant educational materials and other brochures that have been produced. On a local level, the school head authorizes, and sometimes presides over, the club's activities. In addition to the financial support provided to GEEP through PDIs, the Ministry of Health has incorporated GEEP into the National Council for the Fight Against AIDS.
15	Portrays human sexuality as a healthy and normal part of life, and is not derogatory against gender, race, ethnicity, or sexual orientation.	Partially fulfilled	The program considers sex as a normal part of human life and that young people should have access to the information and services they need. Mindful of traditional values, it aims to overcome the cultural barriers that have treated sex as a taboo subject both at home and at school. The program is run on a national level and, as a result, does not discriminate between different ethnic groups. Participants are chosen exclusively for their commitment, dynamism, and open-mindedness. The school program does not take into account the different ideas of sexuality among the different ethnic groups. Homosexuality is not treated in the same way as heterosexuality. It is addressed only as a risk behavior in relation to HIV/AIDS prevention.

	Benchmark	Attainment	Comments
16	Includes monitoring and evaluation.	✓	Each FLE club is monitored through its management reporting, half-yearly visits by a mission from the national coordination team, or a quarterly visit by a mission from the regional center. Only clubs that regularly submit their reports are eligible for GEEP grants.
			The program's success has been measured through two evaluative studies the program's impact (commissioned by GEEP and UNFPA) in 1996 and 2002.
			There are also other, less objective, indications of success:
			• the growing demand from schools for FLE clubs, and
			• testimonials from school heads and the opinions of beneficiaries, which have been collected during studies and school visits by program partners.
			At the beginning of each year, two different meetings are held to review the past year's experiences and share new ideas for the future.
			• A regional meeting is organized for the head of each regional center, FLE representatives, and their local partners.
			• A national meeting also takes place between the national coordination team and representatives from the regional centers.

PART D: ADDITIONAL INFORMATION

Organizations and Contacts

Groupe pour l'Etude et l'Enseignement de la Population (GEEP)
BP 5036
Dakar, Senegal
Telephone: (221) 824-4877
Fax: (221) 825-4714
E-mail: geepop@syfed.refer.sn
Website: www.refer.sn/geep

Contributors to the Report

Program report prepared by El Hadji Habib Camara, an independent specialist education consultant in population, health, and environment issuesand the creation of educational materials.

Edited by Helen Baños Smith.

We appreciate the help of the following people in providing much of the information in this report:

Babacar Fall — GEEP coordinator
Khadidiatou Tall Thiam — GEEP administrator
Ibrahim Senghor — Head of FLE club program
Moustapha Diagne — Minister of Education
Founé Kanoute — Head of COIN-Jeunes club at Lycée Blaise Diagne
A group of four patron supervisors and seven peer educators in Dakar
A group of 3 patron supervisors and 10 peer educators in Saint-Louis

Available Materials

To obtain these materials, please contact ibeaids@ibe.unesco.org or Education for HIV/AIDS Prevention, International Bureau of Education, C.P. 199, 1211 Geneva 20, Switzerland.

Santé reproductive des adolescents (curriculum)
(order number: GEEP01)

Adolescence, sexualité précoce, MST-SIDA pour des comportements responsables (Adolescence, Early Sexuality, STD-AIDS for Responsible Behavior) (manual for peer education)
(order number: GEEP02)

Les jeunes, la sexualité et le VIH-SIDA (Youth, Sexuality, and HIV/AIDS) (manual developed by youth for youth)
(order number: GEEP03)

Report about clubs and activities in Senegal
(order number: GEEP04)

Registration form for club attendance
(order number: GEEP05)

Form for recording club activities
(order number: GEEP06)

Form for recording materials use
(order number: GEEP07)

Form for recording the establishment of a club
(order number: GEEP08)

Promotion de l'éducation à la vie familiale. Didactique des problèmes de population. (Promotion of Family Life Education.. Teaching of Population Problems)
(order number: GEEP09)

Dossiers documentaires et pedagogiques. Livret du professeur. Les problèmes de population. (Documentary and Pedagogical Files. Teacher's Guide. Population Problems)
(order number: GEEP10)

Agenda Education à la Vie Familiale 2001-2002 (Family Life Education Diary 2001–2002)
(order number: GEEP11)

"Stop SIDA/Stop AIDS" (pamphlet)
(order number: GEEP12)

Poster: Children with their teacher
(order number: GEEP13)

Poster: Mother and child
(order number: GEEP14)

Poster: Street painting; fight against AIDS
(order number: GEEP15)

Video: *Le concours théâtrale de lutte contre le SIDA*
(order number: GEEP16)

APPENDIX 1. ORGANIZATIONAL CHART

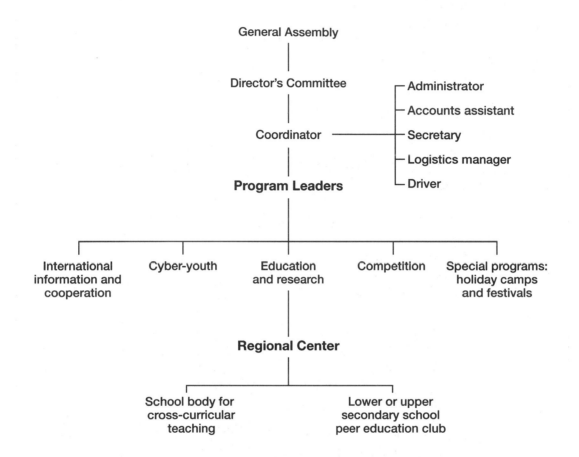

Figure A.1. GEEP Organizational Chart

APPENDIX 2. TRAINING ACTIVITIES AND MATERIALS

Training sessions last between three and five days, and, in general, peer educators and patron-supervisors are trained together.

Information and Sensitization Activities

The awareness marches and sports tournaments are the only activities that deal exclusively with HIV/AIDS issues; all the others deal with a variety of different topics.

Counseling activities are exclusively in the domain of the patron-supervisors and other specialists. Even if the peer educators have received training in this area, they are currently excluded from it.

Types of activities	Leaders	Theme/title	Target
Public conference	Patron-supervisors	Reproduction	Peer educators and pupils
Discussion	Peer educators		
Debate	Peer educators		Peer educators and pupils
Knowledge quiz	Peer educators	Sexuality	Peer educators
March	Peer educators		
Community podium activity	Peer educators	STDs and AIDS	Local community school and local community, young people from the ASC
Sports tournament	Peer educators		Peer educators
FLE festival	Peer educators		
FLE leisure (sketches, role play)	Peer educators		
Holiday camp	Peer educators	Premature pregnancies	Pupils
Essay competition	Patron-supervisors		
Drama competition	Patron-supervisors, social assistant	Reproductive health rights Gender Drugs	
Counseling	School nurse	Prostitution, etc.	Young people from rural areas, students from final-level classes Pupils

Support Materials

The information and sensitization materials, produced by the peer educators under the supervision of experts, are available in French and English.

Object	Type of material	Theme/title	Authors
Education	Training module (2002)	AIDS — gender	GEEP and UNIFEM education team
Education	Training module (1997)	Cross-curricular teaching of population issues	GEEP education team
Education	Information packs Booklet 1	Teaching population issues	Education team
Education	Curriculum (2000)	SRH	Cross-curricular team (doctors, sociologists, educationalists, teachers, and GEEP education team)
Education	Information packs: Booklets 1–7 (1995)	Population issues	GEEP education team
Education	Training module (1998)	Leadership techniques for information and advice centers	GEEP education team
Education	Reference book for FLE and population education (1996)		GEEP education team and other experts
Sensitization	Murals in schools	Pregnancy, HIV/AIDS, and responsible behavior	Peer educators
Information	Pack (2000)	HIV/AIDS	GEEP education team
Sensitization	T-shirt (messages)	ASRH and HIV/AIDS	GEEP education team
Information and sensitization	Manuals (2001)	Young people, sex, and HIV/AIDS	Peer educators and young people from southern African countries
Information and sensitization	Manual (1999)	Adolescents, premature sexual behavior, HIV/AIDS, responsible behavior	Peer educators
Sensitization	Films (1996)	Premature pregnancy	Peer educators
Sensitization	Posters	HIV/AIDS	Peer educators

Object	Type of material	Theme/title	Authors
Information and sensitization	Manual (2000)	Adolescent rights in matters of SRH — let's break the silence	Peer educators
Information and sensitization	Quarterly information bulletin	Special reports on AIDS 11–14	GEEP team
Information and sensitization	Agenda	FLE	GEEP team
Information and sensitization	Video (drama)	AIDS	Peer educators

Summary of Activities in SRH in Saint-Louis Schools, 2001–02

School	Date	Themes	Patron supervisors		Peer educators		Pupils		School authorities		Contributors		Total	Observations
			M	F	F	M	F	M	M	F	F	M		
Lyceé Ameth FALL (ages: 12 to 21 years)	March 23	Premature pregnancy	4	1	40		70	200	3	10	8		1,056	Insufficient time allocated, lack of pedagogical materials
	May 29	Self-awareness HIV/AIDS Premature pregnancy and abortion ASRH, rights and values Materials, the GEEP curriculum	2	1	25		150	80			3		263	
	After school	ASRH	2		25						1	5	33	
Lyceé Cheikh O. F. TALL (ages: 16 to 25 years)	April 14 In class	Talk: Sex and its problems Materials: FLE agenda and SRH materials	1		2		15	25					43	Insufficient time allocated, lack of pedagogical materials
	Study day	Rights of young people in relation to SRH, sex education and young girls, STDs and AIDS	4		6	4	5	10			6		35	
	After school	Talent show on the rights of young people in relation to SRH, contraception, excision, sex education	4		7	10	19	120	5	2	4	12	183	
	In class	Talk: SRH rights and guarantees; sexuality, contraception, STDs, AIDS, hygiene, and abstinence	1 1 1				93 25 70	142 73 112					235 98 182	
CEM Abdoulaye Mar DIOP (ages 13 to 17 years)	March 6	Experimental approaches, communication activity, hygiene	3	3	7	9	20	10					46	
	March 13 after school	Communication in ASRH values — materials: *A Time for Love* (film)	2	2	7	9	20	34					74	
	May 18	Values, sensitization in SRH, poetry recitals, rap	3	3	7	9	80	120	3	3	9	13	250	
	May 19 after school	Prevention and awareness of STDs and HIV/AIDS Supports: *The Shadow Epidemic* (film)	1	0	2	1	3	18	2				27	
CEM Amadou Fara MBODJ (age 13 to 17 years)	May 2	Premature pregnancy, self-awareness, consequences of premature pregnancies, role of parents in society, hygiene, reproductive organs, anatomy	4	0	5	5	177	135	2	1	0	0	347	

School	Date	Themes	Patron supervisors		Peer educators		Pupils		School authorities		Contributors		Total	Observations
			M	F	F	M	F	M	M	F	F	M		
Alfred Doods (age 11 to 13 years)	March 2	Rights of young people in relation to SRH	1	1			16	21					29	
	March 2	Personal hygiene	1	1			16	21					29	
	May 2	Sketch on ASRH	1	1			30	42					74	
Khaly Ousmane Gaye (age 9 to 17 years)	2002	Personal hygiene, infections, and premature pregnancies			1		15	10					26	Lack of pedagogical support, certain taboo terms, insufficient allocated time
		(Same)			1		20	25					6	
		(Same)			1		15	20					36	
		(Same)			1		17	18					36	
Lyceé Charles de Gaulle (18 to 21 years)	March 2	Family planning			1		13	19					33	
CEM Télémaque Sow (age 13 to 16 years)	April 2	STDs and HIV/AIDS: causes, types, treatment, and prevention	4	1	9	5	23	22	1	5	1	5	75	
Université G. Berger (age 19 to 26 years)	February 9	Coeducation and morals at university (dinner-debate)					23	78			1	6	107	
	May 15	Students and sexuality (dinner-debate)					11	70				4	85	
CEM Amadou D. Clédor Ndlaye		Sketch and talent show on AIDS	4		7	8	89	130	10			1	249	
CEM de Gandon (ages 13 to 17 years)	May 11	Film followed by a debate on STDs, AIDS, and premature pregnancy	2	1	7	7					1	7	25	
CREATF (ages 13 to 15 years)	February–May	STDs/AIDS rights, communication between parents and children			4	15	135						154	
Total													3,876	

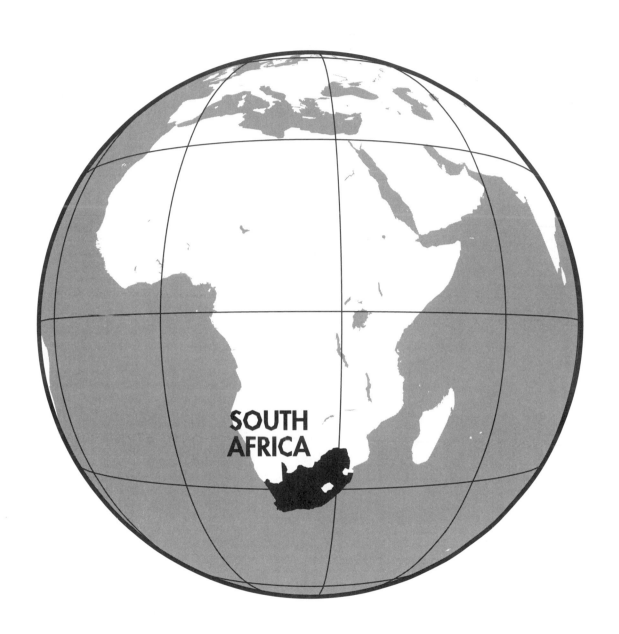

SOUTH
AFRICA

loveLife: Promoting Sexual Health and Healthy Lifestyles for Young People in South Africa

PART A: THE PROGRAM

Program Rationale and History

The idea for loveLife began in the late 1990s, when an organization called Advocacy Initiatives, along with several youth organizations, did a review of research on behavior change in youth. A few of these organizations went on to form a consortium, which included the Planned Parenthood Association of South Africa (PPASA), the Reproductive Health Research Unit (RHRU), and the Health Systems Trust (HST). Initially, this consortium was called the National Sexual Health Initiative (NASHI). In late 1999, this organization was relaunched as loveLife.

I think it makes me feel great... it is difficult with our parents, and the more we see them on the road, the more our parents open up and discuss the loveLife with us.

Girl in rural area

loveLife's objectives are formulated in response to findings that most existing HIV/AIDS education programs have had limited impact on sexual behavior. Surveys show that about 98 percent of South Africans are aware of HIV/AIDS and how it is spread, but condom use among South African males has remained almost unchanged at about 10 percent over the past five years. However, there is a desperate need for effective education on sexual and reproductive health. AIDS is spiralling out of control, one in three women in South Africa gives birth before the age of 18, sexually transmitted infections (STIs) are endemic among young people in large parts of South Africa, and violence, coercion, and abuse are common features of adolescent sexual behavior. loveLife aims to better this situation.

Launched in September 1999, loveLife began with a three-pronged approach. Publications on adolescent sexual and reproductive health (ASRH), relationships, and youth issues were developed and distributed through newspapers and directly to schools, clinics, and loveLife's youth centers. A call center was set up for children and adolescents who needed advice and counseling and for parents who needed advice on how to talk to their children. A radio talk show for young people to phone in and ask experts questions was aired on Youth FM.

In 2000, loveLife expanded into a full media campaign, with billboards and television and radio broadcasts, all aimed at making youth stop and think about ASRH. The call center began to concentrate more on children who had SRH questions but no one to answer them. Youth centers were established where youth could spend free time while learning about SRH issues and discussing relationships under the guidance of trained counselors. The program was also franchised out to other organizations for it to spread farther afield.

In 2001, National Adolescent-Friendly Clinic Initiative (NAFCI) facilities were opened so that youth could have access to SRH care and information in a confidential and welcoming environment. The media campaign and Y-Centers continued to expand, turning loveLife into a household name.

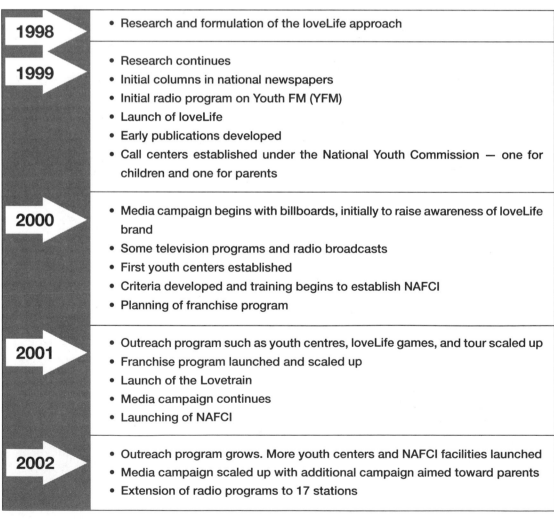

Figure 1. Time Line of Major Program Events

Program Overview

Program Aim

loveLife aims to reduce the incidence of HIV infection and pregnancy among 12- to 20-year-olds in South Africa by at least 50 percent by 2005. It focuses on reducing the negative consequences of premature and adolescent sexual activity by promoting SRH and healthy lifestyles for young people.

loveLife aims to motivate and equip young people to make healthy choices in all parts of their lives. The types of choices that the loveLife program addresses include

- staying in school and pursuing education,
- avoiding illegal drugs,
- respecting yourself and others and rejecting coercive peer pressure,
- not having sexual relations before you are ready or prepared,
- planning for family life and using contraception and protection against sexually transmitted diseases (STDs)if you are having sexual relations, and
- respecting and being faithful to your partner.

Program Objectives

The loveLife program's objectives are to

- target the groups at highest risk,
- deal with the broader context of sexual behavior,
- make condom use a normal part of youth culture,
- sustain education and prevention over many years at a sufficient level of intensity to hold public attention,
- let young people make informed choices,
- encourage young people to share responsibility, and
- encourage positive sexuality.

These objectives are based on the findings of SRH surveys conducted in South Africa as well as international research.

Target Groups

Primary Target Group

loveLife's primary target group is 12- to 17-year-olds.

Secondary Target Group

Adults who interact with young people — for example, health care workers, teachers, parents, and other community members.

Site

loveLife is a national program.

Program Length

loveLife aims to decrease HIV infection and teenage pregnancy among 12- to 17-year-olds by half over the six-year period from 2000 to 2005. To sustain behavior change, the program is planned to continue beyond this initial period for at least 10 years.

Program Goals

Figure 2 shows the main program goals. The program coordinator was unable to rank them because they are perceived to be of equal importance and interconnected. Behavior change is, however, believed to be the cornerstone of avoiding sexual risk and changing sexual health behaviors.

Program Approaches

loveLife works to increase knowledge, change attitudes, and change behavior among youth. The program hopes to achieve this by:

- Offering information and sound advice. This ensures that young people are accurately informed, not just about HIV/AIDS, but also about the issues that surround it.
- Encouraging young people to "talk about it." For example, some billboards are a little cryptic in their message. This encourages youth to discuss issues. Discussion allows them to try and change together, and it helps to internalize the desired behavior changes.
- Encouraging young people to think differently. loveLife's communication strategy seeks to alter the pervasive values and attitudes among adolescents about sex, sexuality, and gender relations. People act according to their beliefs, thus, if we change beliefs, we can change actions.
- Creating a new lifestyle. Internalizing new attitudes requires them to be placed within the context of a lifestyle choice. The idea is to create new behavioral norms for youth. This can be achieved by getting youth "hooked" on loveLife's popular culture.
- Creating a supportive environment. The creation of youth-friendly services (such as clinics) and the formation of positive social networks give youth the confidence to make alternative choices.

In the communication strategy for 2002, the behavior-driven principle "delay" was central. The actual word "delay" was not used in any loveLife media product; rather, media products communicated the principle of delay in fun, interesting ways that resonated with young people.

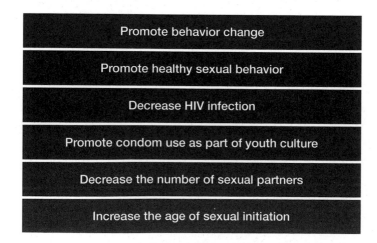

Figure 2. Program Goals Unranked

Components

The loveLife program comprises three main components:

1. a multimedia awareness, information, and education campaign;
2. a social response that puts priority on access and acceptability of quality adolescent (health) services and mobilization of social networks as part of a nationwide program of education, outreach, and support for young people; and
3. research that seeks to understand the dynamics of the HIV/AIDS epidemic and that monitors and evaluates loveLife's activities and outputs.

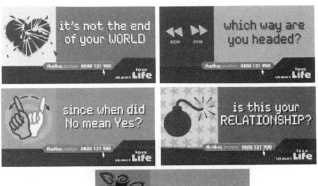

Multimedia Campaign

loveLife has combined traditional marketing techniques with the principles of sound public health education to create a lifestyle brand with which young people will associate healthy positive living. The media campaign is constantly being revised and adapted so that it will retain the attention of young people. It includes a number of different elements. There are four components of the media campaign, each of which is described in more detail below.

loveLife 2002 billboard campaign

Outdoor Campaign

Large billboards are displayed in rural and urban areas. The aim of these billboards is to get young people talking about ASRH issues.

Television

A number of different television programs aimed at youth are commissioned and broadcast by loveLife. Here are three examples of popular loveLife programs:

SEXualMENtality. On December 1, World AIDS Day, loveLife presented *SEXualMENtality* in partnership with the national broadcaster. This was a one-hour documentary about the influence of family, friends, and culture in shaping the attitudes and behavior of young men. It also probed the impact of early sexual initiation, drugs, alcohol, crime, the pressure to conform, and the values and inner thoughts of South African males.

The stories of three different men were told through first-person narrative:

- a graphic artist and convicted rapist who is haunted by his past,
- a restaurant manager who dealt in drugs and sex, and
- a lovestruck student who once tried to kill himself.

I think the colors, when you are walking down the street, catch your attention and it's attractive, and the colors are vibrant.

Girl in rural area

S'camto groundBREAKERS. This is a 13-part reality television series for young people aired on national television. Over a period of 13 weeks, two teams of typical young South Africans compete against each other in the rugged terrain of South Africa.

During the series, the young people work through issues such as team building, conflict, compassion, adversity, and ambition. groundBREAKERS is the quintessential loveLife experience, promoting a new, positive lifestyle for young South Africans that is built on the principles of informed choice, shared responsibility, and healthy living.

S'camto TV. This is a road show that follows the journeys of 16 young people who travel the country talking with other young people about sex and sexuality issues. The focus is on straight, open talk about sex. When the program was evaluated, youth said they found it entertaining as well as credible and truthful. Young people said they would be too embarrassed to watch the program with their parents, so it did not encourage communication between youth and their parents. However, it did encourage young people to talk with each other about topics such as forced sex, decision-making, challenging myths, rape, abortion, and peer pressure. The main achievement seems to have been to create an atmosphere where taboo subjects could be talked about.

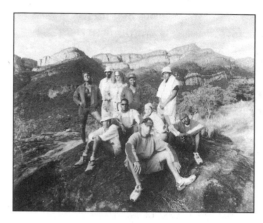

groundBREAKERS

Radio

loveLife, in partnership with the South African Broadcasting Corporation (SABC) and YFM, now works with a total of 17 national and local radio stations, as well as with community radio stations. They have a combined weekly audience of around 30 million. The radio shows cover all 11 official languages and equally penetrate both urban and rural areas. The program formats vary, but are mostly talk shows.

Print

There are a number of different print initiatives.

S'camtoPRINT. This 16-page lifestyle publication is inserted into the *Sunday Times* national newspaper twice a month. The publication is now two years old and is South Africa's largest distributed youth publication, reaching 650,000 youth through the *Sunday Times* with an additional 200,000 copies distributed within loveLife's network of schools, youth centers, franchises, and clinics.

thethaNathi. This eight-page supplement is inserted in the Independent Newspaper Groups publications (*The Star, Pretoria News, Cape Argus,* and *Daily News*) twice a month. thethaNathi was launched in November 2001 as a four-page supplement.

In addition, loveLife produces a set of information and education publications. These are targeted at youth, parents, and decisionmakers:

loveFacts. This information and advice booklet is presented and designed to appeal to young people, using full-color photographs and youth-friendly language. It covers the topics of relationships, puberty, talking about sex, safer sex options, first-time sexual relations, HIV/AIDS, avoiding pregnancy, condoms, contraception, emergency contraception, termination of pregnancy, and STIs.

Tell Me More. This magazine covers a comprehensive range of youth issues and topics around SRH.

Talking and Listening to Your Teenager; Love Them Enough to Talk About Sex. These publications give parents information about youth sexuality and suggestions about how to communicate with their children.

The Impending Catastrophe Revisited. This is a detailed resource book for those seeking information to understand the ramifications of the emerging HIV/AIDS epidemic in South Africa.

loveLife's for us.... This is a survey of South African youth and parents about the effect of the loveLife campaign so far. It is loveLife's most recent publication.

A Social Response: Access to Services and Social Networks

The second component of loveLife's program involves creating an environment that will support behavior change in young people. Figure 3 shows the different components of loveLife's institutional response and how they are linked. These service development aspects of the loveLife initiative are of vital importance. The stimulation of awareness raised through the media has to be reinforced with the provision of services that can meet the demands and needs of youth. Each is discussed in more detail below.

A National Advice and Counseling Service: thethajunction 0800-121-900

A national call center was established to provide a confidential, widely available, and free service for adolescents who need counseling and advice. It was started as a general advice service, but in September 2000, it became a specialized SRH counseling and referral service. This change was made in response to the need expressed by large numbers of callers requesting more in-depth counseling. The name of the help service is thethajunction — *thetha* means "talk" in the Xhosa language. When the thajunction was launched, a separate telephone line called Parent Line was simultaneously established for adults. This was developed in response to the number of calls from parents wanting advice on how to deal with young people's questions and how to deal with adolescent sexuality.

loveLife receives more than 60,000 calls per month. Eighty-five percent of these calls are made from a public telephone. This has provided access to loveLife for youth who do not have a telephone, as well as those who require privacy from inquiring parents or siblings.

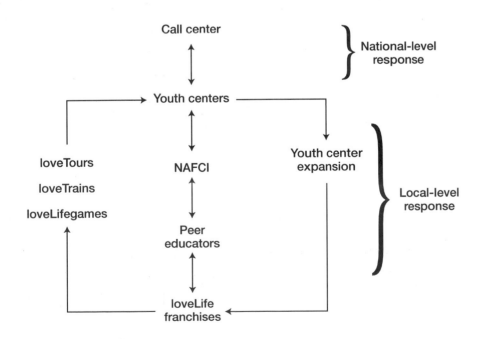

Figure 3. Links in loveLife's Institutional Response

loveLife

Youth centers are a vital aspect of ASRH programs. They provide young people with a place in which they can find quality services for SRH as well as a place where positive lifestyles can be developed. There is a particular need for this kind of service in historically disadvantaged communities. loveLife has established 14 youth centers in South Africa.

These centers offer high-quality clinical services for young people as well as a venue for training (e.g., computer skills), sports and recreational activities (e.g., basketball), and health promotion activities. The youth centers not only provide a service, they also serve as a practical demonstration of the positive lifestyle that loveLife promotes.

NAFCI

The aim of NAFCI is to strengthen the ability of public sector clinics to respond to the needs of young people. The initiative includes education of the public sector as well as a system through which clinics that offer a basic package of adolescent-friendly services can be accredited. These services should include

- appropriate information, education, and counseling on SRH;
- referrals for violence or abuse and mental health problems;
- contraceptive information and counseling and the provision of a choice of methods. including oral contraceptives, emergency contraception, contraceptive injections, and condoms;
- pregnancy testing and counseling;
- counseling and referral for pre- and post-termination of pregnancy;
- information about STIs, including HIV, and about prevention, diagnosis, and syndromic management of STIs, including partner notification; and
- HIV information, pre– and post–HIV test counseling, and referrals for voluntary HIV testing.

NAFCI supports clinic staff in evaluating and improving their services so that they can be accredited for providing adolescent-friendly services. As part of the initiative, clinics are provided with an information center, where young people can have access to resources and information, and a "chill room," where young people can meet and talk and where the peer counselors work.

loveTrain, loveTours, and loveLifeGames

A six-car train and two mobile outside broadcast units (OBUs) travel around the country offering education and services to youth. Community radio tells young people in the area about the arrival of the train, and groundBREAKERS, young people who work as volunteer peer counselors on the train, also visit schools to let the students know. Franchisees (see below) provide follow-up and support after the train and OBU have left the area.

The loveLifeGames are run in association with the United School Sports Association of South Africa. More than 4 million young people compete in sports and cultural events around the country at provincial and national level. Plans are under way to introduce district-level competitions.

Case Study

John Ntsele was a peer educator from the youth center in Orange Farm, outside Johannesburg, before becoming a groundBREAKER on the loveTrain. He told us about his experiences.

Q: What were the highlights of the trip for you?

A: To meet young people and learn from them — to learn about different languages and cultures. The opportunity to visit rural areas. I found there were older people of about 19 or 20 who didn't know about HIV: They'd ask, "What is this virus? What is this AIDS?" They thought condoms were only for people living in town. The work was exciting and also challenging. We often had to improvise and think of other ways to spread the message. I was there not as a professor but as a young person.

Q: What surprised you the most?

A: In Hammanskraal, we had young boys, about 7 to 10 years old, who said, "I used to steal and smoke — but I'm willing to change, but we don't have the resources in our community. What can we do?" I was surprised that children so young were in this situation. I told them about the basketball events on the train. They really liked that and wanted to start their own sports team. I referred them to a youth center in their area, but I wish we had a basketball court we could have left them!

Q: What tips or advice would you give to other groundBREAKERS who were going on the train tour?

A: You need patience, energy, and love — it keeps you going. It's not easy: You have to give 250 percent to make sure you give them the right information — because it's not all about you, it's all about young people. If we can leave one youth center in every place we go, it would really make a difference.

loveLife Franchises

The great demand for information, support, and resource materials from NGOs, community-based organizations (CBOs), churches, and businesses led to the establishment of a network of loveLife franchises. In essence, it is a social version of the commercial franchise idea, but no money is exchanged.

Local youth organizations receive training in the use of popular youth culture as a vehicle for communicating. They are given the loveLife-branded package with resource materials, and they participate in a national franchise network that takes part in loveLife events. In return, the franchises agree to accept the strategies, image, and approaches loveLife uses to achieve its mission. They also agree to conform to a set of standards for the promotion of loveLife and to be partners in the monitoring process. Appendix 1 describes the loveLife franchise holder's core program.

> They talk about our lives, not just products.
>
> *Boy in urban area*

Research

Underpinning all loveLife's work is research and evaluation. A number of publications have resulted from the research undertaken by loveLife over the last few years.

In 2000, a national survey of youth — "Hot Prospects, Cold Facts, Portrait of Young South Africa" — was undertaken. The survey looked at, among other things, how young people in South Africa spend their leisure time, their worries and fears, sexual activity, and knowledge about HIV/AIDS.

Much of the research is packaged in a form that makes it accessible to the public. This is part of the advocacy work of loveLife. In 2001, *Impending Catastrophe Revisited*, a report that helped people understand the scale and ramifications of the escalating HIV/AIDS epidemic in South Africa was published.

PART B: IMPLEMENTING THE PROGRAM

Needs Assessment

No information was available about the needs assessment.

Program Materials

The materials used in the program were described in "Components" above.

Staff selection

loveLife's programs are implemented through a consortium of leading South African NGOs: HST, PPASA, and RHRU.

Staff are employed by the three NGOs to work full- or part-time on the loveLife campaign. The HST employs 47 people, the PPASA employs 125 people, and the RHRU employs 19 people on the loveLifecampaign. There are currently 357 groundBREAKERS volunteers and numerous other volunteers at all levels. Figure 4 shows the management structure of loveLife.

Figure 5 shows how the different program components are organized.

Setting Up the Program

Because the program is so big, describing how to set it up is beyond the scope of this report. For further information, please contact loveLife directly. (See contact information in part D.)

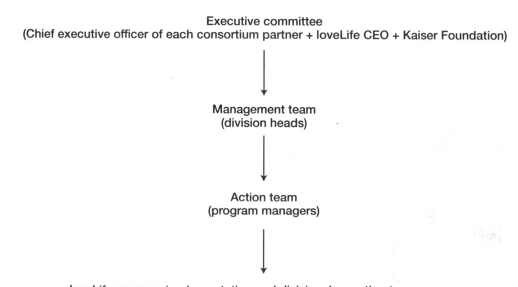

Figure 4. loveLife Management Structure

Program Resources

loveLife has a central office in Johannesburg, where the help lines are based. In addition, the project partners — PPASA, RHRU, and HST — have central offices. PPASA also has a number of provincial offices around the country.

loveLife owns a train and two OBUs. It has also established a number of youth centers around the country.

Advocacy

The publications produced by the research component of loveLife serve to advocate the organization's message. For example, the 2000 national survey of youth, "Hot Prospects, Cold Facts, Portrait of Young South Africa," which was distributed widely in an accessible form, served to raise awareness of the lives of young people in South Africa. This survey looked at, among other things, how young people in South Africa spend their leisure time, their worries and fears, sexual activity among youth, and their knowledge about HIV/AIDS.

The entire program is a model of advocacy in that it promotes ASRH issues and increases awareness of them in the general public. Further, by working in close collaboration with other NGOs and the government, loveLife's messages are being integrated into the foundations of society.

Program Finances

Major funding for loveLife is provided by the Henry J. Kaiser Family Foundation and the Bill and Melinda Gates Foundation. Additional funding is provided by the South African government, the United Nations Children's Fund (UNICEF), and the Nelson Mandela Foundation.

loveLife operates on an annual budget of US$20million (R200 million).

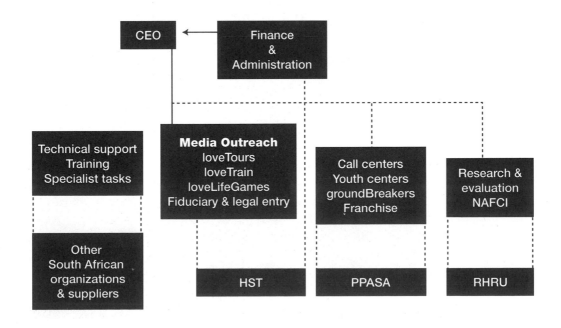

Figure 5. Program Components Organization

PART C: ASSESSMENT AND LESSONS LEARNED

Challenges and Solutions

The recent evaluation of loveLife identified a number of challenges facing the initiative.

Early Days

loveLife was begun only two years ago, and during that time, its visibility and its programs have continued to expand. Many of the key elements of the program are still scaling up, particularly NAFCI. The challenge will be to continue to engage youth with the media awareness campaign while the practical implementation of the program continues.

Many Still Have Not Heard

Sixty-two percent of young people have heard of loveLife, but it is important to remember that currently almost 4 in 10 (38 percent) 12- to 17-year-olds are still not aware of this initiative. This presents both a challenge and an opportunity for those involved in loveLife to continue to broaden and enhance their efforts at getting the word out to other youth.

Although the findings of the recent evaluation show that many youth are aware of loveLife and its overall goals, awareness is just a first step in a long-term process.

Reported behavior change may or may not reflect actual behavior change. Many youth who had heard of loveLife report that it has positively influenced their behaviors. However, the evaluation research conducted so far does not reveal specifically which behaviors have changed. One of the challenges for the research arm of the initiative is to implement a broader, multiyear evaluation that will assess loveLife's impact, including indicators related to adolescent sexual behavior such as delayed onset of sexual activity.

Convincing Parents

Although youth seem open to communication and believe it could help foster safe SRH attitudes and practices, parents seem more reluctant and less convinced that it could make a difference. One of the key challenges will be to convince more parents that open communication about sex and sexuality can in fact ensure that South African youth make healthier choices.

Evaluation

A recent publication titled "loveLife's for us..." includes information from an evaluation of the loveLife initiative.

Please contact loveLife for more information on their evaluation process and results. (See contact information in Part d.)

UNAIDS Benchmarks

	Benchmark	Attainment	Comments
1	Recognizes the child/youth as a learner who already knows, feels, and can do in relation to healthy development and HIV/AIDS-related prevention.	✓	The main value that loveLife seeks to promote is choice. This suggests that they see young people as being able to make wise choices about their sexual behavior. groundBreakers are used to spread prevention messages.
2	Focuses on risks that are most common to the learning group and that responses are appropriate and targeted to the age group.	Partially fulfilled	loveLife is specifically targeted at the 12- to 17-year-old age group. The loveLife program is informed by research with the target group. It is not clear, however, which initiatives and components are directed at the various ages.
3	Includes not only knowledge but also attitudes and skills needed for prevention.	✓	Attitudes, skills, and a supportive environment in which young people can make wise choices are all included in the program.
4	Understands the impact of relationships on behavior change and reinforces positive social values.	✓	The promotion of positive social values in the context of relationships and behavior is one of the main focuses of the program.
5	Is based on analysis of learners' needs and a broader situation assessment.	✓	One of the three main program areas is research. Research informs the media and social response aspects of the program.
6	Has training and continuous support of teachers and other service providers.	✓	Service providers such as clinic nurses and youth workers are trained and supported.
7	Uses multiple and participatory learning activities and strategies.	✓	The program uses multimedia and a variety of activities.
8	Involves the wider community.	✓	The advocacy arm of the program involves the wider community, as does much of the local work at the youth centers.
9	Ensures sequence, progression, and continuity of messages.	✓	Care has been taken to introduce messages developmentally in the media campaign. However, it is possible that children might not see the messages sequentially and could get confused.

	Benchmark	Attainment	Comments
10	Is placed in an appropriate context in the school curriculum.	Not applicable	loveLife does not work in the formal education system
11	Lasts a sufficient time to meet program goals and objectives.	✓	loveLife is aware that mass media interventions in particular need to be sustained at a sufficiently high level for a length of time before they affect behavior.
12	Is coordinated with a wider school health promotion program.	✓	loveLife does not work directly with schools, but its general messages are complementary to the school health program messages. All schools in South Africa do not yet have programs on HIV/AIDS, so in some areas of the country loveLife might be one of the only sources of information on HIV and other SRH issues.
13	Contains factually correct and consistent messages.	✓	Great care is taken to ensure that messages are factually correct and consistent. All initiative are individually researched before implementation. Thorough training is given, but there is some concern that franchises may vary in the messages they convey.
14	Has established political support through intense advocacy to overcome barriers and go to scale.	✓	loveLife advocates its program through its publications. General coverage is so widespread throughout the country that most people are aware of its existence and messages that it is spreading.
15	Portrays human sexuality as a healthy and normal part of life, and is not derogatory against gender, race, ethnicity, or sexual orientation.	✓	loveLife makes efforts to portray sexuality as a healthy and normal part of life.
16	Includes monitoring and evaluation.	✓	Evaluation and monitoring are a critical part of the program. Evaluations have taken place and been published for wider review.

PART D: ADDITIONAL INFORMATION

Organizations and Contacts

loveLife
PO Box 45
Parklands
2121
Johannesburg, South Africa
Telephone: (+27 11) 771-6800
Fax: (+27 11) 771-6801
E-mail: talk@lovelife.org.za
Website: www.lovelife.org.za

Reproductive Health Research Unit
Department of Obstetrics and Gynaecology
Chris Hani Baragwanath Hospital
P.O. Bertsham
2013
South Africa
Telephone: (+27 11) 33-1228
Fax: (+27 11) 033-1227
E-mail: jstadler@rhrujhb.co.za

Health Systems Trust
P.O. Box 808
Durban 4000, South Africa
Telephone: (+27 31) 307-2954
Fax: (+27 31) 304-0775
E-mail: hst@healthlink.org.za

Planned Parenthood Association SA
P.O. Box 1023
Saxonwold
2123
Johannesburg, South Africa
Telephone: (+27 11) 880-1162
Fax: (+27 11) 880-1191
E-mail: ppasa@ppasa.org.za.

Contributors to the Report

The report was compiled by Glynis Clacherty, of Clacherty and Associates, an agency that specializes in participatory research with children and the development of learning materials around children and health. Glynis has worked extensively in the area of HIV/AIDS and children and is based in Johannesburg, South Africa.

Angela Stewart-Buchanan of loveLife assisted in the writing of this report.

Edited by Katie Tripp and Helen Baños Smith

Available Materials

To obtain these materials, please contact ibeaids@ibe.unesco.org or Education for HIV/AIDS Prevention, International Bureau of Education, C.P. 199, 1211 Geneva 20, Switzerland.

Loud and Clear: Tips on Talking to Your Children About Difficult Things!
(order number: loveLife01)

Love Facts: Talk About It
(order number: loveLife02)

Love Them Enough to Talk About Sex
(order number: loveLife03)

Talking and Listening: Parents and Teenagers Together, Find Out How to Make It Easier...
(order number: loveLife04)

Impending Catastrophe Revisited: An Update on the HIV/AIDS Epidemic in South Africa
(order number: loveLife05)

Tell Me More
(order number: loveLife06)

Hot Prospects, Cold Facts, Portrait of Young South Africa
(order number: loveLife07)

Looking at loveLife: The First Year: Summaries of Monitoring and Evaluation
(order number: loveLife08)

"loveLife's for Us..." A Survey of SA Youth 2001
(order number: loveLife09)

Our Story
(order number: loveLife10)

loveLife Franchise
(order number: loveLife11)

S'camto print newspaper
(order number: loveLife12)

APPENDIX 1. FRANCHISE HOLDERS CORE PROGRAM AREAS, ACTIVITIES, AND STANDARDS

Core Program Area	Activity	Standard
Promote the loveLife brand	• Prominently display the loveLife franchise logo. • Distribute loveLife materials; display posters and distribute promotional material at events.	• Logo is displayed where it is visible to the public. • Materials are used and distributed to the appropriate target group according to your plan.

Develop and implement a loveLife action plan	• Communicate loveLife's messages through aspects of youth popular culture (music, sports, recreation, etc.).
	• Develop a peer education and youth leadership element.
	• Implement an SRH and life skills program.
	• Maintain simple records provided by loveLife.
		• Program mix:
		  – basketball or other sport for messaging
		  – drama, music art
		• Peer educators: at lead two groups of 15 to 20 youth aged 12 to 17 years old per year (half male; half female)
		• Community mobilizers: core trained group of 20 community mobilizers aged 18 to 25 years per year (10 male; 10 female)
		• At least two people per organization are trained to run peer education, SRH, and life skills programs.
		• Twenty to thirty youth aged 12 to 17 per quarter participate in workshops. (Peer educators can be recruited from these workshops.)
		• Twenty to thirty youth aged 12 to 17 per quarter participate in loveLife-provided motivational and other youth development workshops.
		• Monthly or quarterly reporting schedules provided by loveLife are submitted.

Participate in national franchise activities	• Encourage young people to participate in nationally coordinated activities organized and paid for by loveLife. • Be willing to participate in research and evaluation. • Be willing to write about your experience and contribute to newsletters and other publications.	• To be negotiated with franchise • Involvement in loveLifeGames • loveTours • loveTrain • Cooperate; provide information; assist with organizational issues. • At least two contributions per year.

Core Program Area	Activity	Standard
Strengthen community's support	Identify key stakeholders to work with to ensure that there is community support for the loveLife initiative.	• Formation of a loveLife task team • Meeting with local health care providers (explore links with NAFCI and/or workshop on adolescent-friendly services). • Parent education training.

Soul *Buddyz*: A Multimedia Edutainment Project for Children in South Africa

PART A: DESCRIPTION OF THE PROGRAM

Program Rationale and History

South Africa needs to ensure that young people have enough information, skills, and a supportive environment to protect themselves from becoming infected with HIV. Because of widespread discrimination against people living with HIV and AIDS, there is an imperative to destigmatize AIDS. Children affected by or afflicted with AIDS need social support. Communities need to be mobilized on a national scale to play this supportive role.

The Soul City Institute for Health and Development Communication was established in South Africa in 1992. It uses the power of the mass media to address the above issues. "Edutainment" (entertainment-education) is seen internationally as a powerful educational tool. Many media educational programs are unable to attract large audiences; edutainment integrates educational issues into entertaining formats that enable health promoters to secure prime-time mass media slots. The power of edutainment rests in its ability to model positive attitudes and behaviors through characters with whom the audience can bond. The characters come to play an integral part in the lives of the audiences, who experience their life lessons vicariously. The ability to attract advertising revenue also allows for partnerships of mutual benefit to develop between broadcasters and health promoters.

> Soul *Buddyz* teaches us...
> we must work hand in hand
> with our friends.
>
> ***Soul Buddyz watcher***

The edutainment approach is particularly apt for South Africa because the reach of media is good: Television reaches about 74 percent of the population, radio reaches 93 percent, and newspapers reach 40 percent.

The Soul City Institute for Health and Development Communication began its work with Soul *City*, a popular, prime-time, weekly television series that deals with health and communication issues through drama. The series was accompanied by a daily radio drama, health booklets, and intensive advertising, marketing, and advocacy work.

Evaluations of *Soul City* consistently show that it is effective at influencing a variety of health issues: It has been shown to convey information, increase debate and interpersonal interaction, and change attitudes, practices, and social norms. Further, it was found to be popular with children younger than age 16, even though the materials were designed for youth and adults. South Africa is a country with a young population: About 40 percent of the population is under 18 years old, with about 13 million children between 5 and 18 years old. Thus, each year, a large cohort of young, vulnerable South Africans become sexually active.

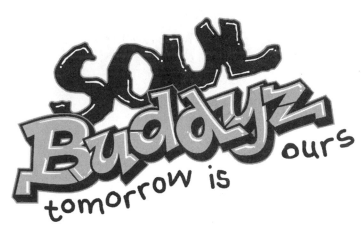

Soul Buddyz logo

In light of this, and the seriousness of the AIDS pandemic, and recognizing the importance of intervening at an early age, the Soul City Institute for Health and Development Communication decided to create an edutainment series, Soul *Buddyz,* for children aged between 8 and 12 years. Soul *Buddyz* focuses from the *child's perspective* on HIV/AIDS, sexuality, and other educational issues of relevance to children. It consists of a television and a radio show with accompanying life-skills print materials for children and parents.

The Soul City Institute for Health and Development Communication is currently developing Soul *Buddyz* 2, which they hope to show on South African television and radio in 2003.

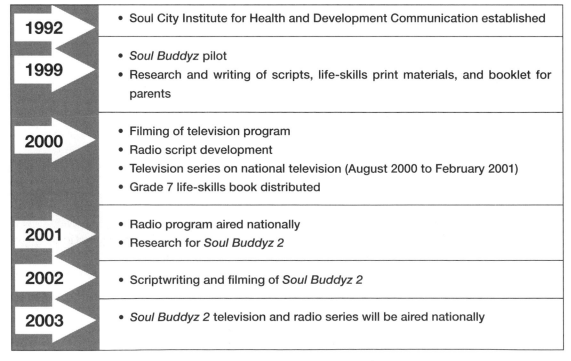

1992	• Soul City Institute for Health and Development Communication established
1999	• *Soul Buddyz* pilot • Research and writing of scripts, life-skills print materials, and booklet for parents
2000	• Filming of television program • Radio script development • Television series on national television (August 2000 to February 2001) • Grade 7 life-skills book distributed
2001	• Radio program aired nationally • Research for *Soul Buddyz 2*
2002	• Scriptwriting and filming of *Soul Buddyz 2*
2003	• *Soul Buddyz 2* television and radio series will be aired nationally

Figure 1. Time Line of Major Program Events

Program Overview

Program Aim

To improve the quality of life of young South Africans through improved health literacy.

Program Objectives

To create a multimedia edutainment vehicle that will be popular with children aged 8 to 12 years. The vehicle will contains key health messages of relevance to this age group and consequently increase health literacy. The vehicle consists of television, print, and radio media.

Target Groups

> *Soul Buddyz teaches us that if you have a problem with a person, violence won't solve the problem.*
>
> *Periurban child*

Primary Target Group

The primary target group is 8- to 12-year-olds of all races, language groups, and socioeconomic groups in South Africa.

Secondary Target Group

Parents and caregivers of children aged 8-12 are also targeted through the television, radio, and print materials created for children, although these are a secondary audience. In addition, a parenting book is specifically designed to assist parents and caregivers.

Site

Soul *Buddyz* is a national project and covers all those who have access to television, radio, and print media.

Program Length

The development of the entire Soul *Buddyz* vehicle was a long one. The initial piloting of one chapter of the book and one episode of the television series took three months. Research, writing of scripts, and filming of the television series took 18 months.

The television series aired on national television from August 2000 to February 2001. Radio development took six months, and the radio program was aired from February 2001 to April 2001. The life-skills book took six months to develop and was distributed to schools in October 2000.

A second series, Soul *Buddyz* 2, is now in development.

Program Goals

The goals of the Soul *Buddyz* program are best summed up in the messages that are embedded in the series. The HIV/AIDS-related messages are both general and specific. The general messages deal with issues relating to self-esteem and gender.

Formative research had shown that these were all areas that children either did not know about, or needed to change their attitudes if they were to avoid risky behaviors and situations. The idea that children can work together, give each other support, and back each other up in positive ways is not often found in programs, yet it can be very empowering. Ultimately, these goals should lead to a better informed, more inclusive and just society.

For more detailed information on Soul *Buddyz* messages, please see South Africa Soul *Buddyz* Appendix 3: Detailed Explanation of Goals.

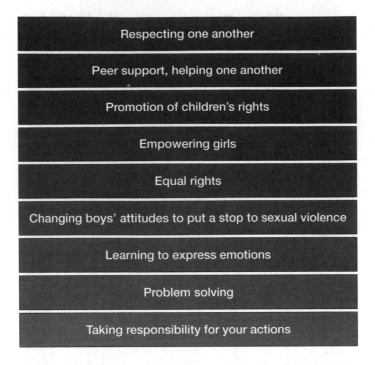

Figure 2. Program Goals (General Message) Unranked

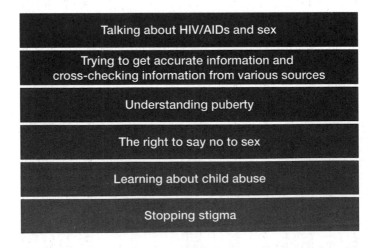

Figure 3. Program Goals (More Specific HIV/AIDS- and Sexuality-Related Messages) Unranked

Approaches

The five principal approaches of the program are

1. promoting healthy public policy,
2. creating supportive environments,
3. supporting community action for health,
4. developing personal skills, and
5. reorienting health services.

I like Soul Buddyz because it teaches me what is right and wrong.

Periurban child

The key aspects of the Soul City methodology are illustrated in figure 4.

Through a thorough formative research process, health and development communication messages are developed and integrated into the edutainment vehicle. Some of these messages deal with HIV/AIDS, youth sexuality, and domestic violence. Care is taken to ensure that the media materials are of the highest quality. The drama portrays realistic situations so that the audience can identify with the modeled characters. Emotions are highlighted in the drama, so as to shape and change attitudes toward gender and the other issues dealt with.

Components

The program consists of six main components, the first five of which are discussed in more detail below.

Things that are on Soul Buddyz happen daily.

Periurban child

1. a television drama series,
2. a radio magazine show,
3. life-skills print materials for children,
4. a parenting booklet,
5. an animated sex education video, and
6. advocacy. (This is discussed in Advocacy in Part b of this chapter.)

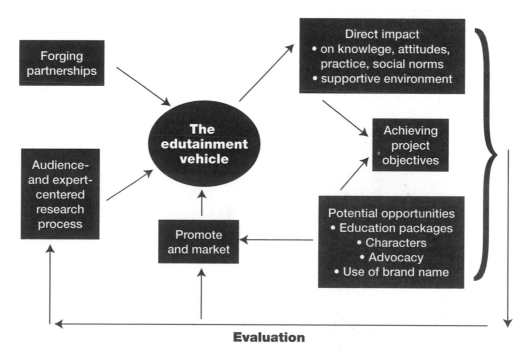

Figure 4. The Soul City Edutainment Model

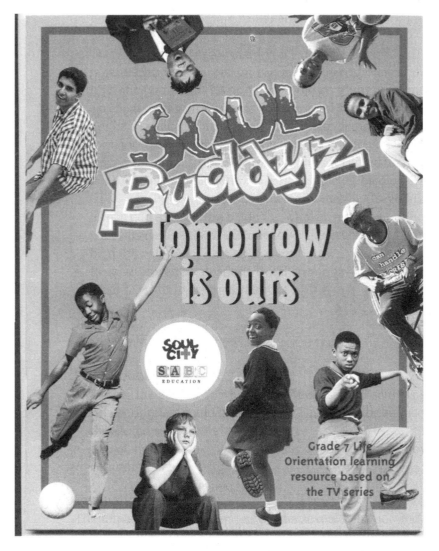

Grade 7 life-skills book

Television Drama Series

The 26-episode television series revolves around the lives of eight child characters (the Soul Buddyz), who deal with various issues such as starting at a new school, being bullied, and having a mother who has AIDS — issues that confront them in their everyday lives. The Soul Buddyz are of mixed race, socioeconomic class, and gender.

The Soul *Buddyz* series uses a number of creative devices to help boost its impact. Each episode unfolds from the perspective of one of the eight Soul Buddyz, whose inner thoughts are conveyed by a voiceover. Each episode also includes a fantasy sequence to illustrate the hopes and fears of children. A rap song in each episode emphasizes the main educational message. At the end of each 26-minute episode, a dozen real children from all over South Africa are shown commenting on the educational issues raised.

NGO services such as the toll-free Childline are often integrated into the Soul *Buddyz* storyline. For example, a plot about sexual abuse showed a child learning how to use the Childline, which provides counseling and follow-up services to children. After each Soul *Buddyz* episode, the Childline number is prominently displayed. Print materials also carry the Childline telephone number.

The Soul *Buddyz* program is multilingual. Each episode is conducted in English, but each child uses his or her own language when at home or talking with their parents or siblings. They also use their home language when using the voiceover technique. The local languages are subtitled (in English) when used. Soul *Buddyz* is thus broadcast in five languages, although about 60 percent is in English.

Soul Buddyz teaches us about life.

Metropolitan child

Radio

The radio component consisted of a 26-episode radio magazine program also called Soul *Buddyz*. The 30-minute magazine incorporated a 10-minute radio drama with child protagonists, a 5-minute dramatized information segment for adults and children, and a phone-in talk show with young presenters and expert guests. This radio magazine program was broadcast in three South African languages — Setswana, North Sotho, and Xhosa — to appeal to a wide audience.

Life-Skills Print Materials

A vibrant life-skills book was distributed to 1 million seventh-grade students (aged around 12 years) in every primary school in South Africa. The life-skills materials, illustrated with pictures of the Soul *Buddyz* characters, cover all the topics tackled in the television series and are designed to be interactive. Each unit begins with a photo comic strip telling the television story in an abbreviated form, followed by true-life stories as told by children. In addition, there are group-based and individual activities for children, educators' notes with ideas for teaching, and contact information for child support organizations. Three informational posters accompany the book.

Parenting Booklet

A user-friendly parenting booklet was distributed through the *Sunday Times,* a Sunday newspaper with the largest na-

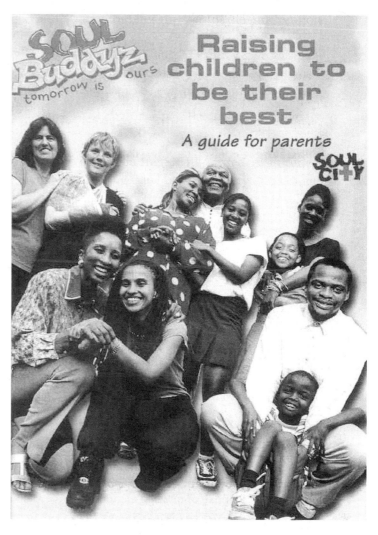

Parenting book

tional circulation of 600,000. It was also distributed through various NGOs in South Africa. The literacy rate in South Africa is relatively high — 81.8 percent of adults older than 15 are literate — but the reading level is not very high. The parenting booklet was thus produced in three languages at a fifth-grade reading level. The booklet covers topics such as communication, discipline, resolving conflict, single parenting, how to build children's self-esteem, and information on how to prevent child accidents. It also describes ways to talk to children about sexuality, HIV/AIDS, and death.

Animated Sex Education Video

Because of the low levels of sexual literacy among South African children, a six-minute, animated, sex education video was produced and integrated into the Soul *Buddyz* television series. The animation helped overcome the problem of showing sexual organs on national television and facilitated an open discussion on the topic.

> It is because our group is united and we care about one another. Sometimes when we are walking around and people try to bully us, my group does not run away and leave others in trouble, we protect each other.
>
> *Periurban child*

The video was incorporated into an episode in which the Soul Buddyz are shown to be confused about sex. A friendly nurse sits them down and shows them the video. The broadcast of

Soul Buddyz — it is real.

Metropolitan child

this episode was the first time such explicit sex education material was ever shown on television in South Africa.

To maximize the usefulness of the animated sex education video, the episode that carried the animation was condensed to a 12-minute segment, and it is sold to schools and parents as a teaching aid. There has been a great demand for this video resource; in the first two months after advertising it, more than 100 videos were sold.

PART B: IMPLEMENTING THE PROGRAM

Soul City has published a comprehensive guide for program managers that describes how to set up an edutainment vehicle like Soul *Buddyz*. The guide, *Edutainment: How to Make Edutainment Work for You: A Step-by-Step Guide to Designing and Managing an Edutainment Project for Social Development,* is available from Soul City (see contact information in Part d).

Needs Assessment

The needs assessment took place in two principal phases. The first phase determined what messages the Soul *Buddyz* program should deliver. The second phase determined whether these messages were being delivered in the most appropriate and effective way for the target audience.

Phase 1

Audience research was conducted nationally with children aged 8 to 12 by specialists in the area of participatory research with children, who made sure that the process was ethical and empowering for children.

A qualitative approach was used in this research. Children working in small groups took part in a number of activities such as drama, drawing, and mapmaking. These activities were designed to give adult researchers a window into the lives of children. The activities were carefully structured around key research questions and were appropriate to the age and stage of development of the children. For example, a true/false game gave an idea of the children's level of knowledge about HIV/AIDS. Another activity involved drawing a girl (or boy) and listing the "good things" about being a girl (or boy) and the "bad things" about being a girl (or boy) around the drawing. The game and drawing then became the focus for a discussion that was tape recorded and transcribed. This audience research was fed into the message design workshops and was referred to by scriptwriters.

Soul Buddyz teaches me about AIDS. Like when one of the boys' mother has AIDS, it shows how a person can cope with AIDS.

Periurban child

Phase 2

Each draft script was shown to groups of children from different environments. Through a process of story reading and discussion, the children commented on the story and the characters. Researchers thus found out if the children understood the messages clearly. In addition, children's language and culture was also added to the scripts. The information was fed back to scriptwriters, who then adapted the scripts.

I think Soul Buddyz teaches kids things that are not easy for parents to talk to their kids about. We black parents, we have a problem — there are things that are not easy for us to talk to our kids about.

Rural parent

Program Materials

The Soul *Buddyz* materials were developed over six months in partnership with the educational branch of the broadcaster, South Africa Broadcasting Corporation (SABC) Educational Television; a number of NGOs, such as Drive Alive, National Association of People Living with AIDS, and the National Council of Child and Family Welfare; and children.

Child involvement in materials development was extensive. Apart from the needs assessment (see above), the use of "true stories" allowed a number of young people to tell their stories to other South African youngsters. In addition, the Soul *Buddyz* logo was developed with children, as were the raps songs profiled in the series. Children have also participated in the making of the radio programs.

Because Soul *Buddyz* is media driven, the target group materials are presented in Components (above).

Staff Selection and Training

Selection of in-house staff is conducted through the usual channels, which include advertising in the media and the use of a specialized employment agency. Selection of service providers is done through a tender or quoting process, where work is advertised in the media and service providers are selected on the basis of expertise and cost-effectiveness.

Training programs are run for service providers when the required expertise is not available. For example, a training program was run for radio scriptwriters and producers. (See Setting Up the Program.)

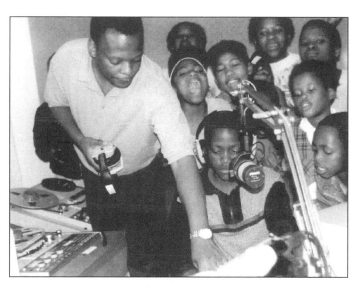

*Children participate in making the **Soul Buddyz** radio programs*

Setting Up the Program

The research process in creating a Soul City intervention is illustrated in figure 5.

Once the final drafts have been produced, they are piloted with parents, teachers, childcare workers, and children across the nine provinces of South Africa. The piloting draws the program developers' attention to any problems in the materials.

For example, the radio pilot, produced by a well-respected production company, used adults to portray children's voices. This alerted the producers that there were no radio programs in South Africa for 8- to 12-year-old children, that radio producers had little experience working with children, and they no experience in producing children's drama. With help from the

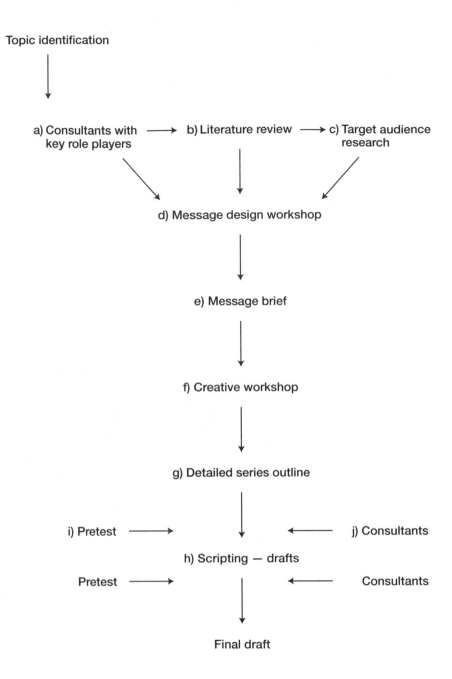

Figure 5. Formative Research Process

British Broadcasting Corporation (BBC), the Soul *Buddyz* project subsequently organized a training program for South African radio producers to learn how to work with children.

Further, the piloting showed that adults needed assistance in parenting skills, especially in terms of communicating with children and how to sensitively handle issues of disciplining. The development of the Soul *Buddyz* parenting booklet was a direct outcome of the pilot process.

Intense advocacy work with the news media also took place to ensure that the messages of Soul *Buddyz* (and Soul City's messages) reached a wide an audience and became socially acceptable. The Advocacy section (below) explains how this was achieved.

Program Resources

The Soul City Institute for Health and Development Communication has an office in Johannesburg. Soul *Buddyz* staff are based there, and all the materials are stored there. Visitors are welcome to drop in and pick up brochures, videos, and so forth.

Advocacy

The Soul *Buddyz* project included an advocacy component with five HIV/AIDS-related focal areas:

- using the news media,
- training NGOs to engage the news media,
- creating resource booklets for journalists on children's rights and HIV/AIDS,
- training journalists in children's rights, and
- launching a campaign for instituting social security privileges for children infected or affected by HIV/AIDS.

> I don't usually talk to my children about everything. I'm very shy, but since I've seen this program [*Soul Buddyz*], I've changed. It has helped me a lot.
>
> ***Parent***

Using the News Media

The Soul *Buddyz* project made use of the news media to profile children's issues among the South African public and policymakers. The news media wrote about reducing HIV/AIDS stigma, promoting care and support, and advocating for sex education among young people (which paved the way for using the animated sex education episode on Soul *Buddyz*). The project expected the explicit, animated, sex education video to create public outrage. Press releases were sent to media newsrooms, coupled with several direct pitches to key journalists.

Specific events were orchestrated for the media to cover. For example, the project set up a viewing of the sex education episode with schoolchildren, inviting journalists to attend. A number of newspaper articles resulted, highlighting the value of early, age-appropriate, sex education as part of a life-skills agenda. The articles emphasized that sex education increases responsible decisionmaking in young people and does not promote promiscuity.

News coverage of the issues dealt with in Soul *Buddyz* thus rose steeply in a number of television and radio talk shows, news programs, and newspaper articles during the Soul *Buddyz* broadcast period.

> *Soul Buddyz* is a bonus. It deals with real-life issues and real-life situations and makes [children] more aware of things which are a reality.
>
> ***Parent***

Training NGOs to Engage the News Media

Soul *Buddyz* conducted a week-long training course for two children's rights advocacy organizations; the National Children's Rights Committee (NCRC) and the National Plan of Action (NPA) for children. The objective of the training was to build capacity within the NCRC and the provincial structures of the NPA to conduct advocacy, with a specific focus on developing skills to deal with the media. An advocacy training manual was developed by the Soul *Buddyz* project and provided to all course participants. The manual provided guidelines on using advocacy tools during campaign planning. Further, a directory of media contacts was developed to assist the NCRC and other child rights advocacy groups to mobilize various media segments in South Africa, especially with respect to children's rights. The directory provided contact details for print, radio, and television journalists in both mainstream and community media.

Resource Booklets for Journalists

A resource booklet on children's rights was produced to assist journalists. The booklet contains succinct information on children's rights initiatives, including the Convention on the Rights of the Child, the African Charter, and South Africa's Constitution. Mechanisms established by the South African parliament to protect children's rights are also detailed.

The booklet examines the role of the mass media in covering children's issues, and it includes several ethical guidelines. The booklet also provides journalists with contact information for children's organizations, including several organizations that deal with HIV/AIDS and children.

> [Soul Buddyz] has changed the way I interact with my friends, parents, and people in the community: I have learnt to be more respectful, and I have learnt to talk about things that are of great concern to me or that hurt me.
>
> **Periurban child**

A second resource booklet for journalists was developed on HIV/AIDS. This contains critical information about the infectious nature of HIV, the epidemiology and prevention of HIV, and information on treatment. It appeared at a critical time (in 2000), when President Thabo Mbeki of South Africa was publicly questioning the link between HIV and AIDS, undermining various prevention and treatment initiatives. This resource book was published jointly with the Department of Health and the South African National Editor's Forum, adding credibility to the initiative.

Training Journalists in Children's Rights

Seven workshops with journalists and key editors were held around the country to coincide with the launch of the children's rights and AIDS booklets. The workshops dealt with issues of children's rights and familiarized journalists with the international, African, and South African institutions designed to protect these rights. They also dealt with ethical issues surrounding media coverage of children's issues, including issues of privacy in the context of HIV/AIDS.

Campaign for Social Security for Children Infected and Affected by HIV/AIDS

Soul City is a cofounder and active member of the Alliance for Children's Entitlement to Social Security (ACESS), a long-term campaign to advocate for comprehensive social security for children. The institute was motivated by recognition of the poverty at the core of many of the health problems covered by both Soul *Buddyz* and the *Soul City* series.

> What I learnt that is interesting is about anger, because sometimes I get fed up and I don't want to communicate with the children when I 'm angry, but from that book, I've learnt that you mustn't. So that you must listen to them when they come with problems, and you must guide them. And when you are angry, you must call them and talk to them so that the problem may be solved.
>
> **Rural parent**

The AIDS pandemic is deepening poverty in South Africa, because it primarily infects the economically active sector of the population. Many children are left without parental support and without access to adequate social security; many of these children face malnutrition, stunting, and a lifetime of negative social and health outcomes.

ACESS activities include lobbying government, building support within civil society, media advocacy, and a process of child participation, to ensure that children's voices are heard in the country's deliberations on this issue.

The campaign links to the Soul *Buddyz* series in a number of ways: First, the story in the second series of Soul *Buddyz* deals with social security and details for children exactly what is available and how to go about getting that security. Second, the social security campaign uses the popularity of the Soul *Buddyz* actors as advocates, to help present materials and make inputs to policy deliberations. Finally, Soul *Buddyz*' television popularity provides the opportunity of access to the press for press releases relating to the campaign.

Program Finances

The total budget for the first series of Soul *Buddyz* was US$2.3 million (R23 million) over three years. Funding was received from The European Union, UNICEF, the National Department of Health, Mobile Telephone Network (MTN), British Petroleum (BP), SABC Educational Television, and Radda Barnen.

Estimate of cost per child/youth: There are approximately 9 million children between the age of six and eight years in South Africa. The evaluation shows that Soul *Buddyz* reached 67 percent of these children. Therefore, the cost per child reached is US$0.38 (R3.80).

For further details, see South Africa Soul *Buddyz* appendix 2: Program Finances.

PART C: ASSESSMENT AND LESSONS LEARNED

Challenges and Solutions

The Soul *Buddyz* experience demonstrates that using edutainment strategies to reach and teach children about difficult topics is possible.

Radio Program

The challenge of creating an entertaining children's radio drama was daunting. As noted previously, there was virtually no prior experience in South Africa in producing children's radio drama. Further, the commercialization of the state media had relegated children's programming to the back burner. The pilot of the Soul *Buddyz* radio magazine on the three radio stations was very successful. The impact of the pilot radio series was measurable, inspiring the other radio stations to participate. The radio stations were pleased with the audience response to the phone-in sections of the radio magazine, and lessons were learned about the appropriate airing times for this type of program (for instance, when children are not in school), and that both adults and children appreciate such programs. As a result of the effectiveness of the first set of Soul *Buddyz* radio broadcasts (in three languages), all nine African language stations are going to produce and air the second radio series, slated for July 2003.

Television Program

The Soul *Buddyz* television program was broadcast in multiple languages with English subtitles. The evaluation results show that this strategy worked well with audience members, and even the younger children had no difficulty in understanding the content. The use of multiple languages is particularly important in a multicultural society in which English is increasingly becoming dominant and children's home languages are being eroded. There was a conscious decision to use multiple languages to affirm children, even though there was a risk of the messages not being fully understood by all. To compensate for this risk, the television series was carefully crafted to be as visual as possible, so that children could understand the stories and messages without understanding each word.

Creating Partnerships

Another major challenge was creating partnerships with key organizations such as the national broadcaster, SABC. Without this partnership, the project would not have been realized. Initiating and building the partnership took time but was essential. It is not only partnerships with big organizations that are important. Small NGOs working in particular fields are also essential. For example, it was important to bring NGOs working on sexual abuse into message design workshops and use them as consultants. This gives the project credibility and ensures that the messages are in line with experience on the ground. Building these partnerships also takes time.

> Since the program [*Soul Buddyz*], these children are now very much open and free to discuss some issues. They go to an extent of getting to their guidance teacher and saying, "Listen, this is something very confidential. I hope you are not going to disclose it." Then they discuss what is on their minds — one, two, three, blah, blah, blah., They are free and open. They can discuss it now."
>
> **Periurban schoolchild**

Distributing and Using Print Materials

Another major challenge has been making sure that the print material was distributed and used in schools. Distribution is a huge challenge in a country that has inherited a legacy of neglected schooling. It was a major challenge finding all the names and addresses of schools in the country and an even greater challenge to make sure that the books got into the hands of teachers.

Funding

Clearly, a project like Soul *Buddyz* needs major funding — this, too, was a challenge. One of the most important lessons learned is that it is possible to implement a project like this in a step-by-step way, by first raising money for a pilot and then using the pilot to raise further funding.

Evaluation

An evaluation of Soul *Buddyz* was commissioned in early 2001; it included a quantitative and a qualitative component, contracted separately to two independent research agencies and coordinated by an independent evaluation coordinator. The purpose was to gauge the audience reach and reception and to investigate the program's impact.

The following groups took part in the evaluation:
- a nationwide-sample survey of 2,000 children aged 8 to 13 years,
- 1,500 parents and caregivers of these children, and
- teachers and principals of the schools the children attended.

The sampling design followed within schools ensured that the sample was representative of school-going children aged 8 to 13 and their parents or caregivers. The sample was also statistically representative of primary, combined, and senior primary schools in South Africa. The response rate (with substitution) was 100 percent for principals, children, and parents, and 98 percent for teachers.

Qualitative interviews (including survey, focus group, structured, semistructured, and in-depth interviews) were used to collect information. This fieldwork was conducted after Soul *Buddyz* was aired on television, and after the life-skills and parenting booklets were distributed. The radio series was still broadcasting on two stations when the fieldwork was conducted.

Statistical analysis of the data collected showed that:

- The majority of 8- to 13–year-old children (of all ethnic groups) had watched, listened to, or used the Soul *Buddyz* life-skills materials. The television series also reached 36 percent of parents or adult caregivers. The Soul *Buddyz* materials were used by 41 percent of rural children. This degree of coverage is high in rural areas, given that the full number of available rural radio stations was not used.

- The material was relevant to the needs of the target audience. They found it enjoyable and educational, and it was supported not just by children, but also by parents, caregivers, and teachers.

- The program encouraged quality discussions among children of issues relating to program topics, including specific discussions on HIV/AIDS and condoms. Furthermore, parents who watched Soul *Buddyz* were more likely to talk with their children about sexual and reproductive health and relationships.

- Exposure to Soul *Buddyz* was associated with increased knowledge, including knowing that people infected with HIV can look healthy.

- Exposure enhanced positive attitudes on a number of youth sexuality issues, including forced or coerced sex. It also encouraged a belief in gender equality, and a reduction of the stigma surrounding HIV/AIDS.

- At the level of community action or social mobilization, many children respondents reported forming support groups. The Soul *Buddyz* support group in the television series undoubtedly inspired some of these. As one schoolboy reported, "We have got a club, we actually made one of our own...I think about seven or eight of us. We watched TV, and we wanted to call it 'survivors.'" At one school, two 10-year-olds managed to successfully motivate for ramps to be built to accommodate children with disabilities. These children did this as a direct result of watching Soul *Buddyz*.

- Adults who watched Soul *Buddyz* increasingly realized that children have rights and can contribute to building a better society. Further, the program helped them to communicate more effectively with children about sexuality and other sensitive topics. More than 90 percent of parents agreed that Soul *Buddyz* made it easier for them to discuss difficult issues with their children.

- Some 94 percent of teachers felt that Soul *Buddyz* had given them a new understanding of the problems faced by children.

For further details of the evaluation results see South Africa Soul *Buddyz* appendix 4: Evaluation Results.

UNAIDS Benchmarks

	Benchmark	Attainment	Comments
1	Recognizes the child/youth as a learner who already knows, feels, and can do in relation to healthy development and HIV/AIDS-related prevention.	✓	*Soul Buddyz* makes extensive use of child participation, which shows a recognition of children's capacity. The formative research is particularly significant. This is done with children and forms the basis of the messages, content, and approach of the final edutainment vehicle. Child actors were used for the filming of the television series. The use of young, unknown actors has contributed significantly to the growth and development of a number of young people. One innovative way of including children was to show them the 26 episodes before airing, and giving them an opportunity to comment on each episode in their own language. These comments were broadcast at the end of each episode as "Buddyz buzz."
2	Focuses on risks that are most common to the learning group and that responses are appropriate and targeted to the age group.	✓	The formative and script-testing research done with the potential target group ensures that the risks most common to the age group and dealt with and that the vehicle is appropriate for 7- to 12-year-olds.
3	Includes not only knowledge but also attitudes and skills needed for prevention.	✓	Through the use of realistic drama on television and radio, the program includes much modeling of attitudes and skills. The grade 7 life-skills book has a strong emphasis on atitudes and skills.
4	Understands the impact of relationships on behavior change and reinforces positive social values.	✓	One of the core themes of the program is the modeling of positive social values such as peer support. The stories that focus on HIV/AIDS look at relationships between adolescent boys and girls and issues such as gender and talking openly with each other.
5	Is based on analysis of learners' needs and a broader situation assessment.	✓	Participatory research was conducted with children. An extensive literature review was conducted. Consultants' expertise was drawn on. This ensured that the program was based on learners' needs and also presented a picture of their broader situation.

	Benchmark	Attainment	Comments
6	Has training and continuous support of teachers and other service providers.	Partially fulfilled	The training of teachers to use the materials in the classroom was undertaken as part of the distribution of the print materials. The evaluation shows that distribution and training are areas that could be improved on.
7	Uses multiple and participatory learning activities and strategies.	✓	The program itself is a multimedia one and therefore consists of a number of different strategies that include film, print, and radio. The grade 7 book, designed to be a classroom resource, makes extensive use of participatory learning strategies. Many of the activities are based on the idea of children taking action to make their lives better. In fact, this is what the *Soul Buddyz* television series models for children.
8	Involves the wider community.	✓	The wider community is involved in the sense the parents are targeted through the parenting booklet. In addition, Soul City forms partnerships with particular NGOs in developing the program. For example, organizations who work with children affected by HIV/AIDS were involved in developing the messages for the television program and reviewing scripts and the text for the book.
9	Ensures sequence, progression, and continuity of messages.	✓	The careful creation of messages is done after the formative research. A "message bible" is given to scriptwriters and directors, and *Soul Buddyz* staff are always on set during filming and recordings to make sure the messages are represented accurately. There has been significant continuity of message through *Soul Buddyz 1* and *Soul Buddyz 2*.
10	Is placed in an appropriate context in the school curriculum.	Not applicable	The National Department of Education is involved in the development of messages and in reviewing the scripts and print material. The print materials are distributed through schools. The grade 7 life-skills book is designed to help teachers deliver the national curriculum.

	Benchmark	Attainment	Comments
11	Lasts a sufficient time to meet program goals and objectives.	✓	The television program consists of 26 episodes that are screened more than once by the national broadcaster. The *Soul Buddyz 1* series was screened three times over a year and a half. The *Soul Buddyz 2* series will also consist of 26 episodes screened weekly and will probably also be rebroadcast.
12	Is coordinated with a wider school health promotion program.	Not applicable	*Soul Buddyz* is at present only a mass media vehicle, although the new *Soul Buddyz* clubs program will broaden the reach into a school health context. The program is not, however, linked in any formal way to a school health promotion program.
13	Contains factually correct and consistent messages.	✓	The messages are developed with experts in the field and are monitored carefully while the series is produced.
14	Has established political support through intense advocacy to overcome barriers and go to scale.	✓	Soul City and *Soul Buddyz* have enormous national reach and political support. They are partially funded by the government.
15	Portrays human sexuality as a healthy and normal part of life, and is not derogatory against gender, race, ethnicity, or sexual orientation.	✓	This is one of the strong messages of *Soul Buddyz.* Many of the stories deal with the issue of healthy sexuality and of nondiscrimination.
16	Includes monitoring and evaluation.	✓	*Soul Buddyz 1* was followed by a large national evaluation that included a quantitative and a qualitative component.

PART D: ADDITIONAL INFORMATION

Organizations and Contacts

The Soul City Institute for Health and Development Communication is an NGO established in South Africa in 1992. It uses the power of the mass media for health and development communication. It has achieved this by creating two ongoing media vehicles that address a variety of health and development issues. The media vehicles are *Soul City,* which is aimed at adults and youth, and Soul *Buddyz,* which is aimed at children aged 7 to 12.

Further information on Soul City and Soul Buddyz can be obtained from

Dr. Sue Goldstein
PO Box 1290
Houghton
Johannesburg 2041, South Africa
Telephone: (+27 11) 643-5852
Fax: (+27 11) 643 6253
E-mail: soulcity@soulcity.org.za

Contributors to the Report

The report was compiled by Glynis Clacherty, of Clacherty and Associates, an agency that specializes in participatory research with children and the development of learning materials around children and health. Glynis has worked extensively in the area of HIV/AIDS and children and is based in Johannesburg, South Africa.

This report was based on an article written by Sue Goldstein, Shereen Usdin, Esca Scheepers, Aadielah Anderson, and Garth Japhet of Soul City Institute for Health and Development Communication. Additional information was provided by Sue Goldstein, the head of Research, and head of the children's series at Soul City.

Edited by Katie Tripp and Helen Baños Smith.

Available Materials

To obtain these materials, please contact ibeaids@ibe.unesco.org or Education for HIV/AIDS Prevention, International Bureau of Education, C.P. 199, 1211 Geneva 20, Switzerland.

Raising Children to Be Their Best: A Guide for Parents
(order number: Soul Buddyz01)

Tomorrow Is Ours (grade 7 life orientation learning resource based on the television) series
(order number: Soul Buddyz02)

APPENDIX 1. STAFF STRUCTURE AND ROLES

This appendix outlines the staffing structure of the Soul *Buddyz* project. It is important to note that Soul *Buddyz* is a project within a larger organization, Soul City. Most of the staff that are indicated as part-time here work for the other part of their time on the *Soul City* project.

An important strategy used by Soul City is to keep the project staff to a minimum and draw on outside expertise. A number of service providers worked on the Soul *Buddyz* project. The main service providers are listed below, with an indication of the work they did.

- research agency: audience research with children,
- film scriptwriters,
- film production company,
- radio scriptwriters,
- radio production company,
- research agency: script testing,
- marketing company: marketing events such as the launch and media marketing,
- advertising agency: advertising the series, and
- research agencies: evaluation.

Staff Roles

Senior Manager (Part-Time)
Overall manager of the project, responsible for fund raising and ensuring that the manager keeps to deadlines. The senior manager also has a coaching role and supports the manager wherever necessary.

Manager
Responsible for the coordination of the series and particularly the involvement of stakeholders and ensuring that everything is kept to schedule. She is also the "keeper of the message" and ensures that the messages that are developed are kept to rigorously throughout the process.

Radio Coordinator
Runs the radio scriptwriting and development process as well as assisting with liaison with the radio stations. This person also coordinates and organizes the training for radio production and oversees the translation processes.

Administrator
Responsible for all administration, including sending scripts to consultants and getting feedback from them. She organizes all the logistics and also assists in the "Buddyz Buzz," as well as in translation.

Researcher

Soul City researches each intervention. In Soul *Buddyz*, the parenting booklet and some of the other aspects of the program are tested with adults. The formative research is done in three parts — with children, adults, and key stakeholders. The Soul City researchers do the formative research with adults. The Soul *Buddyz* manager does the stakeholder research, and the children's research is outsourced to an expert research partner who specializes in that field.

Marketing Manager

Oversees the public relations and advertising campaigns around Soul *Buddyz* (and all other Soul City interventions). He works closely with the Soul *Buddyz* team to ensure that the feel of the campaign is appropriate.

Advocacy Manager

Accompanying Soul *Buddyz* is an advocacy campaign dealing with a particular issue that is dealt with in the program. The advocacy manager develops and runs these campaigns. She also forms alliances and partnerships.

APPENDIX 2. PROGRAM FINANCES

Money spent on	Amount spent (US$)
Research and development (including the pilots)	40,000 (R400,000)
Television	900,000 (R9 million)
Radio	200,000 (R2 million)
Print	550,000 (R5.5 million)
Parenting booklet	100,000 (R1 million)
Public relations and advocacy	200,000 (R2 million)
Staff costs	200,000 (R2 million)
Evaluation	100,000 (R1 million)
Total (based on exchange rate of R10 to US$1)	2.3 million (R23 million)

APPENDIX 3. DETAILED EXPLANATION OF GOALS

The following messages capture what the Soul *Buddyz* series was all about. Beneath each is an explanation of why this message is important.

1. *I am unique and have my own strengths and weaknesses — we are all different and special in our own way. All people are deserving of respect, irrespective of age, gender, religion, race, or state of health or impairment. They have strengths and weaknesses just like you.* This message underpinned the entire Soul *Buddyz* series. Formative research showed that children who were "different" in any way were teased and bullied by others. The message was continuously shown in the composition of the Soul *Buddyz* group, from different races and socioeconomic backgrounds, with different abilities, but friends and supportive and respectful of each other.

2. *It is important to serve the community to which one belongs and recognize that my actions or lack of actions influence and affect others.* This message called for community action around the various educational issues, including AIDS, and promoted the idea of peer-based support. The overarching story was a competition, for which each group of children had to do three community projects and were then visited by a judge who discussed the projects with them. The series culminated in an "International Children's Rights Convention" at which attendance was the prize.

3. *Boys and girls are equal and deserve equal respect. Girls can do anything, though it may sometimes be difficult. Boys are allowed to "feel" and be sensitive.* This message was to uphold the dignity of being a girl in South African society. Formative research showed girls in South Africa felt anxious about the strong possibility of being abused: "I don't like being a girl because I don't want to be raped by gangsters and father," said a 9-year-old girl. An 11-year-old boy said, "When you see her with another man, you beat her." A few episodes were dedicated to this message, showing girls achieving things that many South African children believe is not possible, such as a girl aspiring to becoming a pilot. In addition, great care was taken in every scene not to stereotype gender roles.

4. *I need to identify my feelings and learn to express them in an appropriate way.* Children have the right to dream and hope and to have the space to articulate those dreams and hopes. Children have the right to be worried and have concerns and should be encouraged to express these worries so that they may be addressed.

    Formative research for Soul *Buddyz* showed that children did not know how to express their emotions. Each story was told from the perspective of a child in such a way that the audience could hear the child's inner voice through a voiceover technique. This allowed children to understand in words what the child was feeling and, thus, how to express emotions.

5. *Life is about choices. It is important to realize that your choices will influence your future and can affect others.* A problem-solving approach was encouraged, and children were shown looking for their own answers and trying different solutions. Children were encouraged to take responsibility for their actions.

6. *It is important to communicate about AIDS and sex. It is often difficult to get information about sensitive issues, but it is important to keep trying to get accurate information. Friends and adults are not always right, so cross-check your information with other resources.* Before the series, most children had heard about AIDS, though their knowledge was sketchy. They knew that AIDS was incurable, but believed it involved getting sores and going "mad." Neither the invisible nature of HIV infection, nor its method of transmission, was clearly understood. "If you stand next to them, they infect you — if they have it, then you'll also get it," said a 10-year-old boy.

    Formative research also showed that parents found it very difficult to talk about sex with their children. In a national survey of youth, only 14 percent of 12- to 17-year olds said that they learned about sex from their parents. The story in the series is about a young boy who learns that his mother has AIDS. He then goes through a process of learning the facts about AIDS in a few different ways, one of which (from a school friend) proves to be inaccurate.

7. *My body is my own. It is normal to feel uncomfortable with the changes that happen to one's body at the time of puberty. Children have the right to say no to sex and abuse.* There is a young teenage romance story, starting with a young girl experiencing menarch and finding out the facts about puberty. At the same time, a young boy has a wet dream and has all the myths surrounding this dispelled. There is an additional story of a young girl who has been sexually abused by her uncle. It shows how she is assisted by the "Childline" (a phone help line) and one of her friends to get adult help.

8. *All people are deserving of respect, no matter what race, gender, or religion they are, or whether they have HIV or AIDS.* This Soul *Buddyz* message was designed to address the intense stigma experienced by people living with AIDS in South Africa. Gugu Dlamini, a woman from Kwazulu-Natal province who revealed her HIV-positive status on radio on World AIDS Day in 1998, was stoned to death. Soul *Buddyz* research showed that children had experienced AIDS-related discrimination. The story revolves around a friend of one of the Soul Buddyz who is fired from his job because he is HIV positive. The Soul Buddyz leap to his defense in creative ways and confront this prejudice with protests and information.

APPENDIX 4. EVALUATION RESULTS

Reach of Soul *Buddyz*

After its first season of broadcast, 75 percent of all respondents aged 8 to 13 had heard of Soul *Buddyz*, with 67 percent of the respondents reporting that they had watched, listened to, or used the Soul *Buddyz* life-skills materials. Almost half of the children who watched Soul *Buddyz* on television report that they watched "all or most of the episodes." The Soul *Buddyz* television series also reached 36 percent of parents or adult caregivers.

Soul *Buddyz* was broadcast on the most popular audience channel (SABC 1 at 18h30). This channel often broadcasts programs in languages other than English or features mixed-language broadcasts, which tend to reduce its white audience, thus, the lowest audience was "white" children, 49 percent.

The Soul *Buddyz* materials (including television series, radio magazine, and the two booklets) were accessed by 41 percent of the rural children. This degree of coverage is high in rural areas, given that the full armory of rural radio stations was not used.

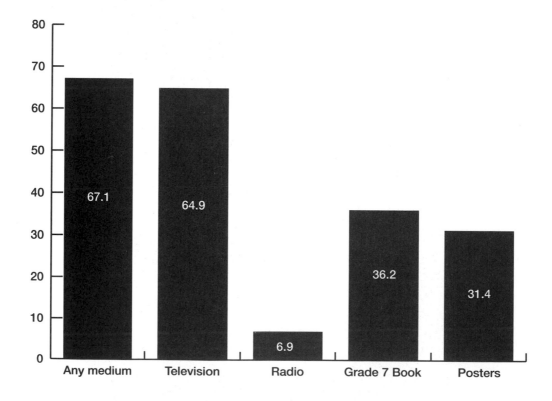

Figure A4.1. Reach of Soul Buddyz Material

Relevance of Soul *Buddyz*

Both quantitative and qualitative analyses indicated that Soul *Buddyz* media materials were highly relevant to its primary target audience. Soul *Buddyz* was very popular among all its target groups, with various sets of viewers experiencing it as enjoyable and educational. In addition to the children, parents, caregivers, and teachers were all highly supportive of Soul *Buddyz*. As a parent said, Soul *Buddyz* is a bonus. It deals with real-life issues and real-life situations and makes [children] more aware of things which are a reality."

Impact on Gender, Youth, Sexuality, and HIV/AIDS

Soul *Buddyz* consistently affected the quality and frequency of discussion of issues among audience members. Some 77 percent of the children who watched the Soul *Buddyz* television series said they talked about the things they saw on Soul *Buddyz* with other people. Parents (and caregivers) who watched Soul *Buddyz* on television were more likely to discuss issues of sexuality with their children (74 percent), compared with parents who had not watched (54 percent) (P = .000). As a rural parent noted, "I like that Soul *Buddyz* teaches kids things that are not easy for parents to talk to their kids about. We black parents we have a problem — there are things that are not easy for us to talk to kids about."

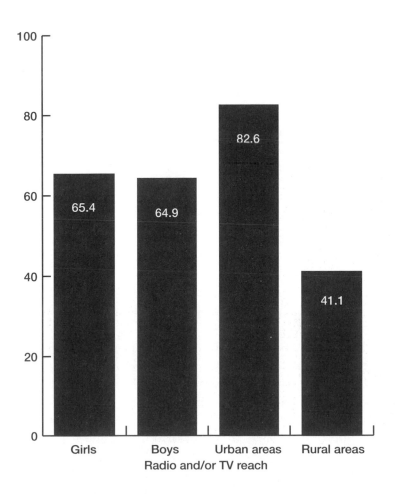

Figure A4.1. Reach of Soul Buddyz *Material, by Gender and Location*

Children exposed to Soul *Buddyz* media materials were more likely to discuss HIV/AIDS, compared with children who were not exposed: Some 80 percent of 11- to 13-year-olds who were exposed to the life-skills booklet reported talking about HIV/AIDS, compared with the 64 percent of the same-age respondents who were not exposed (P = .000). Similarly, some 75 percent of 11- to 13-year olds with high exposure to Soul *Buddyz* television reported talking about HIV/AIDS, compared with the 61 percent of the same-age respondents who were not exposed (P = .000). One young viewer of Soul *Buddyz* noted, [Soul Buddyz] has changed the way I interact with my friends, parents, and people in the community; I have learnt to be more respectful, and I have learnt to talk about things that are of great concern to me or that hurt me."

Exposure to Soul *Buddyz* was associated with increased knowledge as well as positive attitudes on a number of youth sexuality issues. For instance, 67 percent of the boys with high exposure to the Soul *Buddyz* television series disagreed with the statement, "a person has to have sex with their boyfriend or girlfriend to show they love them," compared with 52 percent of boys who were not exposed (P = .002). Similarly, 86 percent of girls who were exposed to the life-skills booklet disagreed with the same statement, compared with 67 percent of girls with no exposure to the booklet (P = .000).

Children exposed to the Soul *Buddyz* television series were more likely to agree with the statement "boys and girls are equal," compared with children with no exposure to the television series. Some 63 percent of 11- to 13-year-olds with high exposure to the television series agreed that boys and girls were equal, compared with 51 percent of children who were not exposed to the television series (P = .001).

Exposure to any of the three Soul *Buddyz* media was positively associated with knowledge about HIV/AIDS, and with the frequency that condom use was mentioned as a way of preventing contracting HIV/AIDS. Eighty-four percent of children with high exposure to Soul *Buddyz* television (whose parents said they never discussed HIV/AIDS with their children) knew what HIV/AIDS was, whereas 67 percent of the same sample segment with no exposure to Soul *Buddyz* on television knew what HIV/AIDS was (P = .05).

Children exposed to *Soul Buddyz* on television were more likely to know that people with HIV can look healthy: 56 percent of 11- to 13-year-olds with high exposure to *Soul Buddyz* on television thought that people with HIV/AIDS can look healthy, whereas 31 percent with no exposure to Soul *Buddyz* on television did (P = .000).

Children exposed to any of the three Soul *Buddyz* media types were more likely to mention consistent condom use as a way of preventing HIV/AIDS than children with no exposure to Soul *Buddyz*. Eighty-six percent of children who did discuss HIV/AIDS with a teacher and were exposed to the grade 7 booklet mentioned condom use as a way of preventing HIV/AIDS, whereas 70 percent of children in the same sample segment, but with no exposure to the grade 7 booklet, did (P = .016).

Qualitative data showed that Soul *Buddyz* messages about care and support for people living with HIV/AIDS came across clearly and effectively. As a young child noted, "Soul *Buddyz* teaches me about AIDS. Like when one of the boys' mother had AIDS, it shows how a person can cope with AIDS." Soul *Buddyz* also seemed to play an important role in addressing HIV/AIDS stigma. Children exposed to the Soul *Buddyz* television series were more likely to say that they were willing to be friends with someone who has HIV/AIDS than were children who were not exposed to the television series. Fifty percent of 8- to 10-year-olds with high exposure to Soul *Buddyz* on television said they are willing to befriend someone with HIV/AIDS, whereas 21 percent with no exposure to Soul *Buddyz* on television were willing (P = .000). Similar trends were observed among 11- to 13-year olds.

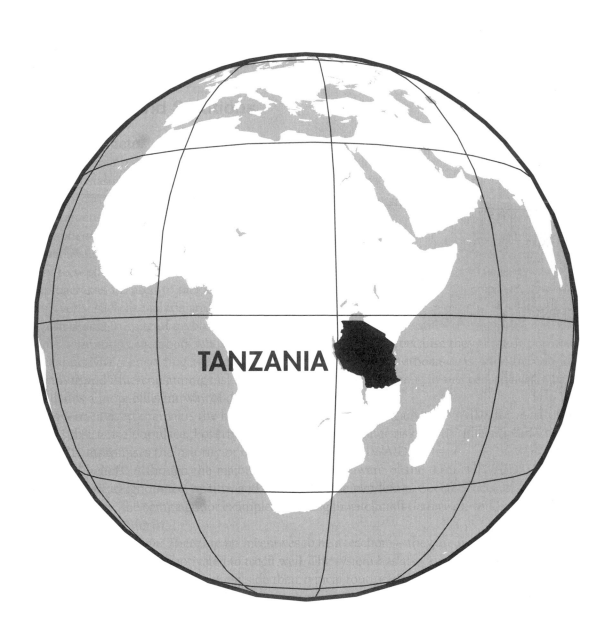

TANZANIA

AMREF, LSHTM, and NIMR: MEMA Kwa Vijana Program

PART A: DESCRIPTION OF THE PROGRAM

Program Rationale and History

Between 1994 and 1998, several baseline studies were conducted in the Mwanza region and neighboring Mara region in Tanzania to look into the status of HIV infection in primary schools. They found that youth in their early 20s were most at risk of becoming infected.

To tackle this problem, the MEMA kwa Vijana program was set up in 62 primary schools in four (of the seven) districts in the Mwanza region in 1999 to target 12- to 19-year–olds, the age just before which they are most likely to become infected. The idea was to equip youth with information about adolescent sexual and reproductive health (ASRH) and get them to think about the consequences of their sexual behaviors. The program title reflects its rationale: *MEMA kwa Vijana* means "Good Things (MEMA) for Young People."

The program is a collaboration between three organizations: the African Medical and Research Foundation (AMREF), the London School of Hygiene and Tropical Medicine (LSHTM), and the National Institute for Medical Research (NIMR) of Tanzania. AMREF designed the program and is responsible for its implementation in collaboration with the Tanzanian Ministry of Health (MoH) and Ministry of Education and Culture (MoEC). NIMR is responsible for designing and implementing the evaluation, looking at both the impact and the cost-effectiveness of the intervention. LSHTM provides technical assistance to both AMREF and NIMR, as well as providing the majority of the funding for the program.

> Setting up an intervention for youth who are at high risk will assist in equipping them with correct information about sex before they start sexual relationships. It also means they will be more likely to practice safer sex. Otherwise, many youth learn from their peers, who also lack the correct information.
>
> ***Program coordinator***

The program involves teacher-led and peer-assisted, participatory, in-class teaching and informal ASRH peer education in clubs and through one-to-one contact. The program also involves youth-friendly SRH services and community mobilization. The program has been set up using an experimental design: The intervention is being conducted in 62 primary schools and 18 health facilities, with the same number of schools and health facilities acting as a control group (see Evaluation below). This design allows scientific measurement of the impact of the intervention program.

So far, the program has reached approximately 17,000 students. The program's future will be determined by the results of the evaluation currently under way (2002) and the availability of funds.

Program Overview

Aim

The main aim of the program is to improve ASRH knowledge and decrease the rate of sexually transmitted infection (STI) and HIV infection and unwanted pregnancies among 12- to 19-year-old youth in Mwanza region.

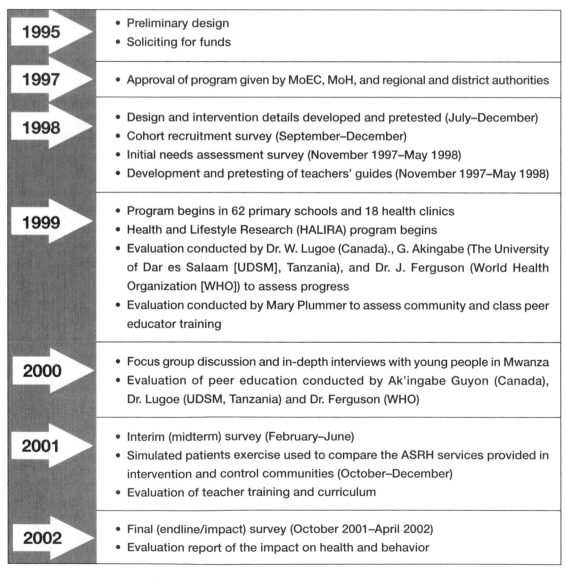

1995
- Preliminary design
- Soliciting for funds

1997
- Approval of program given by MoEC, MoH, and regional and district authorities

1998
- Design and intervention details developed and pretested (July–December)
- Cohort recruitment survey (September–December)
- Initial needs assessment survey (November 1997–May 1998)
- Development and pretesting of teachers' guides (November 1997–May 1998)

1999
- Program begins in 62 primary schools and 18 health clinics
- Health and Lifestyle Research (HALIRA) program begins
- Evaluation conducted by Dr. W. Lugoe (Canada)., G. Akingabe (The University of Dar es Salaam [UDSM], Tanzania), and Dr. J. Ferguson (World Health Organization [WHO]) to assess progress
- Evaluation conducted by Mary Plummer to assess community and class peer educator training

2000
- Focus group discussion and in-depth interviews with young people in Mwanza
- Evaluation of peer education conducted by Ak'ingabe Guyon (Canada), Dr. Lugoe (UDSM, Tanzania) and Dr. Ferguson (WHO)

2001
- Interim (midterm) survey (February–June)
- Simulated patients exercise used to compare the ASRH services provided in intervention and control communities (October–December)
- Evaluation of teacher training and curriculum

2002
- Final (endline/impact) survey (October 2001–April 2002)
- Evaluation report of the impact on health and behavior

Figure 1. Time Line of Major Program Events

Objectives

According to the program coordinator, the program objectives are to

- improve young people's knowledge and skills to avoid sexual and reproductive health risks,
- decrease the prevalence of HIV infection and other STIs among youth,
- decrease the number of unintended pregnancies,
- improve young people's access to youth-friendly SRH services,
- improve adults' attitudes toward ASRH needs, and
- improve adults' skills to respond to ASRH needs.

Target Groups

Primary Target Group

The target group are students in 62 primary schools aged 12 to 19 years (grades 5, 6, and 7) in Mwanza region.

> We appreciate the program because it exposes us to issues which we didn't used to know about. It also allows us to talk freely about things we weren't allowed to before, like mentioning the male and female reproductive organs.
>
> **Youth participant**

Secondary Target Group

The secondary target group are

- students in grades 1 to 4 and out-of-school youth reached during the annual interschools Youth Health Week festivals;
- teachers in the schools where the program is running;
- health workers in the health clinics where the program is running;
- approximately 2,000 out-of-school youth who participate in drama, role plays, and songs, and who are involved in the promotion and distribution of condoms, which they buy and sell at a profit; and
- community members who are exposed to the program.

Site

The program was started and is mainly based in primary schools in the region. It also works in health centers, where it has trained health workers to deliver youth-friendly SRH services.

Program Length

The program has lasted for three years so far.

Program Goals

The list in figure 2 shows how the program coordinator ranked the program goals. The idea is that if young people receive correct information and are taught behavioral and life skills before they engage in sex, they will be more likely to practice safer sex (e.g., using condoms, choosing safe partners, limiting the number of partners, seeking SRH services, etc.) once they become sexually active.

Approaches

Figure 3 shows the program's approaches, ranked in order by the program coordinator.

HIV/AIDS testing and counseling were conducted in 1999 on 10,000 in-school and out-of-school youth (both males and females) who make up the intervention group. They were counseled and tested again in 2002.

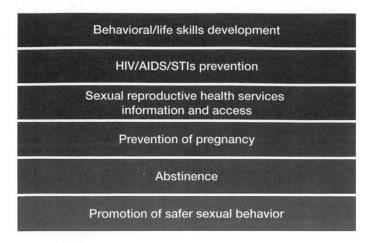

Figure 2. Program Goals Ranked in Increasing Importance by Program Coordinator

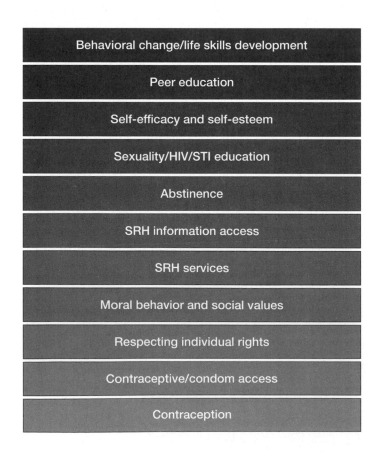

Figure 3. Program Approaches Ranked in Increasing Importance

Activities

The students enjoy drama and role plays most because they can get involved and are given an opportunity to show off their skills. Condom distribution occurs less frequently, because it is done by out-of-school youth on a voluntary basis.

Components

The program consists of four main components:
1. teacher-led and peer-assisted, participatory SRH education and informal peer education,
2. training of health workers to deliver youth-friendly SRH services,
3. condom distribution, and
4. community mobilization.

School Component

Classroom teaching. Each school has approximately three MEMA teachers who have been trained to deliver participatory SRH education. Students in the last three years of primary school are taught about ASRH for one hour per week by these teacher-guardians, who are

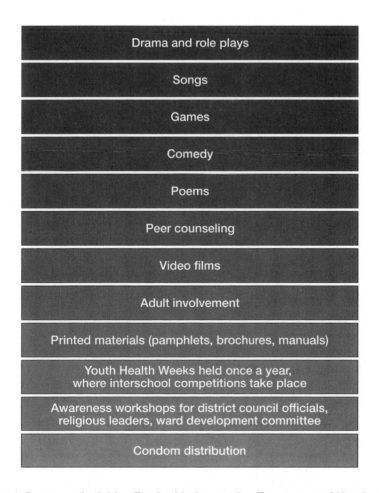

Figure 4. Program Activities Ranked in Increasing Frequency of Use by Youth

assisted by peer educators. The in-class sessions have been developed in partnership with the regional education authorities and aim to enhance adolescents' knowledge and attitudes concerning SRH. They also include a substantial skills-training component designed to assist adolescents in translating attitudes and intentions into behavior.

After school hours, these lessons are followed by drama, songs, role plays, and poems prepared (with help from teachers) by the students. Debate clubs are held twice a month in each school. Younger pupils and out-of-school youth are invited to attend these.

There is a 15-member school committee: two teachers, the ward education coordinator, the village or ward executive officer, a health care worker, and other male and female community members. The committee guides the school by discussing the views, needs, progress, and recommendations reported from all stakeholders (students, teachers, and community members).

Teachers also attend yearly workshops, where they meet with teachers from other schools to monitor and evaluate program progress and exchange ideas and new findings.

The ward education coordinator visits each school three times a month to make sure that the academic subjects and ASRH topics are taught as arranged. They also discuss program progress with the peer educators and teachers. Any problems raised are discussed first by the school committee, and if no resolution can be found, the district education inspector and MEMA kwa Vijana are informed.

> Prior to MEMA kwa Vijana program, we never attended to any pupil. I think they had no confidence in our confidentiality — also, they felt ashamed and feared their parents.
>
> **Public health nurse**

Case Study of a Class Session

The session opens with the teacher asking a pupil to sing a song to "break the ice." The teacher then reviews the previous session through questions — for example, "Who can tell us what we talked about in the last class?" Then the teacher posts the topic of the current session on the board. The pupils are asked to read it and guess what they think will be discussed that day. The topic is then introduced through a short drama enacted by peer educators. Students then form small groups to answer questions in a quiz competition the teacher has posed to them. The students are then given an opportunity to ask questions and review what they have learned that day. Homework questions are given, and the students are asked to discuss them and the lessons in general with others not reached by this session (out-of-school peers, siblings, parents).

Advice. Empathic advice is given, either on demand and or when teachers identify the need, by the teacher-guardian or teachers who have had training in ASRH.

Youth Health Weeks. Youth Health Weeks are held once a year. Students from all participating schools in the district meet and display what they have learned during the year. Members of the community and leaders from the district or regional level are also invited. The aim here is to disseminate messages on HIV/AIDS/STI prevention and raise awareness of ASRH needs.

Health Clinic Component

A program of youth-friendly SRH services has been developed and is being implemented in 18 government-run primary health care facilities. Two health workers per clinic were trained to deliver youth-friendly SRH services with the aim of improving adolescents' access to effective sexually transmitted disease (STD) treatment and family-planning services. It focuses on adolescents' rights to comprehensive services, empathic treatment, respect, and confidentiality.

The trained health workers visit each school once a month to check on the general health of students and exchange news with teachers and the guardians.

Condom Distribution

The project has trained a total of 228 young people (peer condom promoters and distributors [CPDs]) who were elected by their peers to sell affordable condoms in the intervention villages. Condoms are supplied by the project to at least one central distributor in each project community, from whom the CPDs purchase their stock.

Community Mobilization

Community activities are scheduled throughout the year. They aim to raise community awareness of risks to ASRH and mobilize support for the other components of the intervention. These activities are overseen in each community by an advisory committee, which consists of 15 to 22 individuals who were elected by the community themselves at the end of a participatory community mobilization week in late 1998.

PART B: IMPLEMENTING THE PROGRAM

Needs Assessment

The needs assessment was not available. However, the program manager said that the main results revealed that most primary school students began sexual activity by the age of 13 or 14 years. It also found that 5 percent of girls and 1 percent of boys aged 19 years were HIV positive. Many young girls (particularly the poor) were enticed by small gifts into having unprotected sex with older, wealthier men. The men believe that the young and naïve girls are free from HIV infection.

Program Materials

MEMA kwa Vijana has developed its own materials for the teachers and students. The materials are in Kiswahili, and are being translated into English, with publication planned for early 2003. Other materials are adapted from other NGOs, such as Deutsche Gesellschaft für Technische Zusammenarbeit (GTZ), and programs such as Tanzania Netherlands Support for AIDS (TANESA), and so forth.

Target Group Materials

- Guide for peer educators (in Kiswahili) prepared by the Mo E and culture called KINGA;
- health and family life education materialsfor primary school classes 5, 6, and 7 (topics mainly on ASRH); and

- eight GTZ booklets giving answers to the questions adolescents ask most frequently about ASRH:
  - Volume 1 — *Growing Up,*
  - Volume 2 — *Male-Female Relationships,*
  - Volume 3 — *Sexual Relationships,*
  - Volume 4 — *Pregnancy,*
  - Volume 5 — *Healthy Relationships,*
  - Volume 6 — *HIV/AIDS and the New Generation,*
  - Volume 7 — *Drugs and Drug Abuse,* and
  - Volume 8 — *Alcohol and Cigarettes.*

The program is very useful because now the pregnancy rate, absenteeism, and drop out is low. For example, there has been no pregnant pupil for the past two years. Girls are also more assertive and confident. They can just say no to sexual advances, and there are good interpersonal relationships between boys and girls.

Teacher

Additional Materials

Other materials, such as a flip chart on female and male reproductive organs, and posters, booklets, and videos from the National AIDS Control Program and other NGOs, such as GTZ and TANESA, are also used.

Staff Training Materials

Three books, one for each class (grades 5, 6, and 7) have been developed for teachers to use as guides in the classroom:

- a questions and answers book for peer educators that cover common questions asked by young people,
- a teacher's guide used to deliver SRH education, and
- a teacher resource book with detailed information about HIV/AIDS/STI and family planning, including condom use.

Staff Selection and Training

- Initially, the program trained trainers of peers (TOPs) who participated in training their class peers, but these have been dropped in favor of using teachers.
- Senior posts were advertised in the media. Applicants were interviewed and successful candidates employed. Junior staff were recruited from the intervention region through internal and partner advertisement.
- Staff development is ensured through in-house mentoring and capacity-building, attending and presenting at national and international meetings, and access to up-to-date information via unlimited access to the Internet at the workplace.
- This year, the program coordinator has been sponsored to take a one-year course for a master's degree in public health (MPH) in London.

Setting Up the Program

No information was available on how to set up the program.

Program Resources

The program has a spacious office, where books, posters, charts, fliers, pamphlets, and other materials are stored. The office also has a number of computers and printers and a photocopy machine. The program also has four vehicles.

Advocacy

MEMA kwa Vijana involves government officials and community leaders who give their firm support to the program. The government's involvement includes providing policy guidelines for the program and participating in implementing the program (MOEC and MOH, regional and district leaders). Government health facility workers are involved in providing youth-friendly services.

Discussion with the regional education officer for Mwanza and the zonal education inspector showed that they were happy with the program and would appreciate expansion to cover all schools in the region.

Program Finances

Estimates of the cost per participant in the program:

- During the pilot phase (heavy development and monitoring), the cost per primary-target-group youth was US$17 per year.
- The second-year cost was US$ 7.63.
- Annual implementation cost at present is US$1.37 per participant per year.

PART C: ASSESSMENT AND LESSONS LEARNED

Challenges and Solutions

Program Coordinator

- Teacher-led, peer-assisted SRH education is now acceptable and feasible within the regular school curriculum. This was achieved through discussions with educational leaders who agreed to dedicate one hour per week per class for ASRH education. The same is true for youth-friendly health services.
- By targeting parents, ASRH messages can be further integrated into community life.
- ASRH programs need to tap into and build local capacity and infrastructure to promote and sustain peer education.
- Some resistance was noted from religious leaders, especially on condom knowledge and use. This could be overcome if religious leaders are involved right from the beginning of the program. Discussions and demonstrations of condom use in classrooms also remain a controversial issue. This needs to be overcome, especially because it is educationally necessary.
- Building ASRH programs into activities that adolescents identify with (drama, sports, entertainment, and income-generating activities) has broader appeal to young people's needs.

Furthermore, combining ASRH education activities with youth-friendly services and counseling is more likely to result in behavior change.

- The degree of SRH risk an adolescent faces is often indicative of, and is made worse by, important but unmet social and economic needs. Hence, these also need to be addressed.
- It is difficult to train 12- to 19-year-old youth in peer education. However, they can perform excellent drama productions and are good as discussion starters. Therefore, their role should not be to educate directly, but to facilitate better trained, older peer educators.
- Even though condom promotion and distribution has increased in the communities, the youth responsible for distribution used the money earned to invest in other things because they were not earning enough money to realize a decent income. This had the consequence that many CPDs left the program or became very mobile ("searching for life"). The increase in absenteeism and sales inertia made the whole component difficult to sustain. Equipping the CPDs with business skills would not solve the problem; what is needed is for the communities to be more willing to buy and use condoms.
- Regular process evaluations build strong programs by making them proactive and keeping them relevant to emerging needs.

Teachers

Teachers requested that they all be given training.

Peer Educators

- During the annual Youth Health Week, several schools should hold competitions, and the best performers could be rewarded. This would be an incentive for sustaining the status while they learn.
- Use of videos of their performances could be more enjoyable and easily understood by the community and other youth.

Evaluation

The impact of the intervention on the sexual behavior and reproductive health of adolescents will be evaluated by NIMR in early 2003. The final report is expected by October or December 2002. The two principal components are explained below.

Biomedical Impact

The primary outcomes of the trial will be a comparison of HIV, other STIs, and unintended pregnancies between

- a cohort of students in 62 primary schools in 10 communities that were randomly assigned to receive the intervention in phase 1 (January 1999 to December 2002), and
- an equal number of students in 10 comparable communities that were randomly assigned to receive the intervention from July 2003 onward (if the intervention is found to have been effective during phase 1).

The prevalence of HIV, other STIs, and unintended pregnancies was measured when the trial cohort was recruited between August and December 1998, immediately before the introduction of the intervention. An interim follow-up survey was conducted between February and June 2000 (i.e., approximately 18 months after the cohort recruitment survey, and between 13 and 18 months after the start of the intervention in half of the communities). The final follow-up survey will be conducted between October 2001 and April 2002 (i.e., approximately 3 years after the recruitment survey, and between 33 and 40 months after the start of the intervention in half of the communities).

An initial survey (November 1997–May 1998) looking at HIV and STI prevalence was performed in the project communities. (Survey subjects were approximately 9,500 15- to 19-year-olds.) to ensure that the communities were sufficiently similar to be compared, and thus increase the power of the study.

Behavioral Impact

The project is also measuring the effect of the intervention on the SRH knowledge, attitudes, and behavior of adolescents in the same cohort. This is being done using a variety of quantitative and qualitative methods:

- participatory, qualitative study by research assistants who lived in households for seven weeks to study sexual behavior, beliefs, attitudes, and so forth;
- in-depth interviews with program members;
- focus group discussions in villages; and
- evaluation of health clinics by young "simulated patients." (This showed that health workers who had received training as part of the program were significantly less judgmental and more youth friendly.)

Evaluations of other aspects of the program (e.g., teacher/peer educator training, curriculum, etc.) are mentioned in the time line. For further information on these, please contact the program manger directly. (Contact information is given in Part d.)

UNAIDS Benchmarks

	Benchmark	Attainment	Comments
1	Recognizes the child/youth as a learner who already knows, feels, and can do in relation to healthy development and HIV/AIDS-related prevention.	Partially fulfilled	Youth are allowed to express their views freely, and these views are respected. They prepare and conduct drama, role plays, etc. They select their teacher-guardians. However, evidence of their involvement during the design and preparatory stages is not documented.
2	Focuses on risks that are most common to the learning group and that responses are appropriate and targeted to the age group.	✓	Teachers address issues related to the risks in their day-to-day teaching. Stories and drama are built around the risk issues and discussed.
3	Includes not only knowledge but also attitudes and skills needed for prevention.	✓	Skills and attitudes are reinforced. A good number of youth (and especially girls) seem to have the courage to say no to sex when approached. Sexuality is an issue they can now discuss with their peers and teacher-guardian more freely and openly.

	Benchmark	Attainment	Comments
4	Understands the impact of relationships on behavior change and reinforces positive social values.	✓	Positive social values are reinforced. For example, respect for elders, abstinence until marriage, how girls can cope with menstruation when it begins, and giving assistance to the elderly and the sick within the community.
5	Is based on analysis of learners' needs and a broader situation assessment.	✓	MEMA kwa Vijana conducted a needs assessment to determine the needs of the youth. Views were collected and used in the development of training guides.
6	Has training and continuous support of teachers and other service providers.	✓	Schoolteachers, guardians, and the service providers were trained before the program began, and they have an annual workshop to exchange experiences.
7	Uses multiple and participatory learning activities and strategies.	✓	The program fully involves schoolchildren through peer education, drama, role plays, poems, etc.
8	Involves the wider community.	✓	The community is very involved. They are represented at school committees, attend the youth festival week activities, etc. This has tended to improve ASRH communication among students, parents, and community. However, the community should be informed about the actual contents of the program in detail so as to iron out differences — e.g., condom demonstration in class.
9	Ensures sequence, progression, and continuity of messages.	✓	The program builds from simple messages in grade 5, increasing in complexity through grades 6 and 7.
10	Is placed in an appropriate context in the school curriculum.	✓	The program is part of the school curriculum. ASRH subjects are taught during school hours in biology or civic subjects. The MoEC has endorsed the program.
11	Lasts a sufficient time to meet program goals and objectives.	Partially fulfilled	Awaiting results of evaluation.

	Benchmark	Attainment	Comments
12	Is coordinated with a wider school health promotion program.	Not applicable	There is no systematic school health program in Mwanza region.
13	Contains factually correct and consistent messages.	✓	The materials were developed by health experts and are factually correct.
14	Has established political support through intense advocacy to overcome barriers and go to scale.	✓	The regional commissioner, ward counselor, and regional education officer requested scale-up to all schools in the region.
15	Portrays human sexuality as a healthy and normal part of life, and is not derogatory against gender, race, ethnicity, or sexual orientation.	✓	MEMA addresses these culturally sensitive issues. The teachers, peer educators, and guardians faced problems during the first year of the program (in grade 5) because sexuality was not traditionally discussed openly, especially with young people. Youth tend to be more comfortable from the second year onward.
16	Includes monitoring and evaluation.	✓	A large-scale, scientifically designed evaluation has been conducted.

PART D: ADDITIONAL INFORMATION

Organizations and Contacts

Dr. David Ross
MEMA kwa Vijana project director
London School of Hygiene and Tropical Medicine
Keppel St.
London WC1E 7HT, United Kingdom
E-mail: david.ross@lshtm.ac.uk

Dr. Awene Gavyole
Programme coordinator
African Medical and Research Foundation (AMREF)
Lake Zone Programme
P.O. Box 1482
Mwanza, Tanzania
E-mail: gavyolea@amrefmza.org

Mr. Maende Makokha
MEMA kwa Vijana intervention coordinator
African Medical and Research Foundation (AMREF)
P.O. Box 1482
Mwanza, Tanzania
E-mail: maendem@amrefmza.org

Contributors to the Report

Program report prepared by Adeline Kimambo, aided by Ms. Zablon.

Edited by Katie Tripp and Helen Baños Smith.

We appreciate the help of the following people in providing much of the information in this report:

Dr. David Ross — Director
Ms. Bernadette Clephas — Intervention coordinator
Mr. Maende Makokha — Deputy intervention coordinator
Mr. Kenneth Chima — Health learning materials officer
Mr. Godwin Mmassy — Team leader (education)
Ms. Rachel Alex — Youth intervention facilitator
Mr. Joseph Charles — Youth intervention facilitator
Mr. B. J. Mujaya — Regional education officer, Mwanza
Mr. Felix Mwinagwa — Zonal chief inspector for all schools in Lake Zone (four regions)
Ms. Mary Plummer — Social sciences research coordinator

Ms. Anna Mtani — Head teacher, Bugalama Primary School, Sengerema

Ms. Beatrice Venance — Teacher, Bugalama Primary School

12 teachers and students of Bugalama Primary School

Ms. Restituta Kasaka — Clinical officer, Inchange Katunguru Health Centre

Ms. Anastazia Mtebe — Public health nurse, Katunguru Health Centre

Mr. Shadrack Mrutu — Health worker

John Mulunga — Acting ward education coordinator and head teacher of Katunguru Primary School

Available Materials

To obtain these materials, please contact ibeaids@ibe.unesco.org or Education for HIV/AIDS Prevention, International Bureau of Education, C.P. 199, 1211 Geneva 20, Switzerland.

Year 2 Training protocols: Final field versions
(order number: MEMA 01)

Final head teachers' training protocol, February 2002
(order number: MEMA 02)

Protocol for the training of health workers in the provision of youth friendly reproductive health services
(order number: MEMA 03)

Refresher protocol for YFS training for health workers
(order number: MEMA 04)

Chanzo cha Habari 2000
(order number: MEMA 05)

Kinga: Mwongozo wa malezi na ushauri nasaha shule za msingi
(order number: MEMA 06)

Kinga: Elimu ya Afya ya Kujikinga na Magonjwa ya Zinaa na UNIMWI. Kiongozi cha Mwelimishaji Rika. Wizara ya Elimu na Utamaduni
(order number: MEMA 07)

Elimu ya Afya ya Uzazi kwa shule za Msingi: Michezo ya Kuigiza kwa Waelimishaji Rika wa Darasa la 5–7
(order number: MEMA 08)

Elimu ya Afya ya Uzazi Kiongozi cha Mwalimu-Darasa la 7
(order number: MEMA 09)

Elimu ya Afya ya Uzazi Kiongozi cha Mwalimu-Darasa la 6
(order number: MEMA 10)

Elimu ya Afya ya Uzazi Kiongozi cha Mwalimu-Darasa la 5
(order number: MEMA 11)

MEMA kwa Vijana Cohort Recruitment: Self completion questionnaire MALE
(order number: MEMA 12)

MEMA kwa Vijana Cohort Recruitment: Self completion questionnaire FEMALE
(order number: MEMA 13)

1998 cohort recruitment self-completion questionnaire results report
(order number: MEMA 14)

Fourth annual report (Oct 2000- Sept 2001)
(order number: MEMA 15)

Report on a focus group discussion and in-depth interview series with young people in rural
Mwanza, Tanzania, December 2000
(order number: MEMA 16)

Participant observation reports: Jan–Feb 2001
(order number: MEMA 17)

Process evaluation report: Community and class peer educator trainings, Feb 1999
(order number: MEMA 18)

Evaluation report of HIV/AIDS peer education in MEMA kwa Vijana project, Nov 2000
(order number: MEMA 19)

Evaluation of the teachers' training sessions for the MEMA kwa Vijana teacher-led component,
Jan 2001
(order number: MEMA 20)

The MEMA kwa Vijana Curriculum: A review, May 2001
(order number: MEMA 21)

Sexual behaviour among young people in Bunda District, Mara Region, Tanzania; June 2000
(order number: MEMA 22)

Sexual and reproductive health among primary and secondary school pupils in Mwanza,
Tanzania: need for intervention; 1998
(order number: MEMA 23)

MEMA kwa Vijana–Tutawaelimishaje?
(order number: MEMA 24)

National Policy on HIV/AIDS, Nov 2001. Prime Minister's Office
(order number: MEMA 25)

SADC HIV/AIDS strategic framework and programme of action: 2000–2004
(order number: MEMA 26)

APPENDIX 1. STAFF DATA

The number of staff currently working on the program is shown in table A.1.

Until recently, 22 community peer educators worked as volunteers. Until 2001, when payment was discontinued, peer educators receives Tsh5,000 (approximately US$5)per month. Their gender ratio varied over the first three years of the project from 60 percent male and 40 percent female to 75 percent male and 25 percent female. The declining number of female peer educators was due to much higher losses to the program among the females (for example, they moved away to get married, their husbands refused to allow them to continue to volunteer, or they had other domestic commitments).

Table A.1. Mema Kwa Vijana Program

Type	Number	Position	Gender
Full-time, paid	8	Coordinator	F
		Deputy coordinator	M
		Youth facilitators	M & F
		Secretary	F
		Driver (3)	M
Part-time, paid	2	Team leader (education	M
		Team leader (health)	M
Volunteers (peer educators not receiving allowances/incentives)	1,124	Class peer educators	M & F
Volunteers, part-time	62	Head teachers	M & F
	186	Teachers	M & F
Health facility workers	46	Health workers	M & F
Trainers of peers	22	Youth in the community (18–24 years)	M & F

Students Partnership Worldwide: School Health Education Program (SHEP)

PART A: DESCRIPTION OF THE PROGRAM

Program Rationale and History

Students Partnership Worldwide (SPW) has HIV/AIDS programs running in India, Nepal, South Africa, and Uganda, as well as an education intervention being carried out in Zimbabwe that includes medical monitoring. SPW has been working in Tanzania since 1992 and has witnessed the progressively worsening HIV/AIDS situation there. Research was conducted in 1998–99 to see what could be done about this situation. It was found that teaching about HIV/AIDS in secondary schools does not address the urgency or scale of the problem; HIV is not an examinable subject, and teachers do not have the necessary time to dedicate to it. Furthermore, AIDS is mentioned only in biology classes and then in a very formal way.

Consequently, SPW proposed that more HIV/AIDS education was needed in schools and that this education should be nonacademic, nonformal, skills-based, student-centerd, and participatory. SPW also noticed a lack of communication between students and teachers, and proposed that trained peer educators would be better candidates to fill this gap and bridge the void between students and teachers.

Based on these findings, a program was designed in 1999. The idea was to tap into the underused resource of form 6 (the final school year) school leavers in Tanzania by recruiting young, educated, energetic, and enthusiastic Tanzanians to act as peer educators. These young people are aged between 18 and 25 years and work together with foreign (mainly British) youth peer educators, with whom they form a cross-cultural team. The main focus of the program is for the peer educators to discuss adolescent sexual and reproductive health

> Our children especially must be protected against HIV infection. They must be adequately informed, counseled, and empowered early in their lives on how to avoid infection.
>
> ***President Benjamin William Mkapa of Tanzania***

(ASRH) through a one-hour lesson per week during school time, as well as organization and facilitation of numerous school and community health awareness events and festivals.

Iringa region and the rest of the Southern Highlands Zone were chosen as the starting point for the program because the area was found to be severely underprovided by other HIV/AIDS education programs. Iringa is also on the main Tanzania-Zambia highway, which means many truck drivers pass through. (Trucking routes are well-known vectors in the transmission of HIV.) Iringa is also a region with prevalent migrant labor, another factor in the spread of HIV/AIDS. There are also a large number of rural secondary schools, the majority of which are community based. Furthermore, SPW has spent many years building trust and rapport with schools in the area.

The program began in 19 secondary schools in 1999, and a further 16 secondary schools were added in 2002. The three-year demonstration model finished in 2002, and SPW is now planning to scale up the program to Mbeya, Ruvuma, Morogoro, Dodoma, and Rukwa regions. It is hoped that the program will eventually be adopted on a national scale.

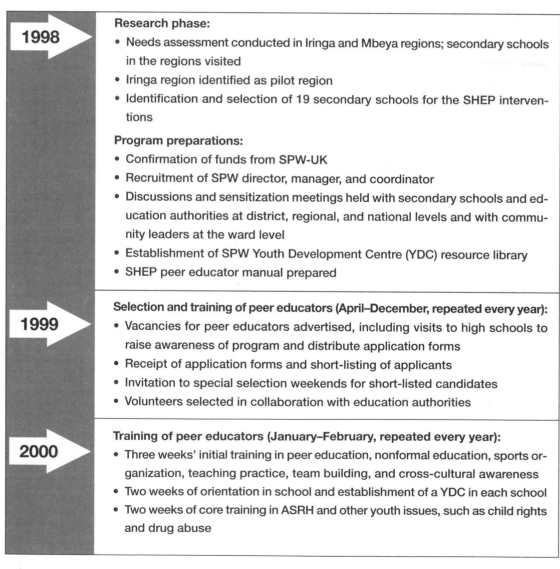

1998

Research phase:
- Needs assessment conducted in Iringa and Mbeya regions; secondary schools in the regions visited
- Iringa region identified as pilot region
- Identification and selection of 19 secondary schools for the SHEP interventions

Program preparations:
- Confirmation of funds from SPW-UK
- Recruitment of SPW director, manager, and coordinator
- Discussions and sensitization meetings held with secondary schools and education authorities at district, regional, and national levels and with community leaders at the ward level
- Establishment of SPW Youth Development Centre (YDC) resource library
- SHEP peer educator manual prepared

1999

Selection and training of peer educators (April–December, repeated every year):
- Vacancies for peer educators advertised, including visits to high schools to raise awareness of program and distribute application forms
- Receipt of application forms and short-listing of applicants
- Invitation to special selection weekends for short-listed candidates
- Volunteers selected in collaboration with education authorities

2000

Training of peer educators (January–February, repeated every year):
- Three weeks' initial training in peer education, nonformal education, sports organization, teaching practice, team building, and cross-cultural awareness
- Two weeks of orientation in school and establishment of a YDC in each school
- Two weeks of core training in ASRH and other youth issues, such as child rights and drug abuse

Figure 1. Time Line of Major Program Events

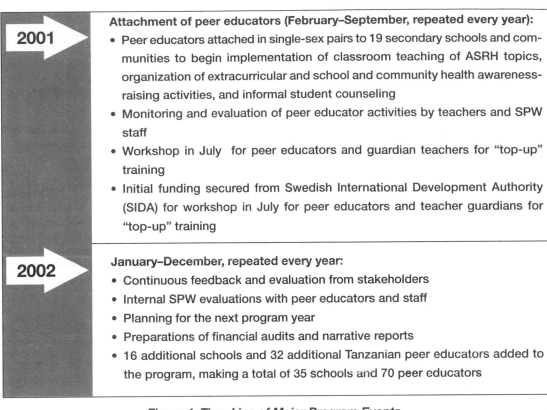

2001

Attachment of peer educators (February–September, repeated every year):

- Peer educators attached in single-sex pairs to 19 secondary schools and communities to begin implementation of classroom teaching of ASRH topics, organization of extracurricular and school and community health awareness-raising activities, and informal student counseling
- Monitoring and evaluation of peer educator activities by teachers and SPW staff
- Workshop in July for peer educators and guardian teachers for "top-up" training
- Initial funding secured from Swedish International Development Authority (SIDA) for workshop in July for peer educators and teacher guardians for "top-up" training

2002

January–December, repeated every year:

- Continuous feedback and evaluation from stakeholders
- Internal SPW evaluations with peer educators and staff
- Planning for the next program year
- Preparations of financial audits and narrative reports
- 16 additional schools and 32 additional Tanzanian peer educators added to the program, making a total of 35 schools and 70 peer educators

Figure 1. Time Line of Major Program Events

Program Overview

Aim

The aims of the program are to create awareness and equip children and youth with correct and appropriate information and skills to enable them to make informed decisions and behave responsibly with regard to their SRH.

Objectives

According to the program coordinator, the program objectives for children and youth are to
- enable the vulnerable group to safeguard their own (reproductive) health;
- promote essential life skills among young people, in particular their confidence and self-esteem; and
- provide wider access to correct, youth-friendly information that highlights the risk factors so that young people can make appropriate decisions on critical issues affecting their well-being. For adults, the program objectives are to
- promote an empathetic awareness of ASRH and give the support young people deserve and require,
- promote an appreciation of the community's SRH status (particularly the threat of HIV/AIDS) and promote appropriate measures to improve it, and

- raise awareness of a range of delicate, yet essential, areas as part of an HIV/AIDS campaign, including children's rights, the social context of HIV/AIDS in Africa, reducing stigma, and improving care for people living with HIV/AIDS.

Target Groups

Primary Target Group

The primary target group is secondary school students (form 1 to 4, ages 13 to 20 years) in 35 schools in Iringa region.

Secondary Target Groups

The secondary target groups are the primary school pupils (standard 5 to 7, ages 11 to 15 years), out-of-school youth (ages 10 to 24 years), and the community at large (all ages). Adults are involved in the program mainly during youth festivals, in which the whole community usually participates.

Site

The program is located in south-central Tanzania in all six districts of Iringa region (Iringa municipality, Iringa rural, Kilolo, Mufindi, Njombe, Ludewa, and Makete). Thirty-five secondary schools are involved in these program.

Program Length

The program lasts for eight months, every year from January to September. The period from September to December is used as an evaluation period and for planning the next year's program. Some secondary schools have received peer educators for three successive years; others, for one or two years.

Program Goals

The list in figure 2 shows how the program coordinator and the implementers ranked the program goals. It is important that the broader social context of HIV/AIDS, rather than just biological facts, be taught. For example, there is a need to discuss such issues as traditional practices and beliefs (e.g., the inheritance of widows, the belief that the traditional doctor can provide a cure for AIDS) and common sexual pressures on young people in rural areas (e.g., sexual harassment and rape, "sugar daddies" or "sugar mummies [adults who prey on young people]," sex for small presents, etc.). There is a need to discuss common myths about HIV/AIDS in rural areas (e.g., condoms do not work, or are infected with HIV as part of a conspiracy; or having sex with a young girl protects a man from contracting HIV).

Approaches

The program director ranked the approaches in order of priority as shown in figure 3.

The program staff believe that the approaches they use are appropriate and suitable to achieve the program goals and objectives because they have seen a marked improvement in knowledge and behavior among the youth.

Activities

Program activities are listed in figure 4.

Components

The program consists of three main components, each of which is discussed in more detail below:

1. classroom activities,
2. extracurricular activities, and
3. festivals.

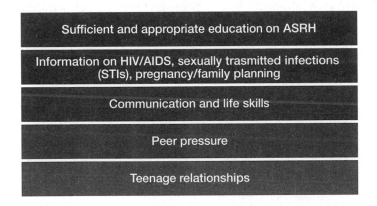

Figure 2. Program Goals Ranked in Increasing Importance by Program Coordinator

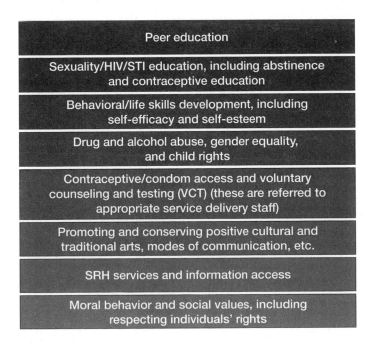

Figure 3. Program Approaches Ranked in Increasing Importance by Program Director

165

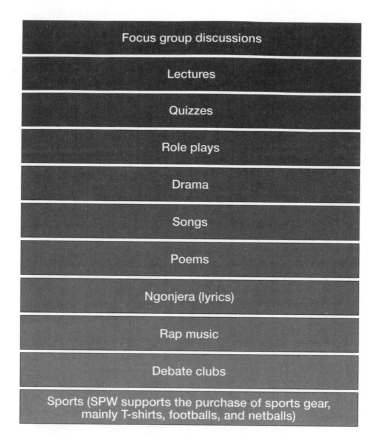

Figure 4. Program Activities Unranked

Classroom Activities

The peer educators are from both Tanzania and foreign countries (mainly the United Kingdom). There are two peer educators per school (usually one Tanzanian, and one foreign, both of the same sex), and they live within the community served by the school. The peer educators are responsible for conducting all the components of the program. In addition, they conduct individual counseling for students when approached and are available to tutor students in academic subjects. They also do the budgeting for festivals.

> Such a mobilization of educated youths must surely represent one of Tanzania's most promising and innovative approaches in the urgent battle against HIV/AIDS.
>
> **Manager of the National School Health Program**

The task of the peer educator is to act as a role model to encourage youth to behave responsibly, have self-confidence, and change their attitudes toward life. They also ensure that youth receive accurate information on ASRH in a fun, nonthreatening environment in which they can open up and discuss their problems.

Each of the schools in the program has one hour per week allocated for ASRH classes, which are run by the peer educators. Each week, a different topic related to ASRH is discussed. These topics include

- communication skills;
- teenage relationships and sexuality;

- STIs;
- HIV/AIDS — its history, symptoms, impact, and other facts and figures;
- facts about pregnancy, including the effects of pregnancy at an early age; and
- family planning.

Each week, various nonformal educational techniques are used to present and reinforce the classroom topics (e.g., a role play about a teenage girl becoming pregnant). Appropriate expert educators (e.g., the National Family Planning Association [UMATI], Population Services International [PSI], UNICEF, doctors, nurses, etc.) also give talks and demonstrations on specific ASRH areas that the peer educators are less qualified to approach, especially condom education and demonstrations. (These experts may also give talks at extracurricular activities and festivals.) At the end of the year, a quiz is held to test the students' knowledge of ASRH.

> The education system teaches history, geography, etc. There is no time for teaching the advantages and disadvantages of social issues not in the school curriculum. SPW fills this gap.
>
> ***Teacher***

Extracurricular Activities

Peer educators organize and participate in a wide variety of extracurricular activities with the aim of both reinforcing ASRH classroom learning and providing students with a platform to perform and keep active. Such activities fall into three broad categories:

1. Expressive performing arts, such as drama, choir, rap, traditional dance, poetry, and so forth, are widely used in schools for both fun and stimulation and as a proven health education method. Peer educators use the arts through cultural evenings; interform, interhouse, or interdormitory competitions; interschool competitions; community shows; and so forth.

2. Youth clubs: Peer educators work with students and teachers to help set up and support student and youth clubs with formal structures. These clubs hold regular ASRH activities, including anti-AIDS messages. The role of the peer educator is as facilitators or advisers to help ensure youth club sustainability.

3. Sports: Peer educators also use sports as an essential component in their approach. They regard sports (football, netball, volleyball, basketball) as a means for youth to lead themselves away from risky sexual behavior and develop self-esteem.

> SPW volunteers teach us about so many things when those responsible to give this education — parents and relatives — cannot. Since SPW volunteers are peer educators, then they touch all issues — even about STDs, teenage pregnancy — without phobia.
>
> ***Child***

Festivals

To take their health objectives to a larger and wider audience, peer educators also plan, organize, and implement many festivals and health awareness-raising activities in their schools and communities. These events are lively, colorful affairs characterized by a carnival-type atmosphere. Typically, the events involve a variety of different health awareness activities, such as expressive arts competitions (drama, choir, dance, etc.), health quizzes, video shows, public marches, candlelit memorial ceremonies, speeches from local leaders, and health talks and seminars given by health workers, students, teachers, HIV-positive speakers, and NGO experts. Generally, peer educators arrange seven or eight such events in every school and local community on the program every year. This makes a total of more than 250 festivals and activities held across all the 35 schools in 2002 alone.

After the festival, an evaluation report is written, signed by the peer educators and the head teacher, and submitted to SPW headquarters.

Case Studies

Malangali Community Seminars

At Malangali, the peer educators spent a week visiting on foot four of the more remote villages in their ward to help choose 25 people from each village to participate in forthcoming community seminars. Many of the village leaders and other people they met with knew the volunteers from previous visits and work that the volunteers had done. As well as identifying the participants, the peer educators also asked each village to prepare a choir on HIV/AIDS and youth and an ngoma dance on HIV/AIDS and drug and alcohol abuse, which they should bring to the seminar. The seminar itself involved nonformal discussions, question and answer sessions, learning games and energizers, as well as clarifications of important HIV/AIDS facts. Interspersed with the seminar sessions, an intervillage choir and ngoma competition took place, providing both entertainment and stimulation for the participants as well as another important educational activity. The winners of the two competitions were given specially prepared mugs, which bore HIV/AIDS messages. The seminar was facilitated by the SPW peer educators and three teachers from Malangali Secondary School who had recently attended a Ministry of Education and Culture (MoEC) training workshop in Mbeya on HIV/AIDS education in schools.

Tosamaganga Secondary School Talent Night

The HIV/AIDS-themed talent night at Tosamaganga was a portrayal of fun learning, set in the beautiful old surroundings of this famous school. Tosamaganga is an all-boys school, and the 600 or so "Tosa Boys" who attended the evening laughed as they learned at the performances. There were interform competitions in comedy, drama, rap, and poetry, all based on the theme, "Underlining the Realities of HIV Infection for Youth in Iringa." There were also other entertainments, including the "Mr. Tosa" and "Mr. Funny" competitions, a fashion show, and bolingo dance contest. On a more serious note, the regional manager of PSI led an inspiring, informative, and open discussion about Youth and HIV/AIDS, culminating in an extended question and answer session about condoms, their use, and the various myths and misassumptions about them. The SPW director further reinforced the evening's theme with an in-depth explanation of the shocking situation of HIV infection in Iringa rural district. The evening culminated in the locally famous anti-AIDS cultural group, Nyota — rappers, dancers, and actors who led the education and entertainment into the small hours of the morning.

PART B: IMPLEMENTING THE PROGRAM

Needs Assessment

A needs assessment was conducted over six weeks by SPW staff. This involved seeking advice and direction from potential stakeholders about the feasibility of the program and the most effective strategies for introducing and consolidating it within the region. The reception afforded to the SPW team was uniformly positive. A lengthy and comprehensive report was produced, recording all meetings convened, advice proffered, and supporting evidence of the region's capacity to deliver an effective demonstration model of school health. The report is available from SPW's offices.

> SPW volunteers and students, we are the same age, which makes a big difference.
>
> *Student*

The program coordinator also said that the program is constantly reviewed in terms of content for the student beneficiaries to ensure that the program addresses their special priorities and concerns, both for them as young people and as young people in different societies. For example, the program emphasizes the social context of HIV/AIDS. In Makete district, there is special emphasis on widow inheritance; in Ludewa district, the special emphasis is on witchcraft beliefs about AIDs, and so forth.

Program Materials

Nearly all materials used by SPW in the SHEP intervention have been provided by and adapted from other NGOs, donors, and government materials. Most of them are in Kiswahili (the national language used by all Tanzanians), and some are in English. Each school sets up its own resource center, in which the materials are stored.

Target Group Materials

The peer educators, guardians, and teachers have no curriculum that is followed explicitly. Instead, they use the available materials to help them plan their lessons. For example:

- publications on HIV/AIDS from the Tanzania National AIDS Control Program (NACP),
- "Towards Responsible Sexuality,"
- *STIs/HIV/AIDS Peer Education Training Manual — a Complete Guide for Trainers of Peer Educators in Prevention of STDs including HIV/AIDS,*
- *WHO Teacher's Guide — School and Health Education to Prevent AIDS and STIs,* and
- "Talking AIDS — a Guide for Community Work."

These materials cover issues of the physiology and psychology of growing up, relationship issues, the psychology and physiology of sex, AIDS and its transmission, contraception, children's rights, gender issues, and substance abuse. For more details see Tanzania SHEP Program Appendix 3: Program Materials.

Additional Materials

Booklets, brochures, leaflets, and flyers, all developed by other NGOs, are also used. These materials convey similar messages to those described above. The materials are distributed to the schools by the peer educators, and they are accessible to all at the YDC in the SPW office.

Sports gear, such as 300 footballs and netballs, jerseys, and T-shirts, is distributed to schools because these items are not available locally.

Staff Training Materials

Although the school staff receive no specific training, they are given a variety of teaching resources that are used for reference. These are also used by peer educators and in the YDC (SPW office). They are listed below:

- *Femina — HIP* magazine (30 copies per school of each edition),
- *Amua* newspaper (30 copies per school of each edition),
- *Sara* comic (UNICEF; 10 copies per school of each edition),
- AMREF — *Vijana kwa Vijana* ("Youth for Youth"; 10 copies per school of each edition),
- AMREF — *Sababu ni moja* (10 copies per school each edition),
- *The State of Education in Tanzania* (Kuleana; one copy per school), and
- various children's rights materials from Kuleana (numerous copies per school).

Staff Selection and Training

Peer Educators

- For each school, there are generally two volunteers — one Tanzanian and one foreign.
- Tanzanian peer educators are recent form 6 school leavers holding "good passes" marks (division 1 and 2) in a variety of subject combinations.

> A speaker from PSI came to give a demonstration on how to use a condom. This is a sensitive area to discuss but PSI knows exactly how to tackle these issues.
>
> *Peer educator*

- Approximately half are recruited from the Highland Zone so that youth can contribute to Highlands development, as well as provide a higher degree of regional sensitivity to the program. The other half come from a wide variety of high schools in different regions of Tanzania.
- The peer educators are recruited according to the following criteria: academic performance at form 6, reference from a previous head teacher, English proficiency, extracurricular proficiency (choir, sports, drama, art, etc.), suitability to be a peer educator (confidence, sociability, assertiveness, creativity, etc.), commitment to nine months on the program, and parental consent to join the program.
- Foreign volunteers have A levels or bachelor's degrees and are selected on criteria similar criteria to those used to select their Tanzanian counterparts. See Tanzania Shep Program appendix 4 for the recruitment procedure.

Both Tanzanian and foreign peer educators receive the same training, carried out by SPW senior staff and invited facilitators from education officers at the district, regional, and zonal levels. The training comes in three phases:

1. Initial training: For three weeks, six days a week, they are taught about:
   - the spirit of volunteerism and teamwork,
   - peer education,
   - language (Kiswahili for foreigners and English fluency for Tanzanians),
   - cross-cultural awareness,
   - gender and development,
   - nonformal education (e.g., drama, group discussions, debates, games, etc.),

- the formal education system in Tanzania, and
- teaching methodologies and practice.

2. Placement orientation: Immediately after the initial training, the peer educators proceed to their placement for the first time. This orientation takes three weeks. Activities during this phase include introductory meetings; teaching practice, observation, and preparation; and extracurricular activities such as games and drama. Peer educators become involved, action plans are prepared, and a baseline survey on the school community is carried out.

3. Core training is carried out by SPW staff, health workers, and staff from UMATI and PSI. It lasts two weeks. Activities include orientation feedback, organizing activities for SHEP, budgeting for activities, further sessions on peer education, ethics, and daily monitoring and evaluation of own work. An ASRH module is explained in detail by qualified health workers.

In addition, a workshop for peer educators and teacher guardians is held for three days at the end of the secondary school summer holidays (June/July) and end of peer educators' holidays. The workshop covers issues that were not covered in previous training and workshops.

> Truly, I have never known an NGO like this, who have the approach of going straight to the villagers and living with them in this difficult environment. I would like to say, "SPW, we need money," but this is not a solution. SPW, do your best to give us knowledge like this, which will endure.
>
> *Villager*

Teacher Guardians
- Each school has one or two guardians.
- The students select the teachers who will be their uardians.
- The guardians receive three days' training on ASRH.
- The role of the guardians is to supporting the peer educators and counseling students.

Staff roles are summarized in appendix 1 to this chapter. Staff data are given in appendix 2 to this chapter.

Setting Up the Program
The following stages were undertaken to set up the program:
- Instruction and guidance were sought from and given by the Commissioner for Education to set up a demonstration model of SHEP in the Southern Highlands.
- Support funding was received from SPW-UK.
- A needs assessment was conducted in secondary schools in Iringa and Mbeya regions in conjunction with the district, regional, and zonal education authorities.
- Iringa region was chosen as the pilot region.
- Nineteen secondary schools were chosen for the SHEP intervention.
- A workshop, overseen by the zonal chief inspector, was held for head teachers, school owners, and government education authorities.
- The program design was agreed upon, based on best practice from other SPW programs.
- The SPW director, manager, and coordinator were recruited and an office was set up.
- The SHEP peer educator manual was prepared.

> SPW is working at a grassroots level on fundamental issues which affect Tanzania, and with the people who are Tanzania's future...our youth....You have my full support.
>
> *Regional commissioner*
> *Iringa region*

Program Resources

There is a main resource center (the YDC) at SPW headquarters. It is a spacious room with tables and benches, and shelves full of training materials. The YDC is open to all youth in Iringa municipality.

Each secondary school on the program has a "mini-resource center" open to teachers, peer educators, and students. Materials available are those mentioned in Staff Training Materials above, as well as pamphlets, festival reports, pictures, flyers, and so forth.

Advocacy

Senior government officials have attended youth events and festivals or had discussed the program with SPW staff. SPW also works in partnership with the local government officers at the district, ward, village, and subvillage levels, who help sensitize communities to the program.

> After the two and a half years of implementation, problems, such as pregnancy among students, have decreased. Youth are more open on ASRH issues. They attend health facilities for services/advice, and they are more assertive and knowledgeable.
>
> *Program director*

SPW works directly in the community, which allows the peer educators to learn about the community's beliefs and attitudes toward HIV/AIDS and share information about the program. The community is invited to the festivals, and formal meetings are also held with head teachers, teacher-guardians, and community leaders to discuss the SPW program.

As well as advocating their program with the government and the community, SPW has also fostered good links with other local, national, and international NGOs working in this field. These NGOs provide many of their materials to the program and give talks in the schools, and SPW has attended their workshops and seminars. They also share their ideas and experiences so as to overlap in their efforts and learn from each other's experience.

Program Finances

Since the establishment of the program funding, approximately US$392,000 has been received from UNESCO, SIDA-Tanzania, the Danish International Development Agency (DANIDA), Elton John AIDS Foundation (EJAF), USAID, The Swiss Agency for Development and Cooperation (SDC)-Tanzania, and SPW-UK. Approximately 16,250 students have benefited from the program. Therefore, the average external financial cost per student is approximately US$24.12 (392,000/16,250). However, it should be noted that 15,000 adults have also benefited, along with an unknown number of other school-aged children and adults in the community.

Please see appendix 5 to this chapter for further details on program finances.

PART C: ASSESSMENT AND LESSONS LEARNED

Challenges and Solutions

Program Director

Using valuable resources: The program uses a much underused resource — young, educated, and enthusiastic local (as well as foreign) people. This approach should be encouraged in all programs because most countries have a large population of young people who can ensure a program's sustainability.

Replicability: The program operates within the government educational system and uses renewable and inexpensive staff. This makes it easy to replicate in other areas and countries. Furthermore, the same approach can be used to tackle not just HIV/AIDS, but other diseases of poverty, such as malaria and tuberculosis.

> Since SPW peer educators have been at Lugarawa Secondary School in Ludewa district, there have been no cases of schoolgirl pregnancy at all in the school.
>
> *Program director*

Advocacy: In spite of involving the wider community, there are still some community members who are against the SPW program because they think it promotes sexual activity. Sensitizing the community and government authorities is an extremely demanding and time-consuming task, yet it is crucial if the program is to succeed. Ideally, what is needed is a more efficient way of doing this.

Poverty: Poverty remains the biggest problem in the fight against HIV/AIDS for most of the rural subsistence populace. Poverty exposes them to a greater risk of HIV infection and immediately compromises the priority or urgency of fighting HIV/AIDS.

Social beliefs: Although the majority of people are aware of the term "HIV/AIDS," there is still widespread ignorance, apathy, and derision of the pandemic. Social beliefs and traditions also complicate the campaign, for example, believing in witchcraft (*kurogwa*), widow inheritance, polygamy, and so forth.

Teacher motivation: There are no incentives to be a teacher — they are poorly paid and ill respected, so they are not motivated to teach well. The system has also, unfortunately, led teachers to expect allowances for any task outside their typical routine. Such an attitude deems any real HIV/AIDS intervention run by teachers at a school level as ineffective and too cost oriented.

Scaling up: The greatest challenge is how to scale up such interventions and ensure that they reach the majority of students (primary, secondary, and tertiary) across Tanzania. An intervention must be effectively and efficiently delivered to make an impact that achieves better ASRH status.. This implies management, training, resources, and consistent sensitization and monitoring. It also implies effective and active collaboration with other sectors (such as health care and social marketers, governments, community leaders, and so on).

Lack of priority: HIV/AIDS education in schools will always come up against more pressing logistical, academic, technical, and social demands and priorities involved in running a successful school. It is therefore critical to get across the equal importance of delivering HIV/AIDS education.

Training: More training of both peer educators and teacher-guardians is needed to increase the impact and effectiveness of the program

Resources: At present, the program is hugely underresourced. Extra staff, as well as funds, would increase capacity and allow the program to work better. The program needs better documentation.

Monitoring and evaluation: Experts are needed to aid in monitoring and evaluation. At present, the staff do not have the technical expertise to carry out a scientific evaluation.

Official committees: The board of trustees is in London only. For more efficient and effective work and commitments on both sides, there should be a locally based body that will at least discuss the program once a year, if not a local board of trustees or advisory and management committee. (Please note: A Tanzanian board of trustees has now been established.)

Peer Educators

Curriculum: At the moment, the ASRH module is fixed in format, content, and approach for all forms. It is necessary for SHEP to produce a form-graded ASRH module (forms 1 to 4) so that as students move up each year, the ASRH module will be both informative and set at a slightly different level for them.

Youth-friendly: Local health facilities need to be youth friendly and have a constant supply of medicine for STIs.

Condoms: Condoms should be made more accessible.

Support: The peer educators need more support and guidance when they come up against difficulties, such as hostility from parents and teachers.

Evaluation

Monitoring and evaluation are carried out by SPW staff, head teachers, and peer educators. A large evaluation is planned for the end of 2002.

Monitoring is done in a variety of ways:

- Weekly record sheets and event-day report forms are filled in by peer educators and head teachers, detailing subjects taught, methods used, extracurricular activities, and community interventions.
- SPW staff hold regular monitoring meetings with peer educators, conduct school visits, and attend activities and events. Problems are discussed and solutions suggested.
- A meeting is held twice a year (one before and one after the intervention) with SPW staff, head teachers, and peer educators to discuss problems and progress.
  Evaluation is also done in a variety of ways
- A health quiz given to students at the beginning and at the end of the program to see how much they have learned.
- Head teachers and school staff write an evaluation report at the end of the program, explaining the impact they think the program has had.

The implications of the evaluation are used to structure the next year's program.

A change in attitudes has been noticed by the peer educators and SPW staff. For example, girls are far more assertive than before and are now willing to discuss issues of gender and ASRH. There has also been a decrease in the rates of teenage pregnancy. Answers from the health quiz indicate an increase in ASRH knowledge.

UNAIDS Benchmarks

	Benchmark	Attainment	Comments
1	Recognizes the child/youth as a learner who already knows, feels, and can do in relation to healthy development and HIV/AIDS-related prevention.	✓	Youth are encouraged to freely express themselves about ASRH issues and all topics taught by the program; their ideas and suggestions are always considered and valued. Program activities are youth led through drama, art, rap, etc. The atmosphere within SPW is that there must be NO GAP and NO BARRIERS between students and volunteers.
2	Focuses on risks that are most common to the learning group and that responses are appropriate and targeted to the age group.	Partially fulfilled	The program addresses the risk behaviors. Peer education is seen as the most effective tool to take into account the specific needs of individuals.
3	Includes not only knowledge but also attitudes and skills needed for prevention.	✓	The program promotes attitudes and behavior change, recognizing that information is not enough. Student attitudes have changed — for example, the students are more assertive in coping with growing-up/adolescent problems.
4	Understands the impact of relationships on behavior change and reinforces positive social values.	✓	One of the objectives of the program is to encourage responsibility in relationships, reinforcing abstinence and saying No to sex before marriage.
5	Is based on analysis of learners' needs and a broader situation assessment.	Partially fulfilled	A health quiz at the beginning of the program identifies weak areas. The same quiz is repeated at the end of the program, so necessary reinforcement and adjustments can be made. Volunteers conduct a community assessment during their orientation week in the schools, health facilities, and community where the school is located.
6	Has training and continuous support of teachers and other service providers.	Partially fulfilled	Peer educators receive training before the start of the program. Head teachers and school guardians are provided with training materials.

	Benchmark	Attainment	Comments
7	Uses multiple and participatory learning activities and strategies.	✓	Multiple participatory learning activities and strategies are used, such as: drama, songs, role plays, poems, debates, and quizzes.
8	Involves the wider community.	✓	The youth events/festivals involve the community by inviting them to participate in the discussions. This exposes them to ASRH issues, which they can take to their homes and the community in general. The issues are also addressed during general meetings of the village.
9	Ensures sequence, progression, and continuity of messages.	Partially fulfilled	The program tries to build from knowledge to action. The same messages are given consistently throughout.
10	Is placed in an appropriate context in the school curriculum.	✓	The program is part of the school curriculum. ASRH HIV/AIDS/STI topics are taught during school hours and appear on the weekly timetable.
11	Lasts a sufficient time to meet program goals and objectives.	✓	The program lasts from form 1 to form 4 of secondary education.
12	Is coordinated with a wider school health promotion program.	✓	School health coordinators at national, regional, and district levels are involved in, and work closely with, the program.
13	Contains factually correct and consistent messages.	✓	All materials used by SPW have been approved by the MoEC and MoH.
14	Has established political support through intense advocacy to overcome barriers and go to scale.	✓	There is political support, from the national level to the community level. The program plans to scale up to other regions in the Southern Highlands. As a result of this political support, more donors are choosing to support SPW, which gives hope for program expansion.
15	Portrays human sexuality as a healthy and normal part of life, and is not derogatory against gender, race, ethnicity, or sexual orientation.	✓	The SPW program portrays human sexuality as a healthy and normal part of life, and it tries to guide students on how to address adolescent and cultural issues.

	Benchmark	Attainment	Comments
16	Includes monitoring and evaluation.	Partially fulfilled	Continuous evalation is done by the volunteers and SPW staff. SPW is planning an external evaluation conducted by technical experts in this field.

PART D: ADDITIONAL INFORMATION

Organizations and Contacts

Jim Cogan
Students Partnership Worldwide
17 Deans Yard
London
SWIP 3PB
Phone: +44 (0) 207-222-0138
Fax: +44 (0) 207-233-0008
E-mail: spwuk@gn.apc.org
Website: www.spw.org

Contributors to the Report

Program report prepared by Dr. Adeline Kimambo, aided by Ms. Zablon.

Edited by Helen Baños Smith.

We appreciate the help of the following people in providing much of the information in this report:

Mr. Craig Ferla — Country director (British)
Mr. Andrew Kalinga — Manager (Tanzanian)
Mr. Jimmy Innes — SHEP coordinator (British)
Mr. Steven Kyaruzi — Assistant SHEP coordinator (Tanzanian)
11 peer educators (8 Tanzanian and 3 foreign)
Mr. L. Lawa — Deputy head teacher, Kibao Secondary School
Six teachers — Kibao Secondary School

Six students (male and female) — Kibao Secondary School
Mr. Ali Athuman Mlanga — Chairman, Kibao subvillage
Mr. Meshack Mlyapatali — Clinical officer, Kibao Dispensary
Mrs. Aurelia Fuluge — Head teacher, Kibao Primary School
Mrs. Maria Ndutule — Acting ward executive officer, Kibao ward
Mr. Salum — Regional education officer, Iringa
Dr. Salum — District medical officer, Iringa rural

Available Materials

To obtain these materials, please contact ibeaids@ibe.unesco.org or Education for HIV/AIDS Prevention, International Bureau of Education, C.P. 199, 1211 Geneva 20, Switzerland.

SHEP Volunteer manual
(order number: SPW01)

SHEP Narrative Report 2001
(order number: SPW02)

Ludewa Youth Festival 2001: A brief report
(order number: SPW03)

Njombe Youth Festival 2001: A brief report
(order number: SPW04)

Iringa and Mufindi Youth Festival 2001: A brief report
(order number: SPW05)

Southern Highlands Demonstration Model: report on first phase research, July 1999
(order number: SPW06)

A documentary record of newsprint media covering SPW Tanzania 2001
(order number: SPW07)

SPW Annual Report 2001
(order number: SPW08)

The questions adolescents ask most frequently about and their answers. Eight booklets in English:
   Vol. 1: Growing up
   Vol. 2: Male-female relationships
   Vol. 3: Sexual relationships
   Vol. 4: Pregnancy
   Vol. 5: Healthy relationships
   Vol. 6: HIV/AIDS and the new generation
   Vol. 7: Drugs and drug abuse
   Vol. 8: Alcohol and cigarettes
(order number: SPW 09)

Maswali waliyouliza vijana kuhusu na majibu yake. Eight booklets in Kiswahili:
  Vol. 1: Kuingia utu uzima
  Vol. 2: Mahusiano kati ya wasichana na wavulana
  Vol. 3: Mahusiano ya kimwili
  Vol. 4: Mimba
  Vol. 5: Usalama katika mapenzi
  Vol. 6: Ukimwi na kizazi kipya
  Vol. 7: Madawa ya kulevya
  Vol. 8: Pombe na sigara
(order number: SPW 10)

Booklets/pamphlets from Kuleana:
  Haki za watoto na wajibu wgo: haki zetu
  Tupate haki yetu ya elimu!
  Wasichana na wanawake wana haki!
  Kulikoni majumbani? Tunataka haki zetu!
  Elimu ni haki ya watoto wote. Je, wasichana wa shule wanaopata mamba?
  "Hatupendi adhabu ya viboko!" Watoto tutimize wajibu
  About Children's Rights
  Zapp magazine. Haki za watoto leo!
(order number: SPW 11)

Pamphlet and magazine from UNICEF:
  Fahamu: Dalili za hatari kwa mwanamke mjamzito
  Sara: Sara anamwokoa rafiki yake
(order number: SPW 12)

PSI pamphlets:
  Tumia Salama Condoms. Jikinge!
  Ukweli Kuhusu Kondom
(order number: SPW 13)

UMATI pamphlets:
  Mapenzi katika umri mdogo ni hatari
  Siri ya Hedhi
  Mabadiliko ya mvulana au msichana wakati: Anapokua
(order number: SPW 14)

TAMWA pamphlet:
  Sheria ya makosa ya kujamiiana, 1998
(order number: SPW 15)

AMREF booklets/pamphlets:
    Yafahamu mabadiliko muhimi wakati wa ujana wako
    Jikinge na magonjwa ya zinaa
    Sababu ni moja: Vijana, ngono na virusi vya UKIMWI/UKIMWI katika nchi tatu za Afrika
    Vijana kwa Vijana: Kuzuia kuenea kwa virusi vya UKIMWI na vijana Kenya
    Je, ukimwi ni ajali?
(order number: SPW 16)

Femina magazine
(order number: SPW 17)

Appendix 2: Staff data
(order number: SPW 18)

Appendix 3: Program materials
(order number: SPW 19)

Appendix 4: Recruitment procedure
(order number: SPW 20)

Appendix 5: Program finances
(order number: SPW 21)

APPENDIX 1. STAFF ROLES

Program Director

Has overall responsibility for all aspects of the Program, in particular
- financial control of budget and expenditure,
- staff recruitment and management,
- fund raising at local and national level,
- liaison with all partners and stakeholders,
- management of media contacts, and
- monitoring and evaluation procedures.

Program Manager

Is responsible for
- personnel management of SPW staff,
- office administration,
- logistical aspects of program (travel, visas, etc.), and
- liaison with relevant government authorities at regional and district levels.

SHEP Program Coordinator

Is responsible for
- recruitment of Tanzanian peer educators;
- training and professional support of peer educators;
- providing leadership and support of peer educators;
- coordination of all school- and community-based health awareness activities;
- program design and development;
- sensitization of all regional, district, and school authorities; and
- assistance to program director in fund raising and budgeting.

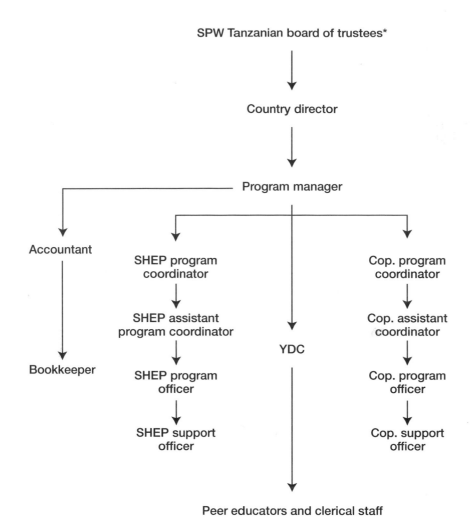

*The Tanzanian board of trustees was established after the preparation of this review.

Figure A.1. Staff Structure

APPENDIX 2. STAFF DATA

Since the commencement of SPW-SHEP program in Iringa, a total number of 154 peer educators have been recruited, 89 Tanzanians and 65 from overseas. At present, there are 49 Tanzanians (30 females and 19 males) and 23 from overseas (17 females and 6 males). Foreign peer educators come mainly from Britain, although three come from Ireland, Australia, and Sweden.

These young people are the backbone of the SHEP in Iringa. Two are placed in each school, one foreigner and one Tanzanian. However, some schools have Tanzanians only. To qualify to be a peer educator, one has to have completed high school. The youth apply for the post, pass an interview, and undergo a six- to seven-week preparatory training course.

Overseas peer educators raise approx. US$3500 to cover airline tickets, health insurance, and U.K. administration, as well as program costs in Tanzania (e.g., training, peer educator allowances, etc.).

Type	Number of staff	Position/title	Gender
Full-time and paid	13	Director, 1	Male
		Manager, 1	Male
		Coordinators, 2	Male
		Asst. coordinators, 2	1 male, 1 female
		Program officers, 2	Female
		YDC coordinator, 1	Male
		Bookkeeper, 1	Male
		Secretary, 1	Female
		Office assistant, 1	Male
Part-time and paid	4	Accountant, 1	Male
		Support officers	Male and female
Peer educator staff, other than peer educators receiving allowances/incentives)	Up to 5	Peer educator support	Male and female
Teacher guardians	1 to 2 per school		Male and female

Total Number of Tanzanian Peer Educators in SHEP 2000–2002

Year	Total	Female	Male	Tanzania total	Tanzania female	Tanzania male	Overseas total	Overseas female	Overseas male
2000	39	19	20	19	8	11	20	11	9
2001	43	29	14	21	14	7	22	15	7
2002	72	47	25	49	30	19	23	17	6
Total	154	95	59	89	52	37	65	43	22

APPENDIX 3. PROGRAM MATERIALS

Author	Title
AMREF	"Know Your Body"
	"Protect Yourself from Sexually Transmitted Infections"
	"Is AIDS an Accident?"
	"The Reason Is One"
	"Youth for Youth"
	"Learning through Experience"
TAMWA	"The Voice of Siti — Empowerment to Women and Other Social Issues"
	"Sex Offences Law 1998"
UNICEF	*Sara* (a comic magazine on youth issues)
	Know the Dangerous Symptoms During Pregnancy (booklet and film)
UMATI	"Sexual Activities at a Tender Age — The Consequences"
	"The Secrets of Menstruation"
	"Body Changes on Boys and Girls at Puberty"
PSI	"The Truth About Condoms"
	"Protect Yourself"
	Amua newspaper for secondary school students provides information about HIV/AIDS prevention, condom awareness, and general ASRH issues

Author	Title
Kuleana	"What Is Happening in Homes" (mistreatment of girls)
	"Girls and Women Have Equal Rights — We Need Our Education Rights"
	"Children's Rights and Their Responsibilities"
	"We Don't Want Corporal Punishment"
	"Education is the Right of All Children — What About Teenage Pregnancies Amongst School Girls?"
GTZ	A series of 8 booklets in both English and Kiswahili on questions adolescents ask most frequently and their answers:
	• *Growing Up*
	• *Male-Female Relationships*
	• *Sexual Relationships*
	• *Pregnancy*
	• *Healthy Relationships*
	• *HIV/AIDS and the New Generation*
	• *Drugs and Drug Abuse*
	• *Alcohol and Cigarettes*
FEMINA	*Femina* magazine mainly consists of health and social life topics.

APPENDIX 4. RECRUITMENT PROCEDURE

The recruitment of Tanzanian peer educators is a long process, covering nine months from April through to December.

- April–May: SPW staff inform head teachers and visit high schools around the country to meet students, explain the program, and leave information about SHEP as well as application forms.
- June–August: Interested applicants send completed application forms to the SPW office in Iringa, where they are studied and filed by SPW staff.
- August–September: Once the National Form VI exam results are published, SPW reviews all received applications and ranks each one on its individual merit to compile a short list of potential peer educators.
- October: Short-listed candidates are sent a letter to invite them to one of two selection weekends, held in Dar es Salaam and Iringa. Their parents are also sent a letter to seek their consent for their child to take a place in SHEP.
- November: The selection weekends are held, involving a range of participatory activities (group work, presentations, drama, debate, etc.) to assess the suitability of each candidate. After the selection weekends, the SPW peer educator selection committee formulates final lists of selected and reserve peer educators.
- December: The final lists are passed to the regional education authorities for approval. All approved candidates are sent a confirmation letter inviting them to join SHEP.

In 2001, a total of 350 application forms were received from recent graduates. Of these, a short list of 80 peer educators were invited to attend one of the selection weekends. Of these, a total of 49 peer educators were recruited.

APPENDIX 5. PROGRAM FINANCES

Breakdown of Funding Sources and Allocation				
	Amount	Donor	Date	Funding required for
Funding 1 (since establishment of the program)	US$4,000 (two grants of US$2,000 each	UNESCO	July 2000 July 2001	Training of peer educators and guardian teachers
Funding 2	US$51,000	SIDA (Tanzania)	July 2001	Covering shortfall between annual budget for activities and actual funds available, also, secondhand vehicle purchase
Funding 3	Approximately US$40,000 (2 grants)	DANIDA (Tanzania)	October 2001– March 2002	Running SHEP in six urban secondary schools. Fund all activities facilitated from secondary school attachments.
Funding 4	US$49,208	EJAF	January 2002	Sponsoring 35 Tanzanian peer educators on SHEP 2002
Funding 5	US$56,210	USAID	April	Running a SHEP in 12 primary schools of Iringa Rural District
Funding 6	US$35,210	SDC Tanzania	May 2002	Preparing and facilitating four district youth festivals
Funding 7	US$157,080	SPW-UK	2000–2002	Contribution from 66 overseas peer educators US$2380.

Year 2001–02 (Last Year) Expenditure

Expenditure	US$ (approximate)
Staff remuneration	49,518
Management, administration, operations	50,100
SHEP	133,389
District youth festivals	35,259
Total	268,263

Management, administration, and operations include: rents; utilities; communications; stationary; office equipment; staff health, travel, and vehicles; publicity and media; profile; personnel relationship and fund raising; staff training; audit expenses; independent evaluations, and so forth.

Estimated Allocation to Each of the Approaches, 2001–02

Approach	Cost in US$ (approximate)
Tanzania peer educator selection	2,779
Training program	30,514
Peer educator set-up monthly allowances	32,532
Sensitization	6,213
School placement visits	5,092
Activity money at placement school	29,555
District youth festival evaluation	35,259
Evaluation	25,074
Total (less miscellaneous and contingency)	167,018

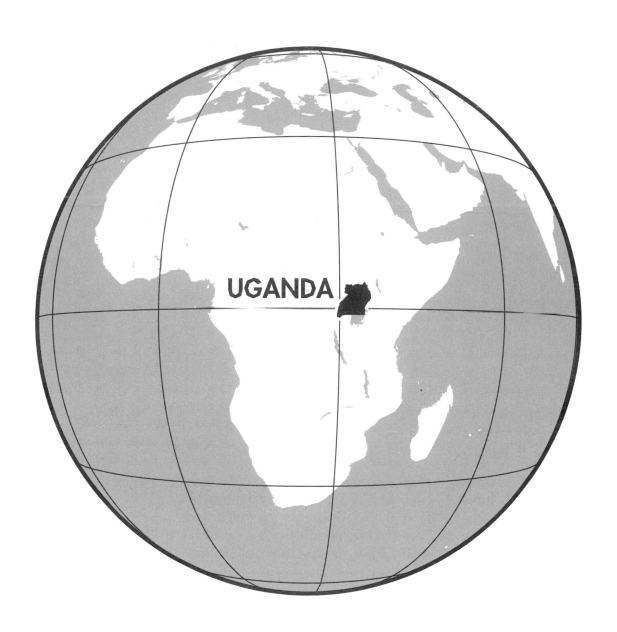

UGANDA

GOAL: The Baaba Project

PART A: DESCRIPTION OF THE PROGRAM

Program Rationale and History

The Baaba project began in January 2001 in response to the sexual and reproductive health (SRH) needs of Uganda identified by the staff of NGOs working with street children and youth in the capital city, Kampala.

Implemented by GOAL (an Ireland-based international humanitarian organization), the Baaba project conducted baseline research into the SRH needs of the street children and youth in Kampala. According to this baseline research, 15 percent of the street children and youth say they have been forced into sex, and 84 percent of the girls in this group have been asked for sex by an adult man. In Kampala, over 70 percent of full-time street children have had sex, yet many do not know how to protect themselves from HIV/AIDS or sexually transmitted disease (STD) infection. Nearly 50 percent of these youth know someone who has had an STD.

Although many of the NGOs working with street children and youth recognize the seriousness of the problem, they are mainly focused on the development and rehabilitation of street children and youth and have a limited capacity to deal with HIV/AIDS issues. Thus, the Baaba project works closely with them to build their capacity and mainstream the subject HIV/AIDS into the existing NGO-run programs for street children and youth.

The Baaba project began with the development of a partnership between GOAL and six NGOs in three Ugandan cities. Later, in 2002, another 6 NGOs were added, to increase the number to 12 NGOs in five cities. The NGOs joining the initiative had identified the need for SRH and HIV/AIDS interventions, were willing to confront HIV/AIDS issues, and were committed to the general development and rehabilitation of street children and youth. Before the project was initiated, a knowledge, attitude, practices (KAP) survey was conducted to identify areas of priority and serve as a baseline for project evaluation.

The project seeks to be sustainable by mainstreaming HIV/AIDS education into ongoing interventions for street children and youth. At present, NGOs plan and manage their own activities with support from GOAL staff. As the project has progressed, planning and implementation of activities have shifted gradually from GOAL to the partner NGOs. This process has strengthened the capacity of member NGOs to establish stronger ownership and leadership within the project. Specifically, some of the Baaba project participants have become trainers of trainers and are involved in training new peer educators. This gradual transfer of responsibilities will lay firm foundations for the complete phase-out of GOAL within a few years.

Program Overview

Aim

The Baaba project aims to promote the SRH of street children and youth by providing training, resources and ongoing technical and financial support to NGOs working with them.

Objectives

The project's objectives are to
- increase awareness and knowledge of HIV/AIDS and other SRH issues among street children and youth and NGO staff who work closely with them;
- empower street children and youth with the skills, motivation, and support to sustain existing safe sexual behavior and change unsafe behavior; and
- reduce the sexual and physical risks that youth are exposed to on the street.

Target Groups

Primary Target Groups

The primary target groups are former and current street children who are younger than age 18 and youth between the ages of 18 and 25.

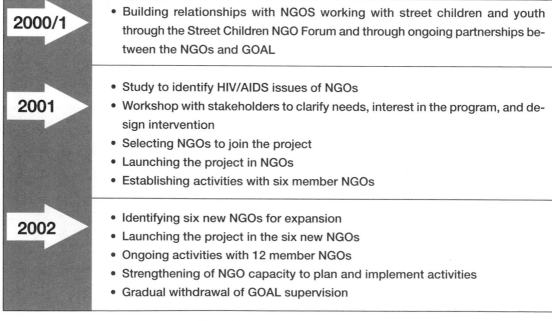

Figure 1. Time Line of Major Program Events

Secondary Target Groups

The secondary targets are

- NGOs who are committed to the general development and rehabilitation of street children and youth. They are supported to mainstream HIV/AIDS issues into their work and build their capacity to effectively address HIV/AIDS.
- Police and other security personnel (military and local defense units) are targeted to enhance their understanding of the situation and the problems and risks to which street children and youth are exposed.

Community leaders are encouraged to have a supportive attitude toward the development and rehabilitation process of street children and youth.

Site

Currently, the project collaborates with NGOs in the towns of Kampala, Jinja, Malaba, Masaka, and Mbale. Project activities are carried out at NGO centers, in the streets, in youth remand homes, and at community venues.

Program Length

GOAL aims to transfer ownership of the project to member NGOs. Increasingly, member NGOs will be responsible for planning and budgeting their own activities, and GOAL will provide resources and training. It is anticipated that this process will take each NGO a couple of years to complete. GOAL's exit strategy is now being designed in collaboration with partner NGOs.

Although the project is fairly new, it is anticipated that street children and youth involved in it will be involved as long as they are living on the streets.

Program Goals

The overall goal is to reduce the vulnerability of children and youth to HIV/AIDS. The project is committed to attaining the goals shown in figure 2.

Approaches

The program adopts a nonjudgmental approach based on the premise that self-efficacy (belief in one's ability to change) is central to behavior change and that the environment in which an individual exists can present significant risks and barriers to behavioral change. It adopts a holistic view of HIV/AIDS prevention and views it within the context of adolescent sexual development. This approach is used in all training, workshops, and seminars for NGO staff and street children and youth. It is aimed at empowering youth, building their confidence, allowing them to make informed decisions, and building their self-esteem. To achieve this, the Baaba project adopted the following:

A Participatory Approach

This allows the generation of ideas from the street children and youth regarding knowledge, attitudes, and practices as well as their skills concerning HIV/AIDS. The Baaba project provides the required information that helps youth to make informed decisions.

One-to-One Counseling Approach

This allows free exchange of information between GOAL staff and the children.

Peer-to-Peer Education Approach

This aims at building the confidence, capacities, and leadership skills of street children and youth who are trained as peer educators through: running project activities, training as trainers, training in project planning and management, occupying respected and responsible positions among their peers, and working as information providers on SRH issues.

Rights-Based Approach

Through this approach, the Baaba project advocates for the SRH of street children and youth through the training of local leaders, police, and child advocates. The street children and youth participate in the advocacy efforts by performing role plays and giving testimonies about the causes and consequences of living on the street. These activities are instrumental in breaking down prejudices about street children and youth.

Partnership Approach with NGOs

The Baaba project works in partnership with member NGOs who meet the priority needs of street children and youth, such as food, education, and shelter.

Activities

Figure 3 shows the Baaba project's activities ranked in order of frequency of use.

Components

The project has five main components:
1. capacity building for peer education and NGOs,
2. advocacy,
3. outreach,
4. HIV Prevention Clubs, and
5. street children and youth–friendly health services.

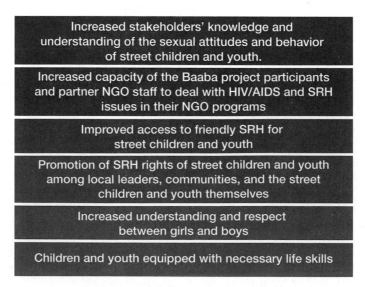

Figure 2. Program Goals Unranked

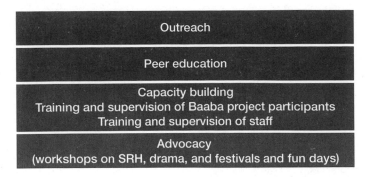

Figure 3. Project Activities Ranked in Increasing Frequency of Use

Capacity Building for Peer Education and NGOs

Under this component, NGO link staff and the Baabas (peer educators) are trained to work on the project.

The Baaba project offers member NGOs regular training sessions on topics of their own choice. The training sessions are held for staff teams from each of the member NGOs, usually in the form of one-day seminars. Previous training sessions have covered topics such as behavior change and participatory research with children. The Baaba project staff also offer backup support to the NGO link staff.

The Baabas are trained in peer education and other skills identified by the Baabas and other youth. The topics include SRH rights and respect for one another.

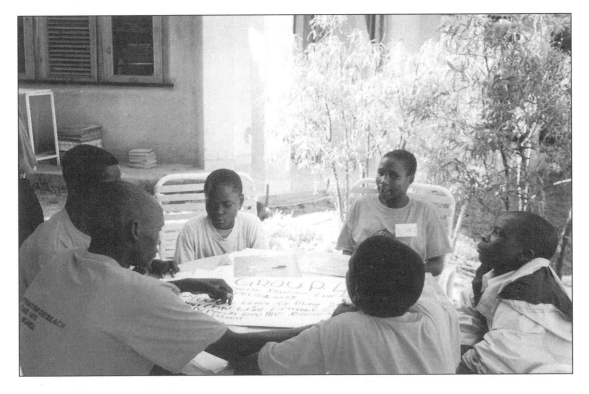

Peer educators working with street children

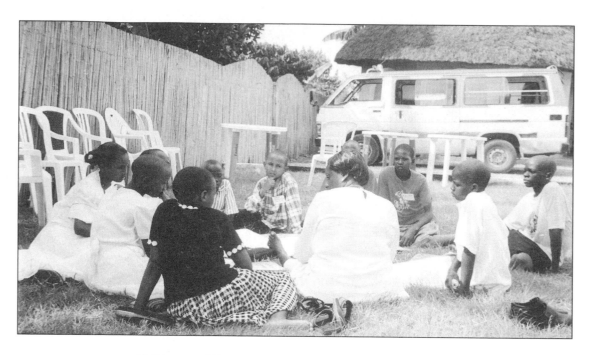

Children and Baabas prepare HIV/AIDS IEC materials

Advocacy

The Baaba project runs workshops on protecting the SRH rights of street children and youth. These workshops target local leaders in areas with high concentrations of street children and youth, as well as those responsible for the safety of children on the street.

The workshop begins by looking at the reasons why children run away to live in the streets, focusing on the role that adults play in driving children away through abuse or neglect. This is followed by sessions on sexual knowledge and behavior of street children and youth in

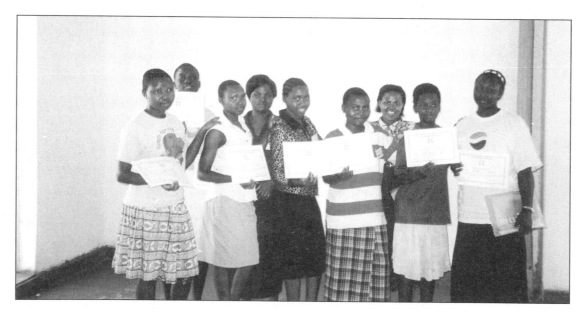

Young girls proudly display their certificates of participation.

Table 1. Participation in Advocacy Groups

City/town	No. of police trained	No. of community leaders/child rights advocates trained	Total
Kampala	50	480	530
Mbale	80	160	240
Malaba	80	70	150
Masaka	78	71	149
Jinja	–	70	70

Kampala, based on findings from the project baseline survey. The Baabas then give personal testimonies, explaining why the children are living on the streets and describing the risks they face, including mistreatment by police, security forces, or adults on the streets. A question and answer session follows.

Baabas then perform a drama or role play illustrating some of these sexual risks and consequences. This is followed by a talk on the SRH rights of street children and youth. In the afternoon, the participants work in groups to look at practical ways in which they, in their roles as leaders or security personnel, can help protect street children and youth. The groups present their strategies during a final plenary session.

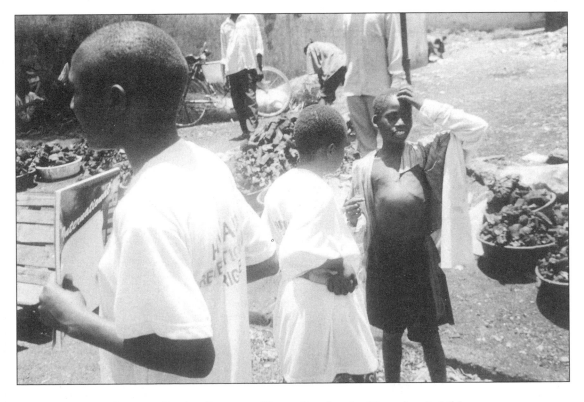

A young Baaba discusses life on the street with a street child.

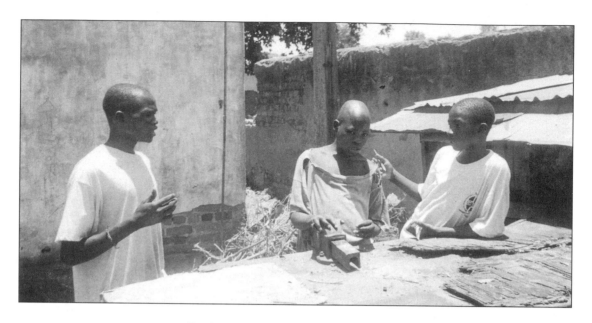

Baabas and youth learn trade skills

The demand for these workshops from member NGOs and local government has been high. Six workshops were held in 2001, and 15 in 2002. Table 1 shows the number of people who have been involved in these advocacy groups.

Outreach

On two evenings per week in Kampala, and on Saturdays in other towns, Baabas from different NGOs accompany the GOAL staff to the streets, to counsel and talk informally about HIV/AIDS and SRH issues with street children and youth. In addition to SRH issues, they talk

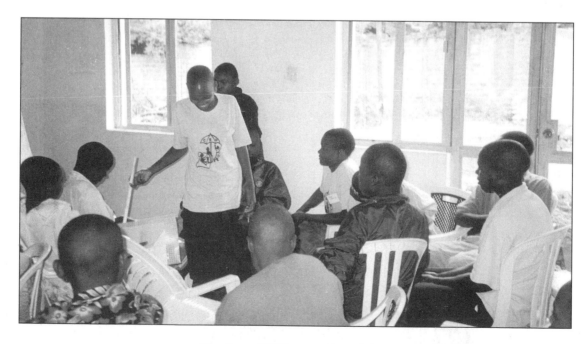

Meeting of HIV prevention club

to street children and youth about going home, getting help from NGOs, and police harassment. An average of 71 youth are met individually or in groups during an outreach session. On average, fivce Baabas participate in each outreach, and each session lasts between one and a half and two hours.

The Baabas also organize outreach seminars for street children and youth and community outreach sessions using drama and sports, targeting communities with a high concentration of street children and youth.

During the first 15 months, 45 sports sessions attracted a total of 1,053 boys and 397 girls. Thirteen Baaba drama shows have been performed for children at Naguru Remand Home, Kampiringisa Youth Prison, and to children on the streets and the local community. After the show, Baabas lead the discussion on HIV/AIDS.

HIV Prevention Clubs and Peer Education

Each member NGO runs an HIV Prevention Club. Clubs meet once every two weeks, and to date, there have been 148 HIV Prevention Club meetings organized by the Baabas, attended on average by 25 to 30 children per session. The Baabas meet once a week within their respective NGOs to plan for club activities. On average, three to five Baabas run the clubs. Club activities include role plays, songs, talks, debates, and sports.

Club activities take place at their NGO centers. On a club day, Baabas usually take 5 to 20 minutes to mobilize the street children and youth. Once all are gathered, the Baabas introduce the theme for the session. Topics include growth and puberty, sexual decision making, peer pressure, drug abuse, condom use, life skills, and preventing HIV/AIDS. Various participatory methods are then used by the Baaba team to explore the theme, including brainstorming, debates, storytelling, role plays, songs, sports, and videos. The key information points are usually drawn from the *Handbook on Sexual and Reproductive Health for Peer Educators* (see Program Materials

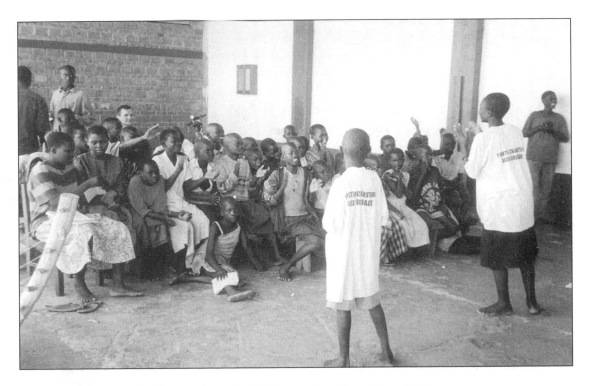

Baabas and street children perform for fellow children

section), although the participants are encouraged to use this only as a guide and avoid regurgitating facts without understanding their meaning. The GOAL staff member or NGO link staff member will wrap up the session by emphasizing the key learning points. After the main session, the Baabas then spend some time discussing issues arising from the session. Each session usually last for about one hour.

Street Children and Youth–Friendly Health Services

A manual summarizing youth-friendly SRH services available to street children and youth in Kampala was developed and distributed to member NGOs. The Baaba project has identified key service providers in Kampala, one in Jinja, and one in Mbale . Service providers in other towns are being identified and links developed. Staff teams at each health center have been trained by the Baaba project in working with street children and youth. The training is mainly to reassure the service providers that street children and youth are just like other children, with the same needs and problems. The youth-friendly services include general SRH services, including STD treatment, HIV testing, contraceptives, and SRH counseling.

The Baabas have visited the clinics so that they become familiar with clinic staff and can feel comfortable with taking other youth there. A referral card system has been established to enable Baabas to refer street children and youth to these health centers during street outreach activities. The number of street children and youth referred through the Baabas is tracked by each service provider.

PART B: IMPLEMENTING THE PROGRAM

Needs Assessment

A baseline study on knowledge, attitudes, behavior, and practices (KABP) of street children and youth was carried out. The purpose of the study was to ascertain the extent to which street children and youth are at risk from adverse SRH outcomes and their needs in SRH information and services.

The baseline study generated information used as
- an advocacy tool for use by NGOs working with street children and youth,
- reference information for interested NGO and government staff, and
- baseline data for evaluation of the Baaba project activities.

The same survey was repeated in 2002.

Methodology

A structured KABP questionnaire (42 items) designed by GOAL was administered to 250 street children and youth (190 of whom were known to the six participating NGOs, 60 of whom were not). For the majority of the questionnaires (213) Baaba project staff helped the street children and youth complete them. The remaining 37 questionnaires were filled in by the participant him/herself.

A total of 186 boys and 64 girls within the age group 10 to 25 responded, with 80 percent of the respondents aged between 13 and 18. Fifty-five percent of the youth who participated in the survey had spent between one and five years on the street. Thirty-one percent were in school, 19 percent were undertaking vocational or business training, and 50 percent were earning a living on the street.

Please see appendix 3 to this chapter for the results of the needs assessment.

Program Materials

The program uses the following materials for the training of the target group and the program staff.

The *Handbook on Sexual and Reproductive Health for Peer Educators* focuses on SRH for young people and is predominantly used in the training of peer educators. It assists peer educators in providing correct and complete information to other young people. It also assists peer educators in planning different educational activities for groups of young people that enable them to

- use the information in their own lives,
- develop their self-esteem,
- develop their communication skills, and
- enhance their ability to defend themselves.

The handbook was developed by Population Concern and Planned Parenthood Association of Ghana. It comprises the following topics:

- Chapter One: Guide to Using the Handbook
  - Preparations and Evaluation
  - How to Do the Activities
- Chapter Two: Changes as We Grow
  - Puberty
  - How Our Bodies Work
  - How Female Organs Look and How They Work
  - Male Sexual Parts and How They Work
  - Wet Dreams
  - Menstruation
- Chapter Three: Self-Esteem
  - Saying How We Feel and What We Want
  - Friendship
  - Peer Pressure
  - Coping with Anger
  - Conflict Resolution Skills
  - Violence

- Chapter Four: Personal and Sexual Relationships
  - Relationships Between Young Men and Women
  - Gender
  - Courtship and Marriage
  - Happy Sexual Relationships
- Chapter Five: Sexual Decision Making
  - Saying No to Sex
  - Sex and Money
- Chapter Six: Sexual and Reproductive Health
  - What is Sexual and Reproductive Health?
  - Sexually Transmitted Diseases
  - HIV/AIDS
- Chapter Seven: Children by Choice, Not Chance
  - How Babies Are Made
  - Ways to Avoid Pregnancy
  - Natural Family Planning
  - Condoms/Contraceptive Methods
- Chapter Eight: Teenage Pregnancy
  - Teenage Pregnancy
  - Coping with Unwanted Teenage Pregnancy
- Chapter Nine: Sexual Abuse
- Chapter Ten: Drug Abuse
- Chapter Eleven: Using Our Local Services.
  - Forced Sex and Rape
  - Child Sexual Abuse

Additional Materials

The Baaba project also uses information, education, and communication (IEC) materials (mainly posters and leaflets) developed by the Ministry of Health, The AIDS Support Organisation (TASO), the AIDS Information Centre (AIC), and the Straight Talk Foundation , to educate the peer educators as well as the street children and youth. Videos are also used to educate the Baabas and to show to street children and youth during outreach and club sessions. Appendix 5 to this chapter is a list of the videos.

In addition, the project has an extensive resource library, which is regularly updated with new materials downloaded from the Internet. The trainers draw upon these resources in preparing tailor-made training sessions. The library has materials from a range of organizations, including Family Care International, Population Council, HIV/AIDS Alliance, World Health Organization (WHO), UNAIDS, Pathfinder International, MEASURE, and Safaids.

Key supporting manuals and materials include

- *Participatory Learning and Action: A Training Guide* (International Institute for Environment and Development [IIED], 1995);
- *Life Planning Skills: A Curriculum for Young People in Africa* (Program for Appropriate Technology in Health [PATH], 1996);
- *You, Your Life, Your Dreams: A Book for Adolescents* (Family Care International, 2000); and
- *Life Skills for Young Ugandans.*

Staff Selection and Training

When the project began, street children- and youth–focused NGOs were approached to see if they would be interested in establishing a link with an HIV/AIDS prevention program for these young people. NGOs could become members provided that they

- work to meet the short- and long-term needs of street children and youth,
- are committed to the long-term development and rehabilitation of street children and youth,
- recognize that street children and youth are at risk of contracting HIV/AIDS, and
- currently lack the capacity to confront HIV/AIDS issues for street children and youth.

In each member NGO, 10 to 20 young people are elected as Baabas by their fellow street children and youth. The Baabas are elected from the different age groups: ages 9 to 12, 13 to 16, and 17 to 25. The Baabas then elect an NGO staff member to be their link staff member to the Baaba project team.

The Roles of Directors of Member NGOs

The chief role of the director is one of encouragement and support in occasionally attending HIV Prevention Club meetings or inter-NGO events to learn how things are going.

In addition, they support the link staff through regular meetings, rewarding them for the extra time they spend on activities and encouraging them to view Baaba activities as an important part of their job. Every six months, directors are invited to a meeting with GOAL staff for feedback on activities and ideas.

The positive aspects of the project described by the member NGO directors:

- Reported STDs among street children and youth have decreased.
- The level of violent or difficult behavior among street children and youth has decreased.
- Self-esteem,sand elf-control among street children and youth has increased.
- Baabas assume positions of responsibility within the NGO and are respected by their peers.
- Baabas acquire leadership skills.
- Street children and youth become social workers for the organization.
- NGO staff have expanded capacity-building and skills development.
- Difficult issues around SRH and HIV/AIDS are being confronted.
- Networking between street children and youth and NGOs has increased.
- NGOs are able to demonstrate to donors that they are confronting HIV/AIDS issues.

The Roles of the NGO Link Staff

Link staff are responsible for

- supporting the Baabas and encouraging respect and cooperation within the Baaba team;
- overseeing the running of the HIV Prevention Clubs with the Baaba chairperson;
- helping the Baabas devise monthly work plans and fill in monitoring forms, as well as mobilizing Baabas for night outreach sessions and preparing for project events;
- escorting Baabas on training days and outings;
  taking responsibility for Baaba project equipment used by their NGO;
- providing support to street children and youth with problems or who have questions that Baabas may not be able to answer; and
- acting as a link between the NGO and the Baaba project. (The project staff rely on the link staff to forward suggestions and feedback from the director or Baabas.)

The Roles of Baabas

Within each NGO, street children and youth elect 10 to 20 of their peers to act as Baabas. The Baabas are trained in peer education for two days. The *Handbook on Sexual and Reproductive Health for Peer Educators,* developed by Population Concern and Planned Parenthood Association of Ghana,[1] is used as the basis for the training. In addition to the handbook, the Baabas are also asked to suggest areas in which they need additional information and skills. Follow-up training sessions are held after four months, during which additional topics from the handbook are covered.

Baabas are responsible for carrying out most of the project activities. These duties include
- running HIV Prevention Clubs, with support from NGO link staff;
- one-to-one counseling of friends and peers between club sessions;
- Completing and filing monitoring forms, with assistance from link staff;
- organizing club sessions and meetings, even in the absence of a Baaba project staff member;
- mobilizing the street children and youth for drama and sport outreach, including planning where and when to hold outreach sessions;
- suggesting new initiatives and ideas to link staff and Baaba staff;
- reporting any challenges and problems to link staff; and
- referring fellow street children and youth to health services.

Setting Up the Program

The establishment of the program involved three stages.

Stage One

The Baaba project manager meets with the NGO director to learn more about the NGO's activities and discuss the proposed project. The director then discusses joining the Baaba project with the rest of the NGO staff. The Baaba team then meets with the NGO staff team to discuss the project.

Stage Two

If the NGO decides to join, the Baaba project team will launch the project. Launching usually involves some fun activities, a short video, and explaining the project to the street children and youth. The young people are then asked to elect the Baabas they would like to represent them, usually by open vote. The Baabas then choose the NGO staff member they would like to act as the link staff. The individual involved and the director must approve the decision. Immediately after the launch, there is a short meeting of the new Baabas and link staff to discuss their roles.

Stage Three

Baaba project staff begin regularly visiting the NGO (weekly visits to NGOs in Kampala and monthly visits to those outside Kampala). The first few sessions usually cover the role of Baabas and life skills, followed by a weekend training. There is an orientation day for the link staff. When the training is completed, clubs and outreach sessions are introduced.

---

1. The handbook was developed by the Population Concern and the Planned Parenthood Association of Ghana, and financed by the U.K. Department for International Development (DFID). Overseas Development Department, Population Concern, Studio 325 Highgate Road, London NW5 ITL, United Kingdom; telephone: +44-20-72418500. Planned Parenthood Association of Ghana, P.O. Box 5756, Accra, Ghana, telephone: 233-21-3045671310369.

Program Resources

The project requires the following inputs:

- project supervisor (20 percent of project time),
- full-time project manager,
- three peer trainers/counselors,
- an arts/drama consultant,
- project office/library.
- venue for events such as drama productions,
- promotion materials,
- stationery,
- training facilities,
- transportation,
- subsidized provision of condoms,
- peer educators' manual, and
- IEC materials, audiovisual equipment, videos.

Youth Involvement

The project relies on the total involvement of both the member NGOs and the street children and youth. The young people are trained as peer educators and are involved in running outreach sessions, weekly clubs, and advising on the development of the project. Baabas are central in the implementation of the project and have put forward many ideas for how the project should be run, and they have taken the initiative in organizing outreach seminars and sports events. They are responsible for reporting on their activities and regularly providing feedback. The project holds regular review meetings with NGO directors and link staff, with Baabas as chairpeople and secretaries. These meetings provide opportunities for joint planning and evaluation.

Advocacy

Advocacy work is undertaken with local leaders, police, and child rights advocates on the SRH and rights of youth. This mainly focuses on their responsibility in protecting street children and youth from abuse, and it takes the form of workshops that include testimonies and drama presentations by street children and youth.

An annual festival of drama, dance, poetry, and music is held on the theme of youth fighting AIDS on the street. This is also a major advocacy tool, which targets a wide audience of policymakers.

The Baaba project is also a member of the Inter-NGO Forum, a network nationally representing NGOs that work with street children and youth. The Baaba project actively supports the advocacy work of the forum.

Program Finances

On average, the total annual cost of the program is US$92,703. The cost per child is US$18.50. Further details of program finances are shown in appendix 4 to this chapter .

PART C: ASSESSMENT AND LESSONS LEARNED

Challenges and Solutions

Overall Approach

- The risk of HIV infection is rarely the first priority of a street child. For this reason, the project did not approach the issues of HIV/AIDS in isolation but also sought to address the material and psychosocial concerns of street children and youth. This was done by working through member NGOs who work to meet these needs, rather than establishing a separate site for activities.
- Living on the street exposes youth to many SRH risks. These risks may be reduced simply by removing young people from the street. Therefore, wherever possible, the project refers homeless youth to NGOs for rehabilitation and resettlement.

Using Street Children and Youth as Peer Educators

- Sustaining enthusiasm without resorting to financial incentives is challenging. This is particularly true for some of the older Baabas who are struggling to survive independently. Alternative motivating strategies have included a theatre trip to see an HIV/AIDS-related play, residential training weekends, and Baaba T- Shirts, mugs, and pens.
- Schedules are erratic, thus, mobilization for meetings requires patience. Because street children and youth are a transient group, turnover of peer educators is high. Sadly, two Baabas have died. High turnover increases training costs and leads to a loss of continuity.
- High levels of supervision and support are required. The project staff meets weekly with the Baabas, either to plan or to supervise a club session. The link staff member within their NGO also supervises Baabas. Ideally, project staff will reduce the level of support gradually. There are signs that the Baaba groups will survive on their own.
- Role play is a popular teaching medium. Baabas use plays regularly within their club meetings. After a drama, dance, song, and poetry festival on the theme of youth fighting AIDS on the street, the NGOs are now taking their plays to the community as part of their outreach strategy.
- Outreach has to be low key. In Kampala, the police and local government discourage obvious assistance to street children and youth. For this reason, the NGOs have decided to take their drama shows to specific venues (such as a remand home) rather than host them on the street.
- The Baabas make effective educators. They understand the reasons why the street children and youth find it difficult to protect themselves against HIV/AIDS. They also serve as role models to their peers.
- Involving Baabas in training local leaders has worked well. Personal testimonies and dramas performed by street children and youth have proven to be powerful in winning over a sceptical audience.
- Many Baabas have developed a sense of ownership of the project. Some have introduced their own ideas for prevention activities, such as community outreach through sport.

Working with NGOs

- Working through NGOs can be challenging. In particular, it is difficult to implement consistent policies when each NGO handles issues differently and deals with slightly different target groups.
- The promotion of condoms had to be handled sensitively. Many of the member NGOs are faith based, and they only reluctantly permit condoms to be discussed. Gradually, with sensitive persuasion, more have agreed to stock condoms. However it is difficult to tell whether the youth feel comfortable with this and are actually able to gain access these condoms.
- The link staff play a crucial role. GOAL relies heavily on the commitment of the link staff in supporting the Baabas and the project in general. On the whole, the link staff are dedicated and encouraging, although some are unable to devote adequate time to supervision.
- NGOs have become united on the theme of HIV/AIDS. Through membership in the project, there has been a discernible rise in the degree of cooperation and information sharing between NGOs.
- Before joining the project, NGO directors and staff have sometimes been concerned that membership will involve a level of commitment beyond their capacity. In practice, the level required is less than originally expected. However, the link staff does need to be prepared to spend time on the project. The project works best in NGOs with a supportive director and an active link staff.

Facing Unsupportive Community Members

- The police were not initially supportive of NGOs assisting street children and youth. They considered assistance given to these young people to be an incentive to keep them on the streets. In addition, they have not offered them adequate protection. In some cases, the police have contributed to the dangers of violence that are faced by street children and youth instead of reducing those risks.

  To change the attitude of the police, the Baaba project has undertaken training with police officers who work in areas with high concentrations of street children and youth. The attitude of the police is now gradually changing, and they are increasingly supportive of the work of the member NGOs.
- Communities often have negative attitudes toward street children and youth. Some of the communities have limited or no understanding of their problems, and they have a lot of misinformation about these youth. Street children and youth are looked on as thieves and violent. Communities have therefore not given the required support to the efforts toward development and rehabilitation of street children and youth. In response to thise constraint, the Baaba project started training sessions within communities. Street children and youth are invited to perform dramas and give testimonies to the communities, aimed at changing their attitude.
- The presence of young people on the street is of a commercial interest to traders and street and market vendors. Street children and youth are a cheap source of labor for many of these merchants. Efforts to rehabilitate street children and youth and remove them from the street are frequently countered by the traders, who discourage these young people from listening to the message of the NGOs. This problem remains a challenge for NGOs and the Baaba project. Continued counseling of street children and youth, as well as the success of those who have been rehabilitated, will help in dealing with this problem.
- The hard-core "mature" youth who have grown up on the streets have significant negative influence over the street children and youth. They tell them what to do and usually advise

them contrary to what the children learn from the NGOs. This also remains a major challenge in the work of NGOs and the Baaba project.

Evaluation

To assess progress, the Baaba project conducted a mini-review with stakeholders (NGO link staff, directors, and Baabas) in October 2001. The methodology adopted during the review was focus group discussion with directors, link staff, and Baabas.

The NGOs reported improved understanding and capacity for HIV/AIDS prevention and control among street children and youth, as well as handling of other issues like their rehabilitation and resettlement. NGOs had started observing positive behavioral change among the street children and youth in their NGOs, such as a reduction in violent behavior, an increase in self-control, and an increase in assertive communication. These changes are attributed to the influence of the Baabas, who have emerged as a respected group among their peers. The Baabas take their positions seriously and have developed their leadership skills and knowledge about HIV/AIDS. They serve as effective role models for other street children and youth. The Baabas say they enjoy their position, and they feel they have learned much about HIV/AIDS, avoiding STDs, peer education techniques, life planning skills, and counseling.

The evaluation led to several changes in approach, which included a shift in focus toward girls living on the street, who were found to be more vulnerable than the boys, and a commitment to train Baabas as trainers of trainers. Other innovations included introduction of a newsletter and an induction pack for NGOs joining the project.

Monitoring

The monitoring strategy has been operational since May 2001. GOAL staff attending Baaba meetings, HIV Prevention Clubs, night outreach, and drama and sports outreach sessions file a brief report after each session. At the end of each month, the NGO completes its monthly summary of activities, and a copy of this is filed at the project office. Every training session is evaluated by participants, and each inter-NGO event is followed by a debriefing session to discuss lessons learned. Monitoring data are collected for the following outputs:

- number of Baabas trained (plus evaluation results from training sessions);
- turnover of Baabas;
- number of meetings, HIV/AIDS Prevention Clubs, and drama practices held by Baabas and topics discussed;
- average and total attendance at meetings and clubs;
- percentage of meetings and clubs supervised by project staff;
- events and activities initiated by Baabas;
- number of street outreach sessions held;
- number of young women and men counseled during the outreach sessions and topics discussed;
- number of street children and youth referred to NGOs during outreach sessions;
- number of NGO staff trained (plus evaluation results from training sessions);
- use of audiovisual and other resources by NGOs;
- number of youth referred to SRH clinics by Baabas and NGO staff;
- number of male and female condoms distributed during night outreach orthrough NGOs; and
- training workshops held by local leaders and evaluation reports by participants.

UNAIDS Benchmarks

	Benchmark	Attainment	Comments
1	Recognizes the child/youth as a learner who already knows, feels, and can do in relation to healthy development and HIV/AIDS-related prevention.	✓	The program adopts a nonjudgmental approach based on the premise that self-efficacy (belief in one's ability to change) is central to behavior change and that the environment in which an individual exists can present significant risks and barriers to behavioral change. It adopts a holistic view of HIV/AIDS prevention and views it within the context of adolescent development. This approach is aimed at empowering youth, building their confidence, allowing them to make informed decisions, and giving them self-esteem.
2	Focuses on risks that are most common to the learning group and that responses are appropriate and targeted to the age group.	✓	The program focuses on problem issues of street children and youth. These include drug abuse (alcohol, glue sniffing, etc.), sexual abuse (defilement and rape), STD and HIV infection, and other risks related to living on the streets.
3	Includes not only knowledge but also attitudes and skills needed for prevention.	✓	One of the objectives the program is to empower street children and youth with the skills, motivation, and support to sustain existing safe sexual behavior and change unsafe behavior. This is done through the peer education approach whereby street children and youth are trained in building confidence, capacities, and leadership skills. Basic life skills needed for prevention are taught, including decisionmaking, negotiating, resisting peer pressure, and condom use.
4	Understands the impact of relationships on behavior change and reinforces positive social values.	✓	The program covers health rights and respect for one another.

	Benchmark	Attainment	Comments
5	Is based on analysis of learners' needs and a broader situation assessment.	✓	The program conducted a baseline study on the SRH needs of street children and youth. The results of the study have been a basis for implementation of activities. In addition, the program uses a participatory approach in implementation of its activities. This allows generation of ideas from the street children and youth with regard to knowledge, attitudes, and practices on HIV/AIDS. This approach enables implementers to understand the information needs of street children and youth which in turn helps in designing appropriate interventions.
6	Has training and continuous support of teachers and other service providers.	✓	The program provides continuous technical support to the NGO link staff and Baabas in the implementation of the project activities.
7	Uses multiple and participatory learning activities and strategies.	✓	The program regularly uses multiple and participatory learning activities in its outreach, club, and counseling sessions. Activities include songs, role play, drama, brainstorming, videos, sports, and debates. Learning strategies include peer education, leadership training for youth, and life skills training.
8	Involves the wider community.	✓	The program involves community leaders, the police, and other security personnel in areas with high concentrations of street children and youth. They are trained in the protection of the SRH rights of street children and youth. In addition, the advocacy work of the project is targeted to the general public, to help them understand the problems and needs of street children.
9	Ensures sequence, progression, and continuity of messages.	✓	The program follows a handbook on SRH for peer educators when training link staff and Baabas. The Baabas use the same handbook when conducting HIV Prevention Club activities. The club activities, which run every week, ensure continuity of messages.
10	Is placed in an appropriate context in the school curriculum.	Not applicable	

	Benchmark	Attainment	Comments
11	Lasts a sufficient time to meet program goals and objectives.	✓	GOAL provides technical and financial support to member NGOs for at least two years, after which the NGOs become responsible for budgeting, planning, and implementing their own activities, using grants provided by GOAL. After two years it is beleived that there will be enough capacity within the member NGOs to meet and sustain project objectives.
12	Is coordinated with a wider school health promotion program.	Not applicable	
13	Contains factually correct and consistent messages.	✓	The messages are basic and based on the facts. The program uses IEC materials developed by the Ministry of Health, AIC, and other organizations.
14	Has established political support through intense advocacy to overcome barriers and go to scale.	Partially fulfilled	The program has carried out advocacy in the communities with high concentrations of street children and youth. The community leaders have been sensitized to the problems of these youth, as well as their rights. Political support has therefore been generated at community level. However, at higher levels, government discouraged obvious assistance to street children because this is considered to be a motivating factor keeping them on the streets.
15	Portrays human sexuality as a healthy and normal part of life, and is not derogatory against gender, race, ethnicity, or sexual orientation.	✓	The program advocates for the SRH and rights of street children and youth. It targets street children irrespective of their ethnic background, gender, and sexual orientation.
16	Includes monitoring and evaluation.	✓	The program has a monitoring and evaluation system in place. Baseline research was carried out as a part of the evaluation, and a review of the project activities is planned this year. Monitoring data are regularly collected on key outputs of the project activities.

PART D: ADDITIONAL INFORMATION

Organizations and Contacts

The Baaba project is an initiative of and is run by GOAL, an international humanitarian organization. It is currently funded by Ireland Aid and the Elton John AIDS Foundation. For further information about the Baaba project contact:

The Baaba Project Manager
GOAL Uganda
P.O. Box 33140
Kampala, Uganda
Telephone: +256 (0) 77-700413
E-mail: goaluga@infocom.co.ug or goalhivaids@infocom.co.ug
or
GOAL
P.O. Box 19
Dun Laughaire
Co. Dublin, Ireland
E-mail: info@goal.ie
Website: www.goal.ie

Contributors to the Report

This report was prepared by David Kaweesa Kisitu, health economist/monitoring and evaluation specialist, Uganda HIV/AIDS Control Project (E-mail: uacp@infocom.co.ug)

It was guided by Nicola Brennan, development attaché, Ireland Aid, Embassy of Ireland — Kampala, P.O. Box 7791, Kampala, Uganda; e-mail: irishaid@starcom.co.ug.

Edited by Katie Tripp and Helen Baños Smith

The following contributed to the report:

Kirstin Mitchell — HIV/AIDS program coordinator, GOAL Uganda
Lysanne Wilson — Project manager, GOAL Baaba project
Juliet Oling — Trainer/counselor, GOAL Baaba project
Monica Nyakake — Peer trainer/counselor, GOAL Baaba project
Tonny Onen — Peer trainer/counselor, GOAL Baaba project
Ochama Jude — Volunteer assistant and former Baaba (Baaba project)
Geoffrey Mananu — Volunteer assistant/peer trainer

Available Materials

To obtain these materials, please contact ibeaids@ibe.unesco.org or Education for HIV/AIDS Prevention, International Bureau of Education, C.P. 199, 1211 Geneva 20, Switzerland.

GOAL Newsletter — Baaba Lessons
(order number: Baaba01)

Peer-Led HIV/AIDS Prevention for Street Children — a Report by GOAL Uganda, April 2001–March 2002
(order number: Baaba02)

GOAL Uganda Newsletter, Volume 1, Issue 1, March 2002
(order number: Baaba03)

HIV/AIDS Prevention for Street Children in Uganda — Questions and Answers for NGO Directors and Staff
(order number: Baaba04)

Appendix 2: Staff Data
(order number: Baaba05)

Appendix 3: Needs Assessment
(order number: Baaba06)

Appendix 4: Program Finances
(order number: Baaba07)

Appendix 5: GOAL Videos
(order number: Baaba08)

APPENDIX 1. BAABA PROGRAM STAFF ROLES

Program Coordinator

The program coordinator is the GOAL HIV/AIDS program coordinator and mainly performs a supervisory role. The program coordinator is employed full-time but spends about 20 percent of her time on the project activities.

Project Manager

The project manager, who reports to the program coordinator, is responsible for the daily management and administration functions of the project.

Peer Trainers/Counselors

There are three peer trainers/counselors, who report to the manager. They are responsible for liaising with the NGO link staff; capacity building of NGO staff members, police, and community leaders; training of Baabas as peer educators; and providing technical support during outreach and club activities.

Project Volunteers

Two volunteers assist the Baaba peer trainers/counselors in carrying out their activities. The volunteers mainly collaborate with NGO link staff and mobilize street children and youth for HIV Prevention Clubs, outreach, and annual inter-NGO festivals. The volunteers help in the running of clubs and outreach sessions and also assist during training activities. One of the volunteers is a former Baaba.

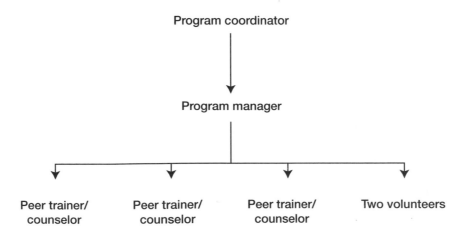

Figure A.1. GOAL: Baaba Project Organization Chart

APPENDIX 2. STAFF DATA

	Number of staff	Position/title	Gender
Full-time and paid	1	Project manager	Male
	3	Peer trainer/counselor	1 male, 2 female
Part-time and paid	1	Program coordinator	Female
Volunteer staff, other than peer educators (receiving allowances/incentives)	2	Volunteers	Male

APPENDIX 3. NEEDS ASSESSMENT

Knowledge	Boys (n = 153)	Girls (n = 59)	NGO (n = 162)	Street (n = 50)	Total
1. When boys grow into men, it is normal to release sperm in their sleep? (% saying yes)	80	81	80	80	80
2. When a girl grows into a woman, do her periods begin? (% saying yes)	70	95	75	82	77
3. A girl can become pregnant the first time she has sex. (% saying yes)	51	59	55	48	53
4. If a boy does not have sex, his penis would stop working and get smaller. (% saying yes)	30	30	27	40	30
5. Can HIV/AIDS be passed on by having sex with an infected person? (% saying yes)	92	98	93	96	93
6. Can mosquitoes spread HIV/AIDS? (% saying no)	54	56	59	40	55
7. It is dangerous to share a meal with someone who has HIV/AIDS? (% saying no)	75	76	80	60	76
8. Can you tell if someone has HIV or AIDS by looking at them? (% saying no)	35	37	40	20	35
9. Is there a cure for AIDS? (% saying no)	78	76	81	66	78
10. Can you say no to a policeman if he demands to have sex with you? (% saying yes)	78	71	82	58	76
11. Do you think it's okay to receive gifts from sugar daddies or mommies in return for sex? (% saying no)	78	59	83	40	73

APPENDIX 4. PROGRAM FINANCES

Item	Year one (Jan–Dec 2001), US$	Year two (Jan–Dec 2002), US$
Equipment	8,202	8,202
Premises	690	3,889
Education, recreation, and sports	15,519	42,360
Local staff costs	18,650	32,600
Expatriate staff costs	2,400	4,200
Transport	9,079	5,209
General administration	4,292	4,439
Total	58,832	92,703

Based on the 2002 figures, on average, the unit cost per child is US$18.50. The total project cost is US$92,703, and the total number of beneficiaries is 5,000.

Project Outputs and Realized Benefits

Number of beneficiaries as of March 2002:

- 137 peer educators (Baabas) have been trained and have benefited through increased knowledge of HIV/AIDS and leadership skills.
- 750 street children served by the 12 member NGOs have benefited through regular HIV/AIDS activities within the NGOs and inter-NGO events.
- 100 NGO staff have benefited from training and support through strengthened capacity to confront HIV/AIDS issues within their organizations.
- An estimated 5,000 street children and children from the community have benefited through outreach activities.
- 1197 local leaders, police officers, and child rights advocates have benefited through the advocacy program.

APPENDIX 5. GOAL VIDEOS

Most of the films are resources from Media for Development Trust, P.O. Box 6755, Harare, Zimbabwe. E-mail: mfd@samara.co.zw.

1. *Dangerous Decisions*
2. *More Time*
3. *Choose Freedom*
4. *It's Not Easy*
5. *Time to Care*
6. *Yellow Card*
7. *Neria*
8. *The Adopted Twins*
9. *Silent Epidemic*
10. *Like Any Other Lovers*
11. *Six Family Planning Methods*
12. *Born in Africa*
13. *Everyone's Child*
14. *Gold Tooth*
15. *Youth Fighting HIV/AIDS*
16. *Sarah the Special Gift*
17. *Sarah the Trap*
18. *Orphans Generation*

Straight Talk Foundation

PART A: DESCRIPTION OF THE PROGRAM

Program Rationale and History

In 1993, UNICEF started a new program in Uganda called "Safeguard Youth from AIDS" (SYFA). The rationale for SYFA was that most campaigns had previously targeted adults: there were few resources or materials produced for children and youth. Therefore, SYFA would address the impact of HIV and AIDS on young people.

There were many reasons to be concerned about the youth: HIV infection among young people was high, parents were often unwilling to discuss sexual reproductive health issues with their children, and there was an acute information gap about sexual reproductive health issues among adolescents and young people.

UNICEF therefore commissioned a newsletter for young people from Uganda-based journalists. The first issue of *Straight Talk*, appeared as a supplement in *New Vision*, a daily Ugandan government newspaper, on October 19, 1993.

Initially *Straight Talk* was designed to target youth between 10 and 24 years of age. As it grew in popularity the writers realized that it was impossible to address such a wide age range in one publication.

Straight Talk therefore narrowed its focus to secondary school adolescents aged 15-19 and in 1998 a newspaper called *Young Talk* was developed for primary school children between 10 and 14 years of age.

In addition to providing accurate information on sexuality, growing up and HIV/AIDS, *Straight Talk* and *Young Talk* also aimed to build children's and adolescents' life skills and to promote their rights. The newsletters provide a forum where young people can write letters about their problems and receive advice from doctors and others who are well informed about sexual and reproductive health (SRH) issues. The newsletters also print responses from other children who may have encountered similar problems or situations.

Straight Talk Foundation became an NGO in 1997. Since then radio shows and school clubs have been developed to help children learn about HIV/AIDS. The Straight Talk School Clubs were initiated in schools to promote peer education among adolescents as well as active

> Teachers did not know their role as far as helping adolescents is concerned..... We are pleased with your efforts for emphasizing good role models among teachers.
>
> *Teacher*

participation in the media interventions through letter writing. This has enabled STF to understand the information needs of young people and be able to respond appropriately.

At present, a new newsletter called *Teacher Talk* is being planned to help teachers understand more about the processes young people go through and how to help them understand more about HIV/AIDS.

Program Overview

STF is an adolescent-driven organization that believes:

- Every person has dignity and self-worth.
- Young people explore their sexuality as a natural part of growing up.
- Adolescent sexual activity brings great risks.
- For all adolescents — and, ideally, for anyone — abstaining from sexual intercourse is the most effective method of preventing pregnancy and HIV/AIDS infection.
- Adolescents have the right to information about SRH and safer sex options, including condom use.
- SRH education does not cause adolescents to be more sexually active.

Aim

The mission of STF is to keep adolescents safe and to communicate for better health. "Safe" means free from infections and unwanted pregnancy, and having skills, education, and values to be a productive adult.

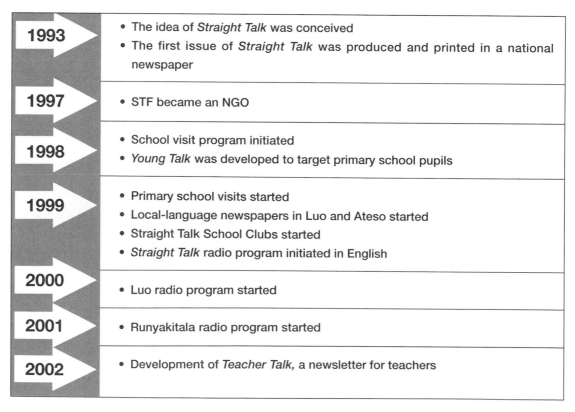

1993
- The idea of *Straight Talk* was conceived
- The first issue of *Straight Talk* was produced and printed in a national newspaper

1997
- STF became an NGO

1998
- School visit program initiated
- *Young Talk* was developed to target primary school pupils

1999
- Primary school visits started
- Local-language newspapers in Luo and Ateso started
- Straight Talk School Clubs started
- *Straight Talk* radio program initiated in English

2000
- Luo radio program started

2001
- Runyakitala radio program started

2002
- Development of *Teacher Talk,* a newsletter for teachers

Figure 1. Time Line of Major Program Events

Objectives
- To increase understanding of adolescent sexual and reproductive health (ASRH).
- To promote safer sex, life skills, and child and adolescent rights.

Target Groups

Primary Target Group
The primary targets for the newsletters are in- and out-of-school 10- to 14-year-olds for *Young Talk* and 15- to 19-year-olds for *Straight Talk*. The radio shows target in- and out-of-school 10- to 24-year-olds, including those who do not speak English and those who cannot read and write. The school clubs are for 10- to 24-year-olds.

Secondary Target Group
Teachers are the secondary targets. They are targeted to improve their communication and understanding of ASRH issues. Communities and the general public are also targeted to educate them about ASRH issues and encourage them to provide information to enable adolescents to make informed decisions.

> Straight Talk, we are proud of you. You have become the "senga." Some of those things you handle, we parents fear to tell our children. You are teaching our children good behaviors. I believe that if young people listen to you, they will be healthy and safe.
>
> *Remarks by the chief administrative officer, Nebbi district*

Site
The STF program covers the whole country. The program distributes the *Straight Talk* and *Young Talk* newsletters to more than 15,000 schools and institutions and 600 community-based organizations (CBOs) and churches countrywide. The newsletters are also inserted as supplements in the *New Vision* newspaper. In addition, they are available from STF's offices in Kampala and from various outlets around the country. Straight Talk School Clubs exist throughout the country, and the radio shows are broadcast on 10 different English-language radio stations and 4 local-language radio stations every week.

Program Length
The radio shows are broadcast once a week and last approximately half an hour. The newsletters come out once a month. Young people who attend the school clubs will, on average, attend for the whole of their secondary schooling, which lasts six years.

Program Goals
STF's program goals are shown in figure 2.

Approaches
STF uses the following approaches to realize its goals:

Provision of information on facts, skills, values, and human sexuality to 10- to 14-year-olds and 15- to 24-year-olds so that they can stay safe is done through mass media interventions. Monthly newsletters (*Straight Talk* and *Young Talk*) provide information responding to the needs of adolescents. In addition, radio "edutainment" (education-entertainment) talk shows, targeted at adolescents and young people, are broadcast weekly.

Promotion of peer–to-peer education and leadership is mainly achieved through the establishment of Straight Talk School Clubs. The club is a voluntary association of boys and girls united by a common interest of promoting their health and the health of their friends. Elected youth leaders, working as a team, lead the club. It is supervised and guided by a patron who is a teacher from the school.

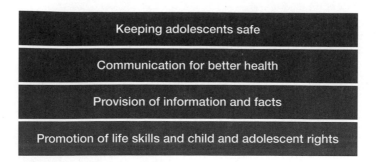

Figure 2. Program Goals Unranked

Promotion of the understanding of adolescent issues by the teachers and parents: *Straight Talk* and *Young Talk* are also circulated to CBOs, NGOs, and churches so that the general public are made aware of the needs of adolescents. Parents are encouraged to read the newsletters to learn what issues are being discussed. In addition, the program targets teachers to sensitize them to adolescents' needs and improve their communication skills with adolescents.

Activities

To make the learning experiences interesting and interactive, Straight Talk School Clubs carry out these activities:

- debates and discussions on topics raised in the latest *Straight Talk* newsletter or STF radio talk shows;
- drama and skits (short plays) depicting the issues affecting adolescents in the school or community;
- health workers invited to lead discussions on the topics chosen by club leaders;
- interclub activities, where one club visits another or joint activities, such as games, songs, drama, and talent shows, are held;
- sports and games organized between clubs and other groups;
- volunteer work, such as painting the school, tree planting, community cleanups; and
- visits to nearby primary schools to help primary pupils read and understand *Young Talk*. (This is done through drama skits, songs, and any other methods the club may find suitable.)

This list of activities is not exhaustive, and members are encouraged to think creatively about the activities that they would like their clubs to conduct.

Components

The program has five main components:

1. *Straight Talk* and *Young Talk* newsletters,
2. "Straight Talk" radio show,
3. Straight Talk School Clubs,
4. school visits, and
5. sensitization workshops.

Straight Talk *and* Young Talk *Newsletters*

STF puts much emphasis on the newsletters being adolescent centred and age appropriate. The newsletters are published in English and local languages.

Straight Talk. Every month, a four-page issue of *Straight Talk* is published. The key *Straight Talk* messages promote

- education about body changes,
- life skills,
- HIV/AIDS and sexually transmitted disease (STD) prevention, and
- safer sexual practices.

> You are really promoting self-confidence, especially among girls.
>
> **Student,
> Sacred Heart, Gulu.**

Straight Talk currently has a monthly print run of 163,500 copies, which are distributed through

- secondary schools (30 copies per school in 1,452 schools),
- institutions of higher learning (20 copies each in 418 schools),
- CBOs, churches, and individuals (7,000 copies),
- NGOs (40,000 copies),
- health facilities (approximately 3,200 copies),
- inserts in *New Vision* (approximately 40,000 copies),
- Straight Talk School Clubs (approximately 4,000 copies), and
- international mailings (approximately 650 copies).

Each month, a main topic is chosen from readers' letters STF has received. The first two pages of the newsletter cover information and life skills related to this topic. These are presented in adolescent-friendly language, with illustrations.

Topics that have been discussed in the previous issues have included

- handling of strangers,
- Hygiene
- talking straight but respectfully,
- making local pads (sanitary pads),
- Saying no to rides from strangers,
- protecting myself against unwanted pregnancy and HIV/AIDS,
- saying a big "no,"
- taking care of myself if I get pregnant,
- family planning,
- babies and HIV/AIDS,
- alcohol and drugs,
- STDs and HIV,
- virginity, and
- sexual abuse, defilement, rape, bullying, teasing.

The third page contains letters written by adolescents giving advice to their peers. The final page contains letters written by adolescents about problems, queries, and situations they have faced. These are answered by experts who advise, guide, and counsel the readers. The letter pages sometimes contain information on available adolescent-friendly services, especially teenage centers, voluntary counseling and testing (VCT) services, and family planning services.

Case Study: July 2002 *Straight Talk*

This issue was dedicated to facts about HIV/AIDS. It began by explaining how prevalence rates among youth were still very high, although they were now declining. The advice given was "keep your safer sex plan, delay sex, or always test for HIV and use condoms". It explained the modes of HIV transmission and the best ways of protecting yourself, including abstinence, asking your partner to get tested and then remain faithful, and always using a condom. It also explained that some things will not protect you, including love, trust, and virginity. The message given was to watch out for statements such as "I love you, we should have sex" or "We cannot use condoms because I love you." It went on to detail things that can put you in danger, such as already having an STD, accepting gifts or money for sex, and alcohol and drugs.

The next part of the newsletter explained what HIV/AIDS does to your body. A story, accompanied by pictures, was told of a young boy whose father had died of AIDS. The story went through the different ways the boy stayed safe, even when he was tempted to do otherwise. The message was that staying HIV free is a lifelong business.

The newsletter ended with letters from readers giving advice or asking questions about HIV/AIDS, all answered in informative and sensitive ways by the *Straight Talk* experts. Information was also provided on where teenagers can go to be tested for and counseled about HIV.

Young Talk. This newsletter is a four-page publication produced for children aged 10 to 14 years. The key *Young Talk* messages promote
- abstinence,
- life skills,
- persistence in school, and
- child rights.

Young Talk has a monthly print run of more than 150,000. The newsletter is distributed through
- primary schools (15 copies each in 12,000 schools),
- sentinel schools (30 copies each in 15 schools),
- institutions (10 copies each in 421 institutions),
- Prevention Training Centres (PTC) tutors (coordinating centers — 10 copies each to 526 centers),
- CBOs, churches, and individuals (approximately 7,000 copies),
- NGOs (approximately 30,400),
- health facilities (aapproximately 16,000 copies), and
- inserts in *New Vision* (approximately 40,000 copies).

Each month, a main topic is chosen from readers' letters received by STF. In some cases, the topic is chosen because of the need to provide particular information to children. The first three pages of the newsletter cover information and life skills related to this topic in a sensitive and appropriate way. The final page contains readers' letters with answers from STF. The newsletter ends with an "agricultural educational" component in which readers are taught something about agriculture. The hope is that in this way, young people will be able to maintain the agricultural skills that are slowly being lost in the country.

Case Study: How to Care for a Sick Mother (April 2002)

The newsletter told a story about Fatuma, a 12-year-old primary schoolgirl whose mother is sick. The story taught children what to do in this situation by describing the various ways Fatuma can help her mother, including bathing her, feeding her, and giving her medicine, while staying in school herself. It also emphasized the importance of the nonphysical aspects of care, such as listening to her mother and showing her empathy, showing her love and care, praying for her, encouraging her, and asking friends and relatives to visit her. It further explained how she can turn to relatives, neighbors, and health workers who can give advice and help on how best to look after her mother.

The second page explained that Fatuma's mother is HIV positive and explains in simple terms what HIV is and what Fatuma must do to not catch it. It also explained the importance of looking after the sick and seeking help and advice from health workers and counselors. The page ended with a snakes and ladders game that tests the reader's knowledge of how to care for and live with someone who is HIV positive.

The third page featured another story, the key messages of which were that we should make friends with lonely children, all children have a right to education, reading improves your skills, and living in war-affected areas can be unsafe.

The final page published children's letters asking questions about ASRH, with answers from STF. The newsletter concluded with an agricultural educational component in which the reader is taught about how and when to weed a garden.

"Straight Talk" Radio Show

The "Straight Talk" radio show aims to reach in- and out-of-school adolescents with STF messages, including those who cannot read and write, those who do not know English, and those who have no access to *Straight Talk* newsletters. It is now produced and broadcast in English on 10 FM radio stations and in 5 local languages on 4 FM radio stations. Two more local-language radio programs are planned to start in the near future.

The show, aired for 25 minutes a week, is hosted by adolescents. Each week, a different ASRH topic is covered, and adolescents are interviewed to give their views on air. An expert or resource person is also featured on the show to give advice to the youngsters. The show runs a quiz, and listeners are encouraged to write in. Prizes, such as a new radio–cassette player, calculators, wall clocks, and T-shirts, can be won by those with the correct answers.

Once a month a "doctor program," dedicated to questions only, is broadcast. Questions that are not answered during the program are responded to by mail.

Topics the radio program has covered include

- condoms
- testing for HIV
- AIDS and stigma
- boyfriend/girlfriend
- negotiating for safer sex
- rape and sexual abuse
- working adolescents
- teachers and students
- personal hygiene

- sugar daddies and mummies
- STD prevention and treatment
- wrong touches
- seeking SRH care
- peer providers
- trust and honesty
- girls have a right to say no
- exercise and diet
- holiday plans
- back to school

- menstruation
- alcohol abuse
- early pregnancy
- peer pressure
- media pressure
- friends
- orphans
- exams
- New Year's resolutions

The radio team also carries out focus group discussions, interviews, and posttests with adolescents from different areas to get the listeners' input and constructive criticism. The radio team also works closely with the newsletters' editorial teams, ensuring that a *Straight Talk* newsletter topic is discussed on the radio every month.

> We don't want to talk to children about sex, and yet the children are dying of AIDS because they are playing sex. We are also the ones who are encouraging early marriages. We do not tell children that it is bad and unhealthy to be married when young.
>
> *Mujje Tukei, chairperson, Anaka Primary School Parent-Teachers Association, Gulu district*

Straight Talk School Clubs

The clubs complement and reinforce the media component. Club meetings are held once a week after school. Any in- or out-of-school 15- to 24-year-old who accepts and abides by the club rules and who has a real interest in working for the club as a volunteer can be a member of a Straight Talk School Club. The aim of the clubs is to:

- help adolescents increase their knowledge and awareness of their sexual development;
- increase adolescents' confidence and skills in reducing risky behaviors and attitudes that may lead to unwanted pregnancy, abortion, and STDs, including HIV/AIDS; and
- organize boys and girls to engage in peer learning activities such as drama, debate, discussion, games, and community cleanups to enable adolescents to develop important life skills that will help them grow into happy, safe, and responsible adults.

The clubs are supervised by a patron, who is usually a schoolteacher. Activities are carried out to make the process of learning more fun.

School Visits

This component of the STF program, which targets secondary schools and tertiary institutions, began in 1997. An STF team made up of youth-friendly doctors, nurses, midwives, counselors, and local resource persons from NGOs visit at least 12 secondary schools per term. The school visits are aimed at reinforcing the "staying safe" message, facts, and life skills advocated by the *Straight Talk* newsletter.

The STF team spends two days with teachers (approximately 15 teachers) and two days with students, drawing up ASRH action plans and personal strategies for safer sex. Various activities, including question and answer sessions and role plays, are used to help students think critically and creatively about the problems they face and the impact of their decisions on their lives. In addition, one-on-one counseling for both teachers and students is provided for those who want it.

Issues addressed during the school visit depend on what the teachers and students want to know, but usually include

- STF: background and objectives;
- adolescence: physical changes, emotional development, adolescent behavior, roles, and responsibilities;
- sexuality and safer sex, including abstinence;
- learning to respect one another;
- STDs, including HIV/AIDS;
- health: menstruation, pregnancy and family planning, planning to stay in school;
- life skills: decisionmaking and communication methods; and
- one-to-one counseling (which is done in the evenings, after the school visits).

Examples of the sorts of issues raised during one-to-one counseling sessions are

- threatened to be killed if no sex;
- teacher trying to coerce student by threatening failure of school subject;
- defiled by a brother;
- having an affair with a sister's husband;
- has no sexual satisfaction;
- boyfriend is threatening to bewitch her if no sex;
- stays with a boyfriend but fears unwanted pregnancy;
- cousin, brother, or guardian demanding sex;
- penis does not get firm erection and finishes quickly;
- parent wants her to get married;
- stepfather threatens to rape her;
- an orphan contemplating getting a sugar daddy;
- mother does not allow her to interact with boys;
- sores on genitals;
- skin rash;
- pain while urinating;
- blood in her urine;
- suspect they are HIV positive;
- had unprotected sex and missed period;
- was raped and has itching in her private parts;
- has made a girl pregnant;
- suspects she is pregnant; and
- prolonged menstrual period.

> I have learnt how to help adolescents overcome their problems. I have also learnt about the different STDs and ways of control and prevention. Above all, I learnt about the importance of guidance and counseling in the course of child development.
>
> *A male teacher in a workshop at Adyel coordinating center, Lira district.*

Sensitization Workshops

Teacher and parent sensitization workshops are held on ASRH and children's rights and responsibilities. The overall objective is to motivate teachers and parents to contribute to the provision of ASRH services. The specific objectives are to

- increase awareness of ASRH and identify ways of meeting the ASRH information and service needs of young people in primary schools,
- develop workable plans of action to meet the ASRH information and services needs of young people, and
- increase communication among parents, teachers, and young people on issues related to ASRH.

> The Straight Talk workshop taught me how to use a condom properly.
>
> *Teacher, St. Joseph Layibi College, Gulu*

Methods used during the workshops include demonstrations, topic discussions, brainstorming, group work, lectures and role plays. Health workers from nearby clinics attend the workshops as facilitators. They raise awareness of ASRH services available in clinics so that young people can be referred to them.

PART B: IMPLEMENTING THE PROGRAM

Needs Assessment

There was no needs assessment carried out before the initiation of the program. The STF project started as an initiative of the SYFA program, which was being funded by UNICEF. SYFA had noticed that

There were high levels of HIV infection among youth (young people make up 40 percent of the population). The prevalence was 30 percent among adolescent girls at prenatal clinics in Kampala in 1991. In addition, the ratio of infection of girls to boys was 6:1; girls were particularly at risk.

Young people can be helped, and information and knowledge can create change and make an impact on young people. Young people can also have an impact on the rest of society.

Society was not ready to give information on SRH issues. Young people therefore faced a knowledge and information gap created by the culture.

Materials, programs, and newspapers produced at the time were targeting adults, and the young people had no reliable source of information.

STF was developed as a consequence of these findings

Program Materials

Target Group Materials

The materials for the target groups include the *Straight Talk* and *Young Talk* newsletters, which are published every month. In addition to the ASRH information, the newsletters also contain information on agriculture, environment, and health, which reinforces their classwork. To motivate adolescents to listen to the radio program, read the newsletter, and to write to the newsletters, STF offers gifts such as school bags, T-shirts, rulers, and radios.

> At first I was negative to StraightTalk. I thought that it was degenerating the morals of children. But now I have seen that it is really necessary.
>
> *Teacher, Uphill Senior Secondary, Hoima*

Staff Training Materials

STF has developed guidelines for the formation and running of Straight Talk School Clubs. They have also developed brochures, pamphlets, and project reports that provide orientation for the staff on the work and objectives of STF. These materials can be ordered. (See Available Materials in part D.)

Staff Selection and Training

Staff must have an interest and experience in ASRH issues. All staff have to be willing and enthusiastic and believe strongly in the aims and objectives of STF. Staff working in the offices do not have any formal training; however, the outreach team receives training in counseling, ASRH communication strategies, and message design. This is done through training workshops organized by other collaborating partners. Staff also receive support if they want to go on short courses relevant to STF's objectives.

Setting Up the Program

How to Set Up a *Straight Talk* Newsletter

Each year, the editors meet to decide on the 12 topics that will be covered over the year in the newsletter. The selection of the topics is guided by letters, questions, and responses received from readers during the previous year. The topics are selected in consultation with the staff of the different programs (school visits, sensitization workshops, radio show).

For each month's newsletter, all letters on that month's particular topic (e.g., condoms) are picked out. The letters are analyzed and grouped into categories. For example, the letters on condoms could be grouped under categories of myths, knowledge about condoms, attitude, and safety. This enables the editorial team to structure the newsletter. Experts write articles on specific topics (e.g., STDs, HIV/AIDS, menstruation, wet dreams, etc.) and also answer the questions published in the newsletter.

> Your key messages have had a drastic impact on the academic performance and behavior of our students. They have acquired positive life skills related to health and, in particular, HIV/AIDS. Now they are agents of behavior change in the community.
>
> *Deputy headmaster and head of science, Buwabwala Primary School, Mbale*

Once the editorial content has been finalized, the draft is passed on to the designers, who format it. The communication director then checks it for quality control and final editing.

The final version is sent to *New Vision* for publication. The newspaper insert is then distributed through *New Vision*. Those to be delivered through the mail are sent to the post office. Those for delivery by STF are delivered to STF local offices for distribution.

How to Set Up a "Straight Talk" Radio Show

The staff of the radio program use information gathered during field interviews to decide on topics to be covered for the year. The topics are finally agreed upon after consultations with the newsletter editorial team because the radio program reinforces the print media interventions.

Field visits are made to various areas in Uganda to conduct group discussions to find out what topics adolescents would like to discuss and where the information gaps exist. Adolescents are interviewed, and their voices are recorded for the program. It usually takes eight days to collect information and materials to produce four to six programs.

The radio team listens to the material recorded in the field and identify the clips to be used in the radio program. The team then agrees on the program's content and writes the script based around the recorded comments. In addition, the team also identifies the professionals who will respond to questions that are raised by the adolescents. This takes about two days.

The presenter is recorded reading the script. The producer then puts together the presenter's voice, interview guests (adolescents and other expert), music, and sound effects. A finished program is dubbed from minidisc to tape and delivered to radio stations.

How to Set Up a Straight Talk School Club

Straight Talk School Clubs can be started by either students or teachers.

A student or student group
- looks for interested peers in their school;
- calls a meeting of 20 to 30 people and forms an executive body of four: chairperson, vice chairperson, secretary, and treasurer;
- asks a friendly teacher or community member to be their club patron; and
- writes a letter to STF requesting recognition of the club.

A teacher

- calls an assembly of all students to explain the objectives of the Straight Talk School Club and the importance of its formation for the youth of the school;
- asks for volunteers and explains to them the nature of a Straight Talk School Club, its functions, and structure;
- circulates a sheet of paper and asks those who want to join to write their names on it;
- proposes to the group to elect club leaders (chairperson, vice chairperson, treasurer,and secretary), taking into account male-female balance. (For continuity purposes, leaders must not come from candidate classes — that is, those who are preparing to take national-level examinations and thus will soon be leaving school.) ;
- arranges the time and place for the next meeting; and
- writes to STF requesting recognition of the club.

> We acquired a lot. We learnt many things about our bodies. After your departure, some of us decided to form a Straight Talk Club
>
> *Maureen Nayebare, student, St. Mary's College, Rushoroza, Kabale*

When the executive committee of a chairperson, vice chairperson, treasurer, and secretary has been elected, they are responsible to the school administration and the club members. Their job is to manage the club, including arranging and supervising meetings and activities and handling club finances. The exeutive committee meets once a week and serves for one year. Decisions are made by a majority vote. They are also responsible for selecting members to visit nearby primary schools to help children read and understand the *Young Talk* newsletter and for keeping records of all club activities.

A teacher-patron chosen by the student group is accepted by the school administration. The patron has no right to dictate his or her religious, political, or other interests to the club. The executive committee can disassociate itself from the patron, should it find this necessary.

Program Resources

No information was available on the program's resources.

Advocacy

Links are fostered with the district education officers, coordinating center tutors, parent-teachers associations members, local councils, and other opinion leaders. They are told about STF's activities and encouraged to tell others about them.

Teacher and parent sensitization workshops are held on ASRH and children's rights and responsibilities.

Program Finances

STF is funded by several development partners including the Danish International Development Agency (DANIDA), United Kingdom Department for International Development (DFID), DSW, EDF, European Union (EU), Swedish International Development Authority (SIDA), Ford Foundation, PSI/CMS, Save the Children Fund (SCF), and UNICEF. The foundation received US$784,917 in 2002.

Please see appendix 4 to this chapter for further details on program finances.

PART C: ASSESSMENT AND LESSONS LEARNED

Challenges and Solutions

Talking to Young People About Their Sexuality

Society largely believes that it is culturally and morally wrong to discuss sexuality issues openly with young people. STF is sometimes accused of "promoting immorality" among young people, and the foundation experiences some problems extending their programs in certain schools. To overcome this challenge, STF endeavors to explain its goals and emphasizes that ASRH education does not cause adolescents to be more sexually active. In addition, STF describes the prevailing situation among adolescents and tries to advocate among members of the community that it is important to understand adolescents and their needs. As a result, STF has built its reputation, and its services are in demand.

> I'm a father of two and also a lecturer. I like the Straight Talk because it tackles a problem we parents cannot handle very confidently.
>
> *John Nayaga Mukasa, senior lecturer, Uganda Polytechnic, Kyambogo*

Increasing Demand for Straight Talk Programs

District authorities, school administrators, and young people are increasingly demanding Straight Talk programs. This is a major challenge, given the capacity and resources available to STF.

Large Turnout for Sensitization Workshops

This forces STF to increase the number of facilitators, which constrains the organization's expenditure framework.

Disparity Between Male and Female Radio Listenership

Eighty percent of "Straight Talk" radio program listeners are male adolescents. Reasons for this disparity have not yet been established. This is a major concern to STF. A study is planned to establish the reasons behind this problem.

Evaluation

STF has a monitoring and evaluation section that is responsible for designing and conducting studies on ASRH. A monitoring and evaluation plan for 2002–04 is being developed.

An evaluation of the *Straight Talk* newsletter revealed that the readership is growing. A total of 2,344 letters were received in 1999, compared with 1,320 received in 1998. About 92 percent of secondary school students read *Straight Talk*. For 25 percent of readers, the strongest influence of *Straight Talk* has been to consider abstinence; for 20 percent, it has been to learn about and consider condom use. Between 20 percent and 52 percent of sexually active adolescents use condoms. *Straight Talk* has enabled students to learn information about SRH issues that teachers are unable to pass on.

Research on *Young Talk* has revealed that the readership is growing. In 1999, 5,111 letters were received from readers, compared with 3,045 in 1998. About 80 percent of primary schoolchildren read *Young Talk*. About 17 percent of *Young Talk* readers were sexually active in 1999 (18 percent male and 16 percent female). In 1998, 27 percent were sexually active. Sexual activity was greater among children in less advantaged schools, reflecting more vulnerability among children with less exposure to appropriate SRH communication, information, and support.

Research revealed that 42 percent of secondary school students now listen regularly to the "Straight Talk" radio show. The listeners are predominantly male (80 percent), judging from the evidence of the letters received about the program. STF is planning to conduct a study to find out why fewer females listen to the program. The biggest influence of the show on adolescent listeners has been educating them about abstinence and safer sex strategies, including condom use and negotiation.

Research work done by STF has shown that teachers and students showed improved knowledge, attitudes, and beliefs about ASRH issues after a school visit workshop. Both teachers and students say they read *Straight Talk* newsletters more and can use it better for discussions. Many students feel encouraged to set up their own Straight Talk School Club.

UNAIDS Benchmarks

	Benchmark	Attainment	Comments
1	Recognizes the child/youth as a learner who already knows, feels, and can do in relation to healthy development and HIV/AIDS-related prevention.	✓	The youth participate in virtually all aspects of this program. Crucially, they are also perceived as being able to offer other youth advice and assistance. They are encouraged to help younger children to read and learn from *Young Talk*.
2	Focuses on risks that are most common to the learning group and that responses are appropriate and targeted to the age group.	✓	The program focuses on the following sexual risks, which are the most common among the young people: HIV/AIDS, STDs, pregnancy, sexual abuse, defilement, bullying and teasing, early or forced marriage. The program also addresses alcohol and drug abuse, as well as managing sexual feelings.
3	Includes not only knowledge but also attitudes and skills needed for prevention.	✓	The program promotes life skills among young people. It provides facts about HIV/AIDS, best methods of protection, things that do not protect you, things that put you in danger. It educates young people on misconceptions and on the realities of life. Some of the life skills promoted include handling strangers, hygiene, talking straight but respectfully, protecting against unwanted pregnancy and HIV/AIDS, children's rights, and many others. STF believes that adolescents have a right to information about SRH and safer sex options including condom use.

	Benchmark	Attainment	Comments
4	Understands the impact of relationships on behavior change and reinforces positive social values.	✓	STF aims to keep young people safe and promotes life skills, education, and values to be a productive adult. These promote positive behavioral change among youth. STF emphasizes abstinence, faithfulness in relationships, and condom use. It promotes respect for parents and encourages youth to follow their religion, to have a purposeful life, and to delay sex as long as it is possible.
5	Is based on analysis of learners' needs and a broader situation assessment.	✓	STF responds to the information needs of youth. The newsletters and radio shows respond to the questions, comments, and demands raised by the young audience. The program employs many adolescents as interns. Also, activities of the school visits are shaped by what the students want to know.
6	Has training and continuous support of teachers and other service providers.	✓	School visits are organized to motivate teachers to effectively contribute to the provision of ASRH services. The visits raise awareness of ASRH information and service needs and also improve the communication skills of teachers on ASRH issues. In addition, STF has embarked on the *Teacher Talk* newsletter, which will regularly update teachers on ASRH issues.
7	Uses multiple and participatory learning activities and strategies.	✓	STF uses different approaches in providing information through newspapers, radio, school clubs, and school visits. Information and guidance are given in a variety of ways, through letters, stories, pictures, role plays, etc.
8	Involves the wider community.	✓	The *Straight Talk* and *Young Talk* newsletters are circulated to the general public through the *New Vision* newspaper. The objective is to let the general public understand the information needs of adolescents and children. In addition, the sensitization workshops reach both teachers and parents.

	Benchmark	Attainment	Comments
9	Ensures sequence, progression, and continuity of messages.	✓	The STF program has been ongoing for nine years, meeting the challenges of ASRH. It tackles issues as they come up and provides information as new interventions and discoveries are made — e.g., on new issues of prevention of mother-to-child transmission of HIV (MTCT) and VCT. There is continuity of the messages every week on the radio programs and every month in the two newsletters.
10	Is placed in an appropriate context in the school curriculum.	Not applicable	
11	Lasts a sufficient time to meet program goals and objectives.	✓	The STF program has been implemented for nine years and continues. This is long enough for the program goals and objectives to be met. The program has greatly contributed to the declining trends in HIV prevalence among the 15- to 19-year-olds, although the achievements cannot be attributed solely to STF.
12	Is coordinated with a wider school health promotion program.	Not applicable	
13	Contains factually correct and consistent messages.	✓	The messages from the program are factually correct and consistent. Resource persons who are qualified professionals in the relevant fields check editorials in the *Straight Talk* and *Young Talk* newsletters.
14	Has established political support through intense advocacy to overcome barriers and go to scale.	✓	The program has political support, especially from the Ministry of Education. The following quote from Professor Apollo Nsibambi, Minister of Education and Sports (1998) is a testimony: "We wish to appreciate the aims of *Straight* and *Young Talk* ... improved adolescent health and support of Universal Primary Education, literacy and persistence in school."

	Benchmark	Attainment	Comments
15	Portrays human sexuality as a healthy and normal part of life, and is not derogatory against gender, race, ethnicity, or sexual orientation.	✓	The program portrays human sexuality as part of human growth, that individuals have to go through. It emphasizes that sex is not necessary for the body to develop, it should not be used for money or material gains, and boys and girls can be friends. The program does not discriminate on the basis of gender, race, or ethnic group.
16	Includes monitoring and evaluation.	✓	The program has a monitoring and evaluation system that focuses on looking at who accesses the newsletters and what questions are asked by youth. Evaluations have also been conduced to determine the SRH behavior of young people and the impact of the school visits program.

PART D: ADDITIONAL INFORMATION

Organizations and Contacts

STF is an NGO promoting communication for better health, to keep adolescents safe. As their mission statement says, "safe" means free from infections and unwanted pregnancy and having the skills, education, and values to be productive adults. For further information, contact:

The Straight Talk Foundation
44 Bukoto St., Kamwoky
P.O.Box 22366
Kampala, Uganda
Telephone: 256-41-543884
Fax: 256-41-534858
E-mail: strtalk@swiftuganda.com
or

strtalk@imul.com
or
strtalk@straight-talk.or.ug.
Website: http://www.swiftuganda.com/~strtalk, www.straight-talk.or.ug
Communications director: C. Watson
Program director: Anne A. Fiedler
Editors: T. Agutu, Betty Kagoro
Project coordinator: Jerolam Omach
Designers: M. B. Kalanzi, D. Lutwama
Photos: H. Mutebi
Publisher: *New Vision*

Contributors to the Report

This report was prepared by David Kaweesa Kisitu, health economist/monitoring and evaluation specialist, Uganda HIV/AIDS Control Project (e-mail: uacp@infocom.co.ug).

It was guided by Nicola Brennan, development attaché, Ireland Aid, Embassy of Ireland — Kampala, P.O. Box 7791, Kampala, Uganda; e-mail: irishaid@starcom.co.ug.

Edited by Katie Tripp and Helen Baños Smith.

The following contributed to the report:

C. Watson — Communications director
Anne A. Fiedler — Program director
Betty Kagoro — Editor
Christine Obbo — Administrator
Moses Owor — Monitoring and evaluation officer
Victoria Nalugwa — Radio program
Jerolam Omach — Project coordinator
Juliet Waiswa — Business manager

Available Materials

To obtain these materials, please contact ibeaids@ibe.unesco.org or Education for HIV/AIDS Prevention, International Bureau of Education, C.P. 199, 1211 Geneva 20, Switzerland.

Straight Talk newsletter, Volume 9, Issue 7, July 2001
(order number: STF01)

Straight Talk newsletter, Volume 10, Issue 3, March 2002
(order number: STF02)

Straight Talk newsletter, Volume 10, Issue 4, April 2002
(order number: STF03)

Straight Talk newsletter, Volume 10, Issue 5, May 2002
(order number: STF04)

Straight Talk newsletter, Volume 10, Issue 7, July 2002
(order number: STF05)

Straight Talk newsletter, Volume 10, Issue 8, August 2002
(order number: STF06)

Young Talk newsletter, Volume 5, Issue 4, April 2002
(order number: STF07)

"Straight Talk Foundation, Audited Financial Statements for the Year Ended 30th June 2001"
(order number: STF08)

"*Young Talk*, Primary Teacher Sensitisation Workshops: Six Months Report, October 2001–March 2002
(order number: STF09)

"Straight Talk Foundation, the School Visits Program Evaluation, August–November 2001"
(order number: STF10)

"Straight Talk Foundation, Guidelines for the Formation and Running of Straight Talk Clubs"
(order number: STF11)

"Straight Talk Foundation, Guidelines on the School Visits Program"
(order number: STF12)

Appendix 2: Staff Data
(order number: STF13)

Appendix 3: Needs Assessment
(order number: STF14)

Appendix 4: Program Finances
(order number: STF15)

APPENDIX 1. STRAIGHT TALK FOUNDATION STAFF ROLES

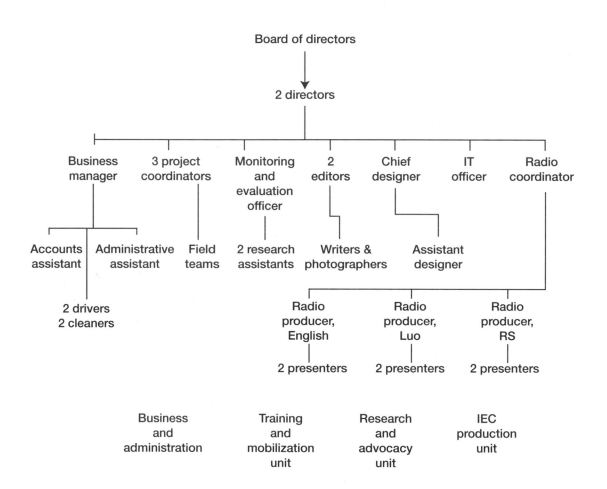

Figure A.1. Summary of Staff Roles

Straight Talk Foundation Organization Structure

Communications Director

The communications director — the head of the media component — guides the design of media interventions, ensures quality control, and supervises the staff working on the media activities.

Program Director

The program director is responsible for policy, planning, program management, and administration, and supervises the business manager; program coordinators, and the monitoring and evaluation officer.

Project Coordinators

There are three program coordinators, one for each of these components:
- secondary school visit program,
- primary school visit program, and
- teacher sensitization program.

The project coordinators are responsible for the planning and implementation of the field activities under their components. They identify the field team members, who handle technical and specialized issues related to youth.

Business Manager

The business manager is the head of finance and administration, responsible for financial management, resource mobilization, human resource management, procurement, and administrative issues. The business manager is assisted by the administrative assistant and accounts assistants and also supported by two drivers and two cleaners. The business manager reports to the program director.

Monitoring and Evaluation Officer

The monitoring and evaluation officer undertakes monitoring and evaluation of STF program activities and provides feedback to the organization.

Editors

There are two editors responsible for putting together the newsletters and coordinating work with writers on the selected topics. They decide on the editorial content of the newsletters and identify the counselors and relevant personnel to answer the questions that are published in the newsletters. The editors also reply to questions that are not published in the newsletters. Writers and photographers assist them. The editors report to the communication director.

Chief Designer

The chief designer is responsible for designing the materials that are going to be published. These include newsletters, brochures, and leaflets. The assistant designer helps the chief designer.

Information Technology Officer

The information technology (IT) officer is responsible for the management and administration of the computer network and helps the chief designer design and format the newsletters.

Radio Coordinator

The radio coordinator is responsible for the overall production of the radio program and coordinates the three subprograms (English, Luo, and the Runyankore-Rukiga/Runyoro-Rutooro). The radio coordinator ensures quality control of the radio programs.

Radio Producers

There are six radio producers, two for each language. The producers look for materials, write the scripts, and put together the program.

APPENDIX 2. STAFF DATA

	Number of staff	Position/title	Gender
Full-time and paid	2	Business managers	Female
	1	Program director	Female
	3	Project coordinators	2 male & 1 female
	1	Monitoring & evaluation officer	Male
	2	Editors	Female
	1	Chief designer	Male
	1	IT officer	Male
	1	Radio coordinator	Female
	3	Radio producers	1 female & 2 male
	3	Radio presenters	2 female & 1 male
	1	Administrative assistant	Female
	1	Accounts assistant	Male
	2	Research assistant	Female
	1	Assistant designer	Male
	2	Drivers	Male
	2	Cleaners	1 female & 1 male
Part-time and paid		Field teams	
		Writers	
	1	Photographer	Male
	3	Radio presenters	2 female & 1 male
Volunteer staff, other than peer educators (receiving allowances/ incentives)	7	Volunteers (no specific time)	

APPENDIX 3. NEEDS ASSESSMENT

Readership Statistics

Variable	2001	
	Young Talk	*Straight Talk*
Readership of the newspapers by the target groups in the last 12 months	81.7%	93.3%
Ever saw YT	95.0%	NA
Ever read YT	92.0%	NA
Proportion that has read an average of 5 (ST) or 4 (YT) issues	50.0%	62.5%
Proportion that has read more than 5 (ST) or 4 (YT) issues	53.4%	51.3%
Reported to have read all 8 issues NA 20.7%		

NA not applicable.
Source: STF evaluation report 2000.

Sexual Practices Among Young People in Uganda Primary Schools

	Male	Female	All
Respondents	644	816	1,460
Age range	10–16	10–17	10–17
Ever had sex	44.6%	16.5%	30.0%
Most common age at sexual initiation	13 years	13 years	13 years

ASRH in Selected Districts

	Male	Female	All
Respondents	719 (43.4%)	936 (56.6%)	1,655
Age range	15–24	15–24	15–24
Ever had sex	54.0%	38.4%	45.2%
Average age at sexual initiation	15.4	15.5	15.5
Who had sex in 2001	69.0%	76.7%	72.8%
Who had sex with more than one person	40.9%	53.0%	30.4%
Used condom first sexual initiation	50.0%	70.5%	60.1%
Consistent condom use this year	76.0	80.2%	78.2%

Source: STF evaluation report 2002.

APPENDIX 4. PROGRAM FINANCES

Straight Talk 2002 Financial Resources		
Expenditure item	Cost (US$)	Sources
Production and distribution of *Straight Talk*	43,750 77,333	DANIDA DFID
Production and distribution of *Young Talk*	39,550 62,867 89,336	DANIDA DFID EU
Local-language newsletter production	48,325	SIDA
Primary school teacher sensitization	10,915 9,999	DANIDA SIDA
Mobilization of primary school teachers	16,590	EU
Equipment (computers, camera, printers, projector, scanner)	3,889 15,000	DANIDA DFID
English-language radio program	37,883	DFID
Local-language radio program	16,485	SIDA
Research, monitoring, and evaluation	18,889 1,167 3,336	DFID SIDA EU
Capacity building (staff training, short courses)	6,667	DFID
Personnel	119,333 14,000 57,188	DFID SIDA EU
Project-running costs	47,000	DFID
Communications	2,100	SIDA
Operations	6,300	SIDA
Operational costs	41,219	EU
NGO meetings	5,845	SIDA
Total	784,916	

Note: Exchange rate as of September 2002, 1 US$ = 1,800USH.

Straight Talk Income and Expenditure: Audited Accounts, 2001

Income	US$
Grants	777,508
Miscellaneous income	6,541
Bank interest	85
Total	**784,134**

Expenditure	
Newsletter production and distribution	
Straight Talk	74,934
Young Talk	129,976
Local-language newsletter	
Health Matters	8,438
Regional visits	17,159
Radio production	47,753
School visits	28,755
Mobilization and development work	
Straight Talk	21,914
Young Talk	38,769
Local-language newsletter	15,057
Monitoring & evaluation	4,573
Administration expenses	79,659
Salaries	102,139
Special activities	33,191
Depreciation	25,429
Audit fees	2,333
Total Expenditure	**630,080**
Surplus for the year	**154,053**

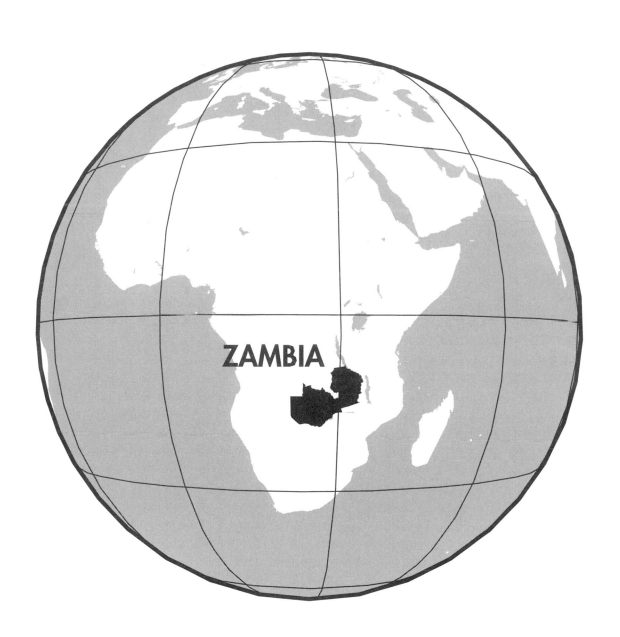

ZAMBIA

Copperbelt Health Education Project (CHEP): The In-School Program

PART A: DESCRIPTION OF THE PROGRAM

Program Rationale and History

The Copperbelt Health Education Project (CHEP) began in January 1988 as a social service project of the Kitwe North Branch of the Rotary Club (a registered charity), with only two members of staff.

Initially, the project aimed to help prevent the immediate spread of HIV/AIDS by raising public awareness of the dangers of the disease and by disseminating information about HIV transmission and how to protect oneself. The project used posters, roadside billboards, leaflets, T-shirts, newspaper advertisements, flip charts, radio and television shows, street theater performances, and discussions with groups of influential members of the community to raise awareness. Even the public trash cans were used to convey HIV/AIDS messages.

During the first two years, CHEP's activities were based on the assumption that people would change their sexual behaviors if they were informed about the disease. However, surveys done toward the end of 1989 revealed that although the general public in the Copperbelt province were well aware of HIV/AIDS as a serious health problem, significant numbers of people still had misconceptions about how HIV is transmitted. In addition, HIV prevalence figures (from the surveys and national data) showed no evidence that people were changing their sexual behavior as a result of greater knowledge about HIV/AIDS.

The CHEP staff decided that as well as increasing knowledge of HIV/AIDS, people also required the motivation and self-confidence to act upon this information. People needed access to services such as professional counseling, HIV antibody testing, treatment of sexually transmitted diseases (STDs), and supplies of condoms. CHEP aimed to provide these through collaboration with social organizations, caregivers, and leaders of public opinion.

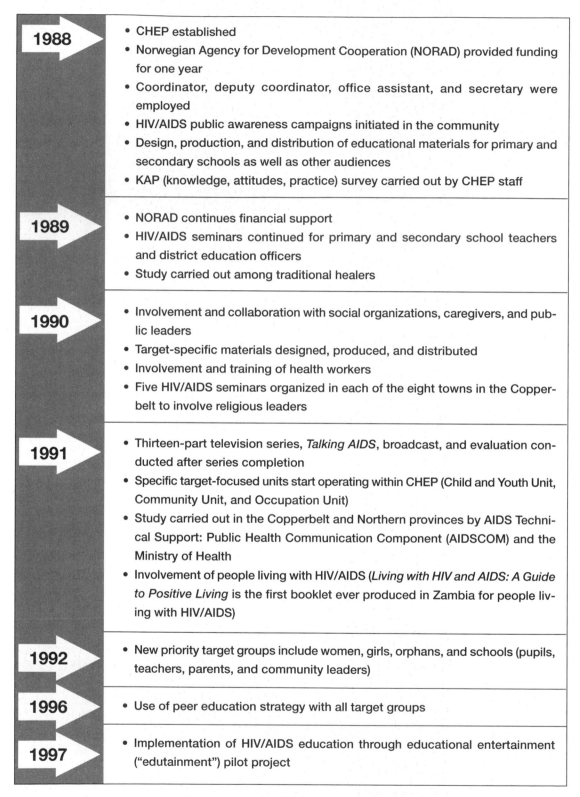

1988
- CHEP established
- Norwegian Agency for Development Cooperation (NORAD) provided funding for one year
- Coordinator, deputy coordinator, office assistant, and secretary were employed
- HIV/AIDS public awareness campaigns initiated in the community
- Design, production, and distribution of educational materials for primary and secondary schools as well as other audiences
- KAP (knowledge, attitudes, practice) survey carried out by CHEP staff

1989
- NORAD continues financial support
- HIV/AIDS seminars continued for primary and secondary school teachers and district education officers
- Study carried out among traditional healers

1990
- Involvement and collaboration with social organizations, caregivers, and public leaders
- Target-specific materials designed, produced, and distributed
- Involvement and training of health workers
- Five HIV/AIDS seminars organized in each of the eight towns in the Copperbelt to involve religious leaders

1991
- Thirteen-part television series, *Talking AIDS*, broadcast, and evaluation conducted after series completion
- Specific target-focused units start operating within CHEP (Child and Youth Unit, Community Unit, and Occupation Unit)
- Study carried out in the Copperbelt and Northern provinces by AIDS Technical Support: Public Health Communication Component (AIDSCOM) and the Ministry of Health
- Involvement of people living with HIV/AIDS (*Living with HIV and AIDS: A Guide to Positive Living* is the first booklet ever produced in Zambia for people living with HIV/AIDS)

1992
- New priority target groups include women, girls, orphans, and schools (pupils, teachers, parents, and community leaders)

1996
- Use of peer education strategy with all target groups

1997
- Implementation of HIV/AIDS education through educational entertainment ("edutainment") pilot project

Figure 1. Time Line of Major Program Events

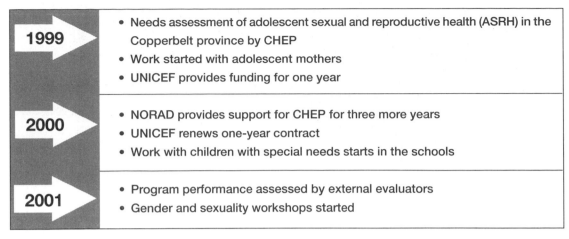

Figure 1. Time Line of Major Program Events

CHEP's main target groups are teachers, schoolchildren, and health workers. Primary and secondary schoolteachers and the district education officers have been involved in CHEP activities since 1988. Schoolchildren have been the primary target group since 1992, and at present, CHEP targets approximately 25,000 in-school youth annually. Health workers were not initially a high priority target group for CHEP. However, since 1990, the project has involved and trained health workers in all eight districts of the Copperbelt province. At the moment, CHEP offers youth-friendly services in four health clinics. In 2001, more than 9,100 youths sought the youth-friendly health services (YFHSs) provided by CHEP.

Program Overview

Aim

The main aim is to ensure that children and youth develop and maintain behaviors that will reduce their risk of contracting STDs and HIV/AIDS and encountering other sexual and reproductive health (SRH) problems. CHEP aims to empower children, adolescents, and youth with life skills to make them more self-confident and able to make better choices. The Child and Youth Unit also endeavors to impart practical skills such as functional literacy and numeracy, which will enable children and youth to venture into gainful employment in the future.

Objectives

The objectives of the Child and Youth Unit are to
- involve young people in planning programs that provide accurate information on sex and SRH;
- enable young people to develop skills to make decisions and communicate about sex and sexual safety;
- promote access to appropriate services for young people to act on decisions regarding sex, their sexuality, and SRH;

In 1982, when I first arrived in Zambia, AIDS was virtually unknown. It was not until 1985 that the first case of AIDS was officially identified in Zambia.

My training was in clinical medicine, but like many other health professionals, I felt increasingly frustrated by the impotence of modern medical science in the face of HIV....

Finally, I decided to abandon clinical medicine, which I had practiced for several years, to devote myself instead to the prevention of AIDS. Together with a few close friends and colleagues, and with support from the National AIDS Prevention and Control Program and NORAD, I formed the Copperbelt Health Education Project (CHEP).

V. Chandra Mouli, founder of CHEP

- promote a supportive environment by addressing negative gender roles, inequalities, cultural norms and expectations, and other socioeconomic conditions, to enable young people to make healthier choices about their SRH;

    - develop support systems for young people that will enable them to improve their risk perception, and develop and maintain safe sexual behaviors to reduce their risk of STD/HIV infection;
- establish YFHSs and strengthen existing ones; and
- reduce gender disparities between boys and girls by addressing gender roles, relations, and inequalities that hinder sexual communication and the practice of safe sex.

> Youths are a window of hope on the one hand, but they are also at great risk of HIV infection. More than two decades into a mature epidemic, we are wiser than we were before, realizing that young people are not passive recipients of information and skills but are active participators, policy definers, and key informants.
>
> *Executive director*

Age- and Gender-Specific Objectives for In-School Youth Aged 9 to 13 years (Primary School)
Overall objective: Improve knowledge and skills of young people to deal with emerging sexual feelings and risky situations.
Specific objectives:
- to increase accuracy of knowledge on sexually transmitted infections (STIs), HIV/AIDS, sex, and SRH through "Games for Life," peer education, and peer counseling;
- to empower them with appropriate skills to deal with emerging sexual feelings and risky situations through peer education and counseling, by developing their decisionmaking and communication skills, and by advocacy for the protection of child rights.

Age- and Gender-Specific Objectives for In-School Youth Aged 14 to 19 Years
Girls. Overall objective: Reduce risk of HIV/STD infection among young women.
Specific objectives:
- to increase the number of young women who have access to SRH services by strengthening networking and referral systems;
- to increase the number of girls who are able to protect themselves from unwanted pregnancy, STIs, and HIV by using appropriate skills. (This can be done through peer education and counseling and by using the multimedia communication package.)

Boys. Overall objective: Reduce risk of HIV/STD infection in young men.
Specific objectives:
- to improve communication, manual (i.e., condom use), and decisionmaking skills;
- to increase ASRH knowledge and improve attitudes toward sex, sexual health, sexuality, and gender roles, relations, and inequalities that hinder sexual health.

Target Groups

Primary Target Group
- preschoolchildren aged between 3 and 6,
- primary schoolchildren aged between 6 and 13,
- secondary and high school youth aged between 14 and 19,
- college and university youth aged between 18 and 35, and
- children with special needs aged between 6 and 15.

Secondary Target Group
Head teachers, teachers, and lecturers in all learning and training institutions, health workers, policemen, parents, and community leaders.

The Occupational and Community Units in CHEP target these groups directly (as a primary target). The Occupational Unit targets health workers, police officers, and civic leaders. The Community Unit targets parents and other community members.

Site

The in-school program is mainly based in rural and urban schools in the Copperbelt province. Most activities are extracurricular and take place after the school hours or during school holidays. However, some particpating schools have allowed the peer educators to work with students in the formal setting of the classroom. In addition, six schools have "Youth-Friendly Corners" in schools, where trained peer educators offer information and counseling on SRH and HIV/AIDS. These services on school premises are open to everybody.

Some activities, such as Games for Life and edutainment, take place in the communities, because these activities are provided to both in-school and out-of-school youth. The YFHSs take place in four health clinics. Trained peer educators from the out-of-school program provide these services for both in-school and out-of-school youth.

The program takes place in 4 preschools, 11 primary schools, 7 secondary schools, 4 colleges, and 1 university.

> Talking about HIV/AIDS facts alone is not enough. Young people need to understand and assimilate a whole range of life skills to cope with their daily life pressures.
>
> They also need to be helped to appreciate the links between HIV/AIDS and issues of gender and sexuality.
>
> *Edward Mupotola,*
> *coordinator for the CHEP*
> *in-school program, May 2002*

Program Length

The average length of club attendance is four years, and the maximum is around eight years. However, children can participate from preschool up to college or university. The participation of youth in other program components, such as Games for Life or edutainment, is voluntary, so the length of attendance can be from one time to several years.

Program Goals

As shown in figure 2, the in-school program mainly focuses on ensuring that children and youth form and maintain behaviors that reduce their risk of contracting STDs and HIV. This is primarily done by teaching life skills, such as decisionmaking, negotiation, communication, problem solving, and survival skills. Other goals are abstinence and pregnancy prevention.

At present, most of the CHEP staff recognize that most of the young people have some basic knowledge of HIV/AIDS prevention and transmission, although this knowldge is sometimes inaccurate or inadequate. Information dissemination continues to be a major focus, but the primary goal now is to improve young people's SRH-seeking behavior and increase their risk perception of STDs and HIV transmission while offering young people opportunities to learn new psychosocial life skills.

Abstinence is the only preferred sexual behavior for pupils younger than 15 years. Pupils older than 15 are also encouraged to abstain from sex. However, if they are sexually active, they are helped to have positive attitudes toward safer or low-risk sexual behavior.

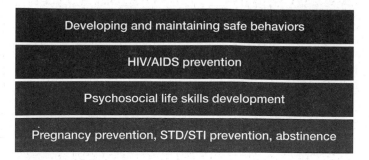

Figure 2. Program Goals Ranked in Increasing Importance

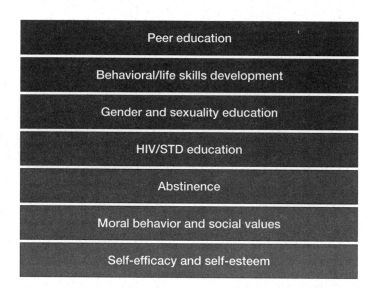

Figure 3. Program Approaches Ranked in Increasing Importance by the Program Coordinator

Approaches

The program coordinator ranked the primary approaches according to importance, as shown in figure 3.

Peer education is the main approach used in the in-school program. CHEP believes that changes in behavior patterns and attitudes will be achieved only through a participatory approach to learning.

The program implementers — the volunteers and peer educators, and especially the CHEP staff — have found that peer education is a very effective and appropriate approach to use with young people. In preschools and primary schools, older children (volunteer youths who are usually secondary school secondary leavers or graduates) plan and implement the club activities. In the primary schools, the child-to-child approach is also used, with the children being encouraged and expected to teach other children about the information they have learned.

Since 2001, CHEP has incorporated a rights-based approach in all programs. Additionally, the rights of women and children have been addressed in several training workshops. These include girls' right to refuse sex, right to be respected when they say no, right to be sexually active or not, right to marry or not, right to be free from coercion or force, and right to start, maintain, or end a relationship.

Activities
Various activities are used in the CHEP program, as shown in figure 4.

Components
The in-school program consists of five main components:
* Anti-AIDS Clubs,
* HIV/AIDS education through entertainment (edutainment),
* HIV/AIDS education through sports and games (Games for Life),
* Sara Communication Initiative, and
* YFHSs.

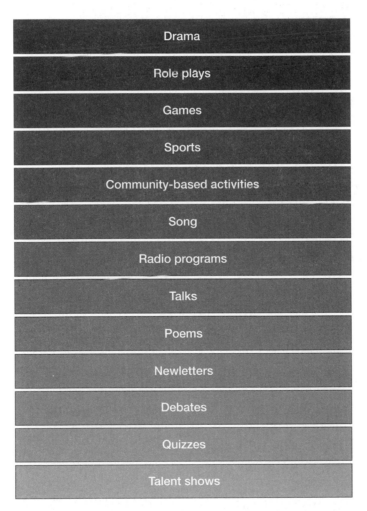

Figure 4. CHEP Program Activities Unranked

Anti-AIDS Clubs

The CHEP in-school program directly supports Anti-AIDS Clubs in 4 preschools, 11 primary schools, 7 secondary schools, 4 colleges; and 1 university in the Copperbelt province. The Anti-AIDS Clubs are run by several different organizations, such as the Family Health Trust and Society for Family Health. CHEP also periodically assists other schools by providing information, education, and communication (IEC) materials.

The Anti-AIDS Clubs are extracurricular activities. However, some of the schools where CHEP operates have allocated slots during school hours for peer educators to teach pupils in all the grades on a regular basis.

> Attitude change is a slow process.... The positive information the we peer educators give to other pupils will make someone want to change from the "bad" person that's/he was to one with good morals.
>
> **Peer educators from Helen Kaunda Secondary School Anti-Aids Club**

The number of the regular Anti-AIDS Club members for each club varies significantly, depending on the size of the school. The club meetings usually take place twice a week. For example, in some schools, the club meets once a week during the morning period and once a week during the afternoon period. This is done to provide all pupils an equal opportunity to join the club, whatever their class schedule.

The number of the peer educators per school also varies (an average of 30 per school). The peer educators run the club activities with the help of a matron or patron and the CHEP volunteers and field officers, who visit the clubs regularly. The peer educators use interactive methods, such as drama, focus group discussions, debates, role plays, picture codes, sketches and poems to work with their fellow students on issues related to SRH. In addition, six schools also have Youth-Friendly Corners, where all the students (not only the club members) are provided with information (printed materials and flyers) and counseling.

The curriculum for Anti-AIDS Clubs follows mainly the curriculum used in the peer educators' training. However, the club members themselves decide on what topics should be covered in each club session. They are taught assertiveness techniques, decisionmaking, survival and negotiation skills, and forms of sexual pleasure other than sexual intercourse. They also discuss issues related to gender and sexuality.

Edutainment

A number of innovative, youth-friendly, and cost-effective strategies have been used to effectively reach youth. One of these strategies is edutainment, a form of education through entertainment.

The general aim of edutainment is to provide young people with an alternative method of receiving HIV/AIDS education. Edutainment activities include debate, drama, and quiz; talent shows, musical concerts, and sports.

The debates, drama, and quizzes mainly focus on HIV/AIDS, STD prevention, and promotion of SRH. The pupils are provided with an opportunity to freely discuss important life issues that they would not normally talk about in classrooms. These activities usually take place once a year in school halls.

In addition, bimonthly talent shows have been held in two towns, Kitwe and Ndola. The guiding themes for these shows have been youth health promotion and youth development. Young people are given an opportunity to develop and design their own songs and visual artistic presentations to share with their peers. CHEP officers are always present at these gatherings to ensure accurate messages and help dispel rumors, misconceptions, and myths attached to HIV/AIDS and other SRH issues.

Games for Life

Games for Life is an education program designed to provide HIV/AIDS and SRH education to both in-school and out-of-school youth and children through sports and games, such as football, netball, volleyball, chess, and badminton in a youth-friendly atmosphere. Games for Life activities are organized by trained peer educators at the project sites.

The goal of Games for Life is to provide health education and information to vulnerable children and youth. Positive behavior change and life-changing commitments can be promoted through active participation in sports.

The games are run on a league basis or as a tournament. The first league runs from February to June, and the second league begins in August and ends in November each year. The league finalists receive prizes of health education materials, chlorine, toothpaste and toothbrush, or T-shirts.

> I thought and believed that my private organ [penis] would shrink if I am not practicing sex with girls, hence, I will be impotent and not be a man enough. Now I know that it is not true but mere myth and misconception. I can still delay sex and wait for the right time.
>
> **Anti-AIDS Club member**

Sara Communication Initiative

In Sub-Saharan Africa, many of the rights of children, particularly adolescent females, are not recognized and protected by families and communities. African girls have fewer educational opportunities and are often exploited in the labor force. They lack opportunities to develop psychosocial skills, and they are also often victims of sexual abuse. These factors have led to a growing incidence of STIs, including HIV/AIDS, among young females.

In an effort to address these issues, UNICEF has been implementing a program called the Sara Communication Initiative (SCI). SCI is an edutainment strategy that seeks to harness the drawing power of popular entertainment to convey educational messages. Sara is a cartoon character who emerges from the various impeding circumstances that she faces as a dynamic role model for the adolescent African girl. (For more details on SCI, please see appendix 1 to this chapter.)

CHEP has initiated SCI in 30 schools in the Copperbelt province. Fifteen CHEP volunteers, with the help of the coordinator, held 750 sessions between January and June 2000. Schools were then left to decide whether they wish to establish Sara Clubs. After the sessions in 2000, three secondary or high schools decided to establish Sara Clubs, which are still very active.

Youth-Friendly Health Services

The YFHSs are aimed at increasing needy young people's access to SRH services through improvements in health-seeking attitudes, behaviors, and practices. The aim is to ensure early diagnosis and effective treatment of STDs and ultimately the prevention of these diseases. YFHSs provide information, education, and communication on HIV/AIDS.

CHEP has established YFHSs in four health clinics in the Copperbelt province, with approximately 10 peer educators/counselors in each of the clinics.

The services provided by the trained peer educators and the clinic staff include counseling, STD/HIV/AIDS information dissemination, SRH education, psychosocial life skills, and information on anatomy and biological and physical developments during adolescence.

There is a great demand for these services. In 2001, 9,143 young people (3,767 females and 5,376 males) attended the YFHSs, compared with 7,500 males and females attending in 2000. There has also been an increase in the number of the boys and girls reporting STDs in the YFHSs. For example, in 2000, the average number of suspected STD cases per month was 132 per clinic. In 2001, the figure was 308 cases per clinic per month.

Case Study: Ms. Mwale's Story

After the death of her boyfriend, Ms. Mwale (a fictitious name) decided to go for voluntary counseling and testing (VCT). She was counseled and had her blood tested. The test showed that she was HIV positive. "I was devastated and confused. I thought that this is the end of me.... I knew of course that I was not the one who caused my infection...that brought a lot of anger in me and I was at the brink of getting depressed."

After some counseling at the YFHS, she decided to break the silence. "Due to counseling, I decided to let my family know about my test results. I was still scared because I was not sure about their reaction.... I did tell them anyway." As expected, her family, especially her parents, received the news with mixed feelings. They asked her not to tell anyone about her HIV status.

"I did not like my parents' idea. I had this thing in me that continually urged me to help my fellow young people to avoid infection or to accept it if infected.... I could not remain silent; I had to broaden my disclosure circle. I decided to tell one of my best friends..."

Ms. Mwale's first public disclosure was at a YFHS workshop, where about 40 participants listened to her moving stories. Many asked her how it was possible to be happy as a lady with the virus in her. With calm and determination, she said, "HIV infection is the battle of the mind, never let your emotions overrule your thinking ability. Talk to the virus everyday, and you will be feeling better. After all, there is a possibility of living more than 15 years."

Today, Ms. Mwale is one of the peer counselors that are helping other youths to understand and know how to prevent HIV infection, STDs, and unplanned teen pregnancies. Ms. Mwale has become a role model among youths in the community. However, her parents have been unhappy with their daughter for disclosing her HIV status to the community.

Source: CHEP, "Narrative and Financial Reports for the Period January to December 2001"

PART B: IMPLEMENTING THE PROGRAM

CHEP's in-school program includes various different strategies and components, as described above. Each of them can be developed and implemented separately to suit the needs of the children and youth in different settings.

Before and during the implementation of the activities, the Child and Youth Unit and the entire CHEP organization have carried out several baseline studies.

Needs Assessment

CHEP has conducted many KAP surveys since its inception. Assessments have been carried out for in-school youth during the years 1991–92, 1998, 1999, and 2001. The last survey, conducted in 2002, looked at knowledge, attitudes, skills, and habits (KASH). However, results of this last survey are not yet available.

In March 1999, CHEP staff carried out a needs assessment of ASRH in the Copperbelt province. The specific objectives were to

- establish appropriate health programs to meet the health needs of the youths,
- educate and counsel youths on important topics related to SRH,
- train peer educators in ASRH,
- reduce and prevent the SRH problems affecting adolescents, and
- conduct basic research in ASRH.

A cross-sectional study of randomly selected in-school and out-of-school youth was conducted. The study sample included 94 in-school youths from four schools from grades 8 to 12 (the majority were 16 to 18 years old, from both genders) and 86 out-of-school youths (the majority were 19 to 21 years old, from both genders).

Data were collected from in-school youth by use of a structured, self-administered questionnaire and structured interviews with both open- and closed-ended questions. Focus group discussions were used with the out-of-school youths. The data collection tools were pretested with 10 in-school youths to assess the ability of the tools to yield valid information.

The results of the study are shown in table 1.

The results from the assessment are encouraging because they indicate that youth are willing to discuss SRH issues with adults and people outside their peer group. CHEP also discovered that health needs can be addressed through STD clinics and counseling service. The results from the study were used to address specific program needs and to develop the program. A copy of the needs assesment is available. Please see Available Materials at the end of this chapter.

> There is a very high standard of confidentiality at this clinic. People do not know what you have come for. The youths [peer educators] are good and they have taken our parent's roles because they discuss with us important and sensitive issues.
>
> *A YFHS client*

Program Materials

Materials development has been an ongoing process. CHEP uses and adapts some materials that have been developed by other organizations, such as UNAIDS, UNICEF, the United Nations Development Programme (UNDP), the Southern Africa AIDS Information Dissemination Service (SAFAIDS), the United States Agency for International Development–Zambia Integrated Health Program (USAID/ZIHP), the Family Health Trust (FHT), the International HIV/AIDS Alliance, and the Ministry of Health. However, many organizations have also come to CHEP to collect their materials, and have adapted them.

Most of the materials are produced in English rather than local languages. According to the unit officer, English is used in CHEP materials because most of the people who are literate can read in English.

> The key step in changing children's and young people's attitudes is getting to understand their risk perceptions, habits, thoughts, feelings, and actions towards sexual health. We have learned from previous KAP [knowledge, attitudes, and practice] and KASH [knowledge, attitudes, skills, and habits] surveys that there exist a clear disconnect between their beliefs, thoughts, and actions.
>
> *Edward Mupotola, coordinator of the CHEP in-school program*

Target Group Materials

Brochures
Several brochures have been developed by CHEP for use with the target groups.

Assertiveness; Decision and Choice Making; Self Control; Self-Awareness, Self-Esteem, Self-Actualisation and Self-Confidence; and *Shyness* are aimed

Table 1. Needs Assessment Results

	In-School	Out-of-School
Main age group	16–21 years	16–20 years (58%)
Married	0/94 (77%)	25/86 (29%)
Had experienced sexual intercourse	34/94 (36%)	52/86 (60% incl. 29% married)
Engaged in first sex at what age (including those not engaged in sexual intercourse)?		
4–9 years	6/53 (11%)	0
10–15	22/53 (42%)	20/60 (33%)
16–21	23/53 (43%)	35/60 (58%)
No. of sexual partners (including those not engaged in sexual intercourse), including kissing:		
1	21/53 (40%)	30/60 (50%)
2	5/53 (9%)	10/60 (17%)
3	2/53 (4%)	7/60 (12%)
4 or more	14/53 (26%)	11/60 (18%)
Ever used condoms (including only those engaged in sexual intercourse)	24/34 (71%)	52/60 (87%)
Familiar with sex education	74/94 (79%)	56/86 (65%)
Discuss sex education with others	82/94 (87%)	66/86 (77%)
Appropriate cadre to teach sex education:		
Relatives	9/94 (10%)	2/86 (2%)
Teachers	8/94 (9%)	7/86 (8%)
Health workers	51/94 (54%)	60/86 (70%)
Peers and friends	18/94 (19%)	6/86 (7%)
Anybody	5/94 (5%)	10/86 (12%)
Not stated	3/94 (3%)	1/86 (1%)

at building the life skills of readers, improving their assertiveness, self-control, and ability to make good choices.

Stepping Stones Strategy: Information that You Need for Full Enjoyment of Your Life provides information about the Stepping Stones program offered by CHEP to families, companies, communities, and religious groups.

Games for Life is a brochure that gives general information on CHEP and the Child and Youth Unit. It also explains the Games for Life program, how the sports activities are organized, and the lessons learned from Games for Life.

Child and Youth Focused Unit gives information about the unit: the objective, target group, activities, achievements, challenges, and contact details.

Explaining CHEP gives general information on the organization, such as the mission statement, main goals, strategies, activities, and contact details.

Some of these brochures are available. Please see Available Materials at the end of this chapter.

Booklet

What Everyone Should Know About STD (Sexually Transmitted Diseases) is a 12-page booklet that gives information about STDs and HIV/AIDS, how they are and are not spread; how to know whether a person has an STD; what to do when an STD infection is suspected; how to prevent oneself from contracting STDs and HIV/AIDS; and where to get condoms.

This booklet is available. Please see Available Materials at the end of this chapter.

Fact Sheet

"Check Your Facts!" gives answers to some of the questions about HIV/AIDS. The questions include:

- What is HIV?
- How does HIV affect the body?
- What is AIDS?
- What is the HIV test?
- How do you get infected with HIV?
- What is high-risk behavior?
- How is the virus not transmitted?
- Can mosquitoes spread HIV?

> Young people have negative attitudes towards VCT [voluntary counseling and testing]. Most of them think that if you were diagnosed as HIV positive, you would "lose market," i.e., everyone will look down upon you.
>
> **Edward Mupotola, coordinator of the CHEP in-school program**

This fact sheet is available. Please see Available Materials at the end of this chapter.

The *Gender and Sexuality Toolkit* (International HIV/AIDS Alliance–ZIHP 2001) is a guide that provides several tools to facilitate interactive, participatory discussion with young people of issues related to gender and sexuality. CHEP has organized several workshops for youth, teachers, and peer educators using these toolkits.

Staff Training Materials

- *Gender and Sexuality Toolkit* (see above).
- *Manual for Peer Education Training:* CHEP has developed a training manual for peer education training. This manual is used in all peer education training with youth and adults.
- *Peer Education Modules 1–10:* These modules have been developed by the University of Zimbabwe and University of Zambia.
- *Training for Transformation:* A training program for community workers that was developed in Zimbabwe, based on the seminal thinking of Paulo Freire on developing critical awareness, along with developing the skills needed for a new society, especially relationship skills.
- *Stepping Stones*: A 1995 peer-based training package by Alice Welbourn about HIV/AIDS, gender issues, communication, and relationship skills. According to the *Stepping Stones* concept, when people undergo a series of training modules, it progressively builds their self-confidence and assertiveness. As they become more self-confident with increased levels of training and knowledge, they are able to speak more openly about their private lives, including aspects of sexuality and reproduction.
- *Participatory Approaches in HIV/AIDS Community Work: A Facilitator's Guide:* This guide, developed in Zimbabwe, provides basic information on the history and principles of participatory approaches and facilitation skills. It explains several participatory tools that can be used in HIV/AIDS education, including comprehensive guidelines on their particular uses.

Various other manuals are also used in staff training. Please contact CHEP (contact information in Part D of this chapter) for further information on these titles:

* *Zimbabwe's AIDS Action Program for Schools;*
* *Life Skills Education in Schools,* published by the World Health Organization (WHO)–Global Programme on AIDS (GPA) in 1994;
* *The Oxfam Gender Training Manual — Life Skills and Development,* also published in 1994;
* *School Health Education to Prevent AIDS and STDs,* a resource package produced by WHO and UNESCO in 1994.

Staff Selection and Training

CHEP's own staff conduct most of the training for its program implementers (peer educators, matrons and patrons, health workers, and counselors). However, some training workshops for health workers are conducted in collaboration with the district health management team (DHMT) , and with the Zambia Counselling Council for counselors' training.

The health workers' and peer educators' training usually lasts one to two weeks, and the counselors' training lasts around six weeks. CHEP organizes several different training workshops for its staff and for members of the wider community.

Training of Peer Educators

Training workshops for peer educators usually last one to two weeks. After the initial training, a follow-up training is usually provided after six months.

The peer educators are trained using the peer education manual developed by CHEP and the *Peer Education Modules 1–10* developed by the University of Zambia and University of Zimbabwe project support groups (PSGs). Peer educators are trained in these topics:

* introductions to peer approaches,
* basic facts on HIV/AIDS and STDs,
* condom use,
* family planning,
* care and treatment of persons living with HIV/AIDS,
* community norms of "ideal" images of boys and girls,
* sex and sexuality,
* adolescence,
* risk assessment of HIV/AIDS,
* life skills (problem solving, decisionmaking, critical thinking, creative thinking, interpersonal relationship skills),
* assertiveness,
* school outreach and its elements, and
* participatory and interactive methodologies.

Gender and Sexuality Workshops

Since July 2001, CHEP has organized several gender and sexuality workshops for students, teachers, and peer educators. Training lasts one to two weeks. Approximately 150 people have been trained. The trainers are CHEP staff that have been trained in gender and sexuality issues. The training takes place in schools and communities, at least twice a month.

Facilitators' Guide to Participatory Practice in HIV/AIDS Work: Gender and Sexuality in Young Men's Lives provides several toolkits to facilitate interactive, participatory discussions with young people about issues related to gender and sexuality. Even though these tools were originally developed to be used with young men, CHEP has found that most of them are suitable for use with both sexes. The toolkits were developed by the International HIV/AIDS AllianceZIHP.

An example of how one of the toolkits is used is described below:

Toolkit No. 5: Gender Boxes

Aim: To understand the costs and benefits of conforming to or resisting gender stereotypes.

Instructions:

- Discuss the profiles of a number of "typical" young men and young women (including factors such as age, class background, social status, ethnicity, educational level, employment status, marital status, sexual identity, rural/urban location, religious affiliation, and so on).
- Break into smaller groups to work on one typical young person each. Ask each small group to
  - Draw the outline of a body on the ground or large piece of paper and draw a box around this body outline. This is the gender box.
  - In the box, write, draw, and mark all of the gender stereotypes about this person (including how he or she should look and behave, his or her roles, responsibilities, and expectations, and so on).
  - Outside the box, write, draw, and mark all of the things that will be said to this person and will happen to this person if he or she steps "outside the box" — in other words, if the person does not conform to the stereotype.
- Bring the groups back together to share their gender boxes. Discuss and write up the costs and benefits of staying inside or stepping outside these gender boxes.
- Lead a general discussion of gender stereotypes, their influence on SRH, and how stereotypes can be challenged to improve SRH.

Questions to discuss:

- What are the main differences between the gender boxes for men and for women?
- How are gender stereotypes affected by other factors?
- How are people pressured to conform to gender stereotypes?
- What are the main costs of staying "in the box"? How different are these for men and for women? How do these costs relate to SRH?
- What are the main benefits of stepping "outside the box"? How different are these for men and for women? How do these benefits relate to SRH?

CHEP educators, field officers, peer educators, and supervisors receive training and refresher courses regularly. They are also able to attend various other courses according to their needs and interests. These courses include "Training for Transformation," "Stepping Stones," "Peer Counseling," "Participatory Approaches in HIV/AIDS Community Work," "Youth-Friendly Health Services for Health Workers," and "Matron/Patron Training for Teachers."

CHEP holds in-service training sessions once a month for all full- and part-time staff. The staff members who have attended different workshops share their new learning with the other staff. As a result of this in-service training, the project staff are well informed in number of technical areas of HIV/AIDS prevention and community work.

Setting Up the Program

Because the CHEP in-school program has so many components, describing how to set up each of them is beyond the scope of this report. For further information, please contact CHEP's Child and Youth Unit officer or the coordinator for in-school programs. (See contact information in part D of this chapter.)

Program Resources

CHEP has a resource room, open during working hours to everyone who is interested in CHEP educational materials. This room contains different books, reports, leaflets, videos, and so forth that are mainly related to SRH and general health.

Understanding the audience, or target group, and involving them in the process of designing health messages and materials is the key to successful health education. When planning any new materials, we first ask ourselves five basic questions:

1. To whom are the materials directed?

2. What behavior are we trying to change, and in what way?

3. What information does the target group require?

4. What emotional appeal will be most likely to strike a chord with the target group?

5. Through which communication channel, or combination of channels, can the information be communicated to the target group?

The responses to these questions determine the contents and presentation of the materials, and the ways in which they are disseminated to the various target groups, whose knowledge, attitudes, and behaviors we are trying to influence.

V. Chandra Mouli,
founder of CHEP

Advocacy

Advocacy has been a critical part of CHEP's strategy since its inception . The knowledge, attitudes. and skills of the wider community are seen by the program staff as important factors that affect and influence the sexual behavior of the children and youth in these communities. Therefore, their involvement is important in forming safe sexual behaviors among youth.

The Child and Youth Unit has carried out advocacy campaigns on specific issues such as prevention and mitigation of child pornography, teacher-pupil sexual relationships, abolishment of school fees for primary education, formation of community schools for vulnerable children, and child labor. These campaigns have targeted political leaders, civic leaders, police officers, teachers, school administrators, and the public, including young people themselves. The other two program units that form the CHEP project also actively involve and target civic leaders, traditional chiefs and leaders, police, traditional healers, and religious leaders.

CHEP is a member of the district AIDS force organized by the DHMT. Members from several other organizations and the government participate in meetings to share their plans and ideas related to HIV/AIDS work.

Program Finances

The total budget for 1996 was US$347,250, including a UNICEF contribution of US$50,000. IEC work (support services, IEC programs, and mass media) accounted for 68.5 percent of the total amount. The remaining amount was allocated to meeting the following costs: overhead (18 percent), capital equipment and maintenance (8 percent), monitoring and research (1.5 percemt), and conferences and meetings (4 percent).

CHEP's main cooperating partners are NORAD, Christian Aid, the Canadian International Development Agency's (CIDA) Southern African Training Program (SAT) program, UNICEF, the Netherlands, and the Zambia Educational Capacity Building Program (ZECAB). The support from NORAD, Chrisitian Aid, and the Netherlands is long-term, renewable after successful implementation of each three-year plan. The other donors' support is on a yearly basis.

Costs per child per year were not available.

PART C: ASSESSMENT AND LESSONS LEARNED

Challenges and Solutions

- At the beginning of the project, the messages were based on fear creation, as in many other countries. However, the staff realized very soon that this kind of message served to strengthen the stigma associated with HIV/AIDS, thus discouraging people from coming forward for testing or admitting their HIV status to their sexual partners. The fear-based messages also had the unintended effect of leaving many people anxious, afraid, and even angry because they were unable to respond effectively to the threat posed by AIDS to their own health and survival. Such messages may also have reinforced the negative feelings already harbored by many people toward those already infected with HIV/AIDS. The messages based on fear creation were withdrawn and new messages that promote positive values and attitudes were produced.

- In the beginning, CHEP messages were based on one-way communication. The needs of the targeted groups were neither researched nor taken into account. Later, CHEP became more sensitive and responsive to the needs of the public through direct, interpersonal contact. This was possible, for example, through question and answer sessions during workshops and teaching sessions. The project became aware of what people in various groups already knew about HIV/AIDS and how they felt about the disease. It also became clear that there were large and important differences from one group to the next concerning their knowledge, concerns, and fears about HIV/AIDS. Thus, CHEP started to tailor the contents and presentation of the materials to the knowledge, concerns, and fears of particular audiences — target groups — rather than to the public in general. Involving the audience or target group in the process of designing health messages and materials (for example, by pretesting) is the key to successful health education.

- Training youth as peer educators and including them in the executive committee of the Anti-AIDS Clubs from each grade in each school ensures continuity of the club activities, even after graduation of the upper grades.

- Lack of incentives, either financial or nonfinancial (T-shirts, badges, certificates, transport logistics, etc.) can result in loss of volunteer peer educators, especially among the out-of-school youth and school graduates.

- CHEP conducted a countrywide survey of the Anti-AIDS Clubs in Zambia (but not in their own clubs). This survey found that rather than getting across vital education to schoolchildren as hoped, these clubs tend to marginalize young people in schools and encourage stigmatization among young people.... A significant failing of Anti-AIDS clubs is that they do not reach enough of the young people at highest risk of contracting HIV. One problem is that patrons often select for membership those pupils who they feel already exhibit the "best" behaviour (e.g., they do not engage inany sexual activities). While these young people can undoubtedly benefit from membership and act as positive role models to their peers, it is also vital to include pupils who are currently at higher risk of getting infected with HIV and other STIs.

- Since CHEP intervened in the school Anti-AIDS Clubs, with a strategy of holding HIV/AIDS sessions in each and every class (in some of the schools) and holding workshops with teachers on facilitating HIV/AIDS sessions, all the pupils are getting involved in the fight against HIV/AIDS. The Anti-AIDS Club members are more able to share information with pupils who are not members and circulate materials evenly.
- Youths like youth-friendly health education programs. This is made evident by Games for Life, in which youth have actively participated in football, netball, and other sports. Because of this, young people are more willing to come to CHEP's center to seek information on health education.

Evaluation

The Child and Youth Unit undertakes continuous monitoring and evaluation of activities. The youth are actively involved in the planning, monitoring, evaluation, and all aspects of or research related to their activities. The unit ensures that the work on activities is reviewed weekly. The peer educators report their activities to the unit officer by filling out weekly monitoring sheets.

CHEP carries out monitoring and evaluation at three levels: program effectiveness, process effectiveness, and impact effectiveness. Both quantitative and qualitative research methods are used, involving observation, focus group discussions, questionnaires, individual interviews, and so forth. CHEP's programs and approaches are constantly reviewed and adapted as an outcome of this work.

Annual Participatory Planning Review Meetings

Each year, CHEP's staff and cooperating partners come from all over the Copperbelt province to hold their annual participatory planning review meeting. These meetings are held to review the annual activities and strategies undertaken by CHEP in preventing and mitigating the impact of HIV/AIDS on the Copperbelt populace. The meetings discuss successes, challenges, and opportunities for growth as well as the weaknesses of the organization. The main aim of these meetings is to plan appropriate strategies for the next year.

Baseline Study, 2001

One of the fundamental requirements of CHEP's donors is continuous monitoring and evaluation of the impact of CHEP's activities on its target groups. This calls for continuous reexamination at the end of the activity period of the indicators for measuring performance of programs. In addition, it is in CHEP's interest that it appraises the impact of its activities, identifying the best practices learned from the activities, with a view to improving performance and further maximizing the impact of its health education and community development programs among the vulnerable and marginalized groups in the Copperbelt province.

Therefore, CHEP commissioned Bravo Development Corporation Limited to conduct a baseline study of the key programs implemented by its three units. The overall objective of the study was to improve CHEP's planning, monitoring, and evaluation systems through review and development of qualitative and quantitative performance indicators for its activities. The results of the study will be valuable benchmarks that would make the three CHEP units more focused in their continued implementation of health education and other community-based development initiatives in the Copperbelt province of Zambia.

Please see appendix 2 to this chapter for CHEP's monitoring plan for both in-school and out-of-school youth.

UNAIDS Benchmarks

	Benchmark	Attainment	Comments
1	Recognizes the child/youth as a learner who already knows, feels, and can do in relation to healthy development and HIV/AIDS-related prevention.	✓	Youth are actively involved in the program at different stages: They participate in the CHEP's annual participatory review meetings; their ideas are incorporated in the final program plans; all the program activities are planned and carried out by the trained peer educators, with the help of the trained matrons or patrons and the CHEP staff; they are involved in the materials development, and they have been actively involved in monitoring and evaluation of the program activities.
2	Focuses on risks that are most common to the learning group and that responses are appropriate and targeted to the age group.	Partially fulfilled	The objectives and the strategies of the program are age- and gender-specific (since 2002). Gender issues related to SRH have been well addressed through gender and sexuality workshops and SCI.
			The program also targets preadolescents (preschool and primary schoolchildren), emphasizing behavior formation by encouraging values and skills conducive to safe sexual practices in the later years.
			The needs of the sexually active youth under age 15 years are not well addressed, do not receive information on safer sexual practices, such as condom use. (The baseline studies and the observations made by the peer educators and other staff clearly indicate that some of the youth start sexual activities sooner than the age of 15 years.)
			Peer pressure is commonly discussed with the young people. The youth have cited it as a very common problem affecting their behavior. The life skills taught aim at helping the children and youth to deal with everyday pressures (including peer pressure) they experience.
3	Includes not only knowledge but also attitudes and skills needed for prevention.	✓	The program addresses knowledge, attitudes, and skills in trying to help young people form healthy sexual behavior patterns. The main focus of the program is on attitude change and new skills taught to children and young people include assertiveness, self-awareness and self-confidence, decisionmaking, negotiation, communication, problem solving, and refusal skills.

	Benchmark	Attainment	Comments
4	Understands the impact of relationships on behavior change and reinforces positive social values.	✓	CHEP recognizes the impact relationships can make on behavior change. The project encourages youth and children to change their behavior through peer education, debates, discussions, etc., which help to enforce positive social values and also encourage young people to work together.
5	Is based on analysis of learners' needs and a broader situation assessment.	✓	CHEP'S in-school program bases its strategies and activities on the needs of the children and youth. The program regularly carries out KAP and KASH surveys and needs assessments to find out the actual SRH needs and problems of youth.
6	Has training and continuous support of teachers and other service providers.	✓	All the peer educators have received training in peer education, which usually lasts between one and two weeks. After the initial training, a follow-up training is usually provided after six months. Almost all the peer educators interviewed had received three or more trainings. All staff are trained and then receive refresher courses and additional training. Facilities are also provided so that staff can meet to discuss the program's progress, and offer each other advice and support.
7	Uses multiple and participatory learning activities and strategies.	✓	Most children and youth in Zambia lack entertainment facilities. CHEP has responded to this need by designing the edutainment and Games for Life programs. Most of the learning methods used by the peer educators are interactive and participatory. They include drama, debates, picture codes, role plays, focus group discussions, quizzes, poems, songs, and counseling.

	Benchmark	Attainment	Comments
8	Involves the wider community.	Partially fulfilled	The involvement of the wider community in the program activities is actively encouraged. According to the coordinator, behavior formation and change happen within the community. The knowledge, attitudes, and skills people in the community have, or do not have, obviously have implications for children's or youth's behavior. Thus, involving the wider community in the SRH program supports change in the community. However, the in-school program does not directly target the wider community. This is partly because other projects focus specifically on this area. In addition, other CHEP programs target directly the members of the wider community (community leaders, civic leaders, leaders, and members of religious groups, etc.)
9	Ensures sequence, progression, and continuity of messages.	✓	There appears to be continuity in the messages promoted. A wide variety of materials that children can use are provided so that they can continue to build on their knowledge.
10	Is placed in an appropriate context in the school curriculum.	Not applicable	HIV/AIDS is not yet part of the school curriculum in all schools in Zambia, so the work done by CHEP is in some areas the only exposure children have to information on HIV/AIDS.
11	Lasts a sufficient time to meet program goals and objectives.	✓	The entire CHEP program has been in existence for 14 years. The objectives and strategies have changed over time. New target groups have been included, such as orphans, children with special needs in schools, and adolescent mothers.
12	Is coordinated with a wider school health promotion program.	Not applicable	The CHEP approach does not yet seem to be completely coordinated into the wider school health program. At present, most CHEP activities are complementary to school programs and initiatives.
13	Contains factually correct and consistent messages.	✓	The IEC materials, other materials, and contents of the workshops are regularly updated, developed, and adapted according to the feedback from the courses and results of the surveys and evaluations.

	Benchmark	Attainment	Comments
14	Has established political support through intense advocacy to overcome barriers and go to scale.	✓	CHEP collaborates actively with other local, national, and international organizations and government offices, such as CINDI (Children in Distress Project), Friends of Street Kids, the Salem project, Catholic Diocese, the Society for Family Health, the Lions Club, FACT Mutare (Zimbabwe), Heart and Lung Association of Norway, DHMT, and the National AIDS Council.
15	Portrays human sexuality as a healthy and normal part of life, and is not derogatory against gender, race, ethnicity, or sexual orientation.	✓	According to the program coordinator, sexuality is portrayed as a concept that takes into account all aspects of people's sexual lives, including desires, identity, fears, and past histories. Issues related to sexuality are discussed in the peer educators' training workshops as well as in other trainings. Homosexuality is discussed with peer educators during their training (respecting each other's sexual identities and sexual and reproductive rights).
16	Includes monitoring and evaluation.	✓	Monitoring and evaluation of the program and its impact take place regularly, i.e., the peer educators from schools record their activities on a weekly basis; the unit monitors quarterly all its activities (using the monitoring plan); and CHEP has both midterm and annual review workshops.

PART D: ADDITIONAL INFORMATION

Organizations and Contacts

Contact persons:
Mr. Alick Nyirenda, CHEP executive director
Mrs. Evelyn Lumba, Unit officer for the Child and Youth Unit
Mr. Edward Mupotola, Coordinator for the in-school program

CHEP office location:
8 Diamond Drive
Kitwe, Zambia
CHEP postal Address:
P.O. Box 23567
Kitwe, Zambia
Telephone: +260-(0)2-229512
Fax: +260-(0)2-222723
Cell phone: +26096901965
E-mail: chep@zamnet.zm
or
alick@zamnet.zm
Website: http://www.chep.org.zm

Contributors to the Report
This report was prepared by Anne Salmi, M.A., Education and International Development: Health Promotion. Anne is an independent consultant living and working in Zambia (e-mail: annesalmi@yahoo.com).

It was guided by Michael J. Kelly, M.A., Ph.D., Educational Psychology. Michael has worked extensively on HIV/AIDS prevention in Zambia and is currently based at the University of Zambia (e-mail: mjkelly@zamnet.zm).

Edited by Katie Tripp.

Thanks to all CHEP staff, especially:
Mr. Nyirenda Alick, executive director
Mrs. Theresa Simwanza, office administrator
Mrs. Evelyn Lumba, unit officer and manager for the Child and Youth Unit
Mr. Mupotola Edward, coordinator for the in-school program
Ms. Chileshe Cecilia, field officer for the in-school program
Twelve Anti-AIDS Club members and the matron from Matete Primary School
Four peer educators from Helen Kaunda Secondary School
Fourteen CHEP volunteer peer educators

Available Materials

To obtain these materials, please contact ibeaids@ibe.unesco.org or Education for HIV/AIDS Prevention, International Bureau of Education, C.P. 199, 1211 Geneva 20, Switzerland.

Baseline Survey, October 2001
(order number: CHEP01)

"Needs Assessment of Adolescent Reproductive H — Copperbelt Province — Zambia"
(order number: CHEP02)

Working with Young People: A Guide
(order number: CHEP03)

Person to Person: Communication in HIV/AIDS Prevention (peer approaches)
(order number: CHEP04)

"Peer Education Training Workshop for In-School Youth 2001"
(order number: CHEP05)

Peer Education Training Manual
(order number:CHEP06)

Participatory Approaches in HIV/AIDS Community Work: A Facilitator's Guide
(order number: CHEP07)

"Report on the Annual Participatory Review Meeting"
(order number: CHEP08)

"Annual Participatory Review Workshop, November 1999"
(order number: CHEP09)

"Evaluation of HIV/AIDS Education Through Entertainment" (Edu-tainment Initiative), July 2001"
(order number: CHEP10)

"Annual Planning Meeting 2002:Child and Youth Focused Unit"
(order number: CHEP11)

Annual Report 2000: Child and Youth Focused Programme
(order number: CHEP12)

Narrative and Financial Reports for the Period January to December 2001
(order number: CHEP13)

All Against AIDS: Strategies for Hope
(order number: CHEP14)

Pamphlets:

"What Everyone Should Know About STDs"

"Prevention, Care, Openness: Community Focused Unit"

"Self Control: Owning Yourself"

"Shyness: No! They Will Laugh at Ne..."

"Explaining CHEP"

"Decision and Choice Making"

"Young People First"

"Young People: A Force for Change"

"Games for Life: Fighting Against AIDS the Sportive Way"

"Check Your Facts!"

Men Against AIDS"

"Self-Awareness, Self-Esteem, Self-Actualisation, Self-Confidence"

(order number: CHEP15)

APPENDIX 1: THE SARA COMMUNICATION INITIATIVE

The Sara Communication Initiative (SCI) uses a multimedia approach within the wider context of social mobilization, advocacy, and program communication. The existing package consists of an animated film, a comic book, a user's guide, a brochure, a poster, and a radio series about the "Sara" character's activities. This multimedia effort seeks to address discrimination against women in access to education, health, and social services and enhance the development of girls' psychosocial skills.

Before SCI's creation, a needs assessment was carried out in eastern and southern Africa. Several problems of adolescent girls were identified.

The overall goal of SCI is to promote child rights and support their implementation and realization, with special emphasis on adolescent girls in eastern and southern Africa and in other parts of Sub-Saharan Africa, where the materials are found to be acceptable and appropriate.

The main objectives of SCI are to
- support advocacy for the reduction of existing disparities,
- support social mobilization processes for girls,
- support the development of a positive symbol and dynamic role model for girls, and
- communicate specific messages on
  - rights,
  - education, and
  - health and nutrition.

The themes and rights highlighted in the seven-episode Sara series are
- *The Special Gift:* on girls staying in school and their right to education and nondiscrimination;
- *Sara Saves Her Friend:* on sexual harassment and HIV/AIDS; the right to protection from sexual exploitation, abduction, and violence; and the right to health and education;
- *Daughter of a Lioness:* on female genital mutilation and the right to health and protection from harmful traditional practices;
- *The Trap:* on "sugar daddies," HIV/AIDS, and the right to protection from sexual exploitation and abuse;
- *Choices:* on teenage pregnancy and continuing education, positive adolescent relationships, avoiding HIV/AIDS, and the right to education and health;
- *Who Is the Thief?* on domestic child labor, the right to protection from harmful and exploitive labor, and the right to education; and
- *The Empty Compound:* on breaking the silence about HIV/AIDS and care of orphans, and the right to life and maximum survival and development.

APPENDIX 2: MONITORING PLAN

Program components	Implementation indicators	Information source	Frequency
Advocacy	Number of schools implementing SRH and HIV/AIDS education	School project records	Quarterly
	Number of communities participating in youth prevention activities	Peer educator records	
Training	Number of trained peer educators who are active	School project records	Monthly
	Number of trained matrons and patrons who are active	School	
Peer education activities	Number and type of informal activities implemented	School project records	Monthly
	Number and type of formal activities implemented		
	Number of target groups reached (male and female) and type of activity		
	Number and type of IEC materials given out		
Organizing other services (VCT, STI, treatment, condoms)	Number of young people referred from schools and Youth-Friendly Corners to clinics	Youth-Friendly Corner records	Monthly
	Number of young people treated for STIs	Clinic records	
	Number of young people counseled on safer sexual practices	School project records	
	Number of young people who receive condoms		
	Number of young people counseled on sexual abuse/ violence or referred to the police victim support unit		

APPENDIX 3: STEPS FOR AN ANNUAL PARTICIPATORY REVIEW MEETING

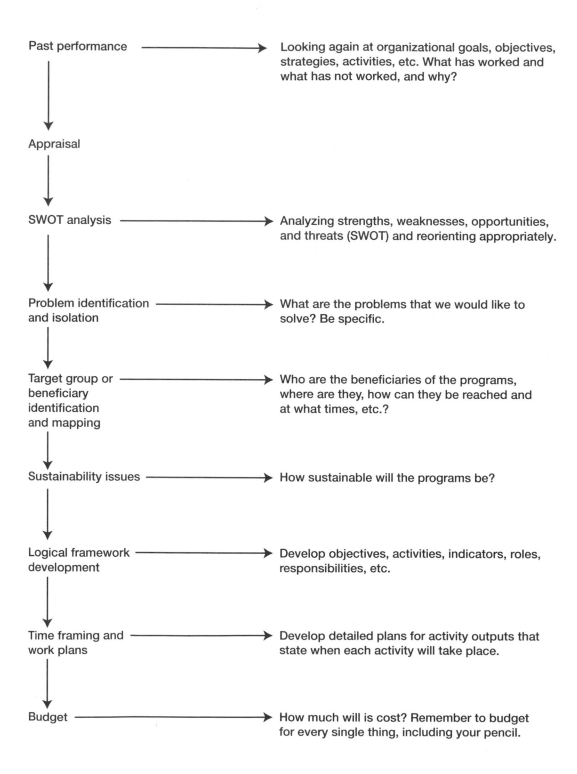

Past performance → Looking again at organizational goals, objectives, strategies, activities, etc. What has worked and what has not worked, and why?

Appraisal

SWOT analysis → Analyzing strengths, weaknesses, opportunities, and threats (SWOT) and reorienting appropriately.

Problem identification and isolation → What are the problems that we would like to solve? Be specific.

Target group or beneficiary identification and mapping → Who are the beneficiaries of the programs, where are they, how can they be reached and at what times, etc.?

Sustainability issues → How sustainable will the programs be?

Logical framework development → Develop objectives, activities, indicators, roles, responsibilities, etc.

Time framing and work plans → Develop detailed plans for activity outputs that state when each activity will take place.

Budget → How much will is cost? Remember to budget for every single thing, including your pencil.

PPAZ, FLMZ, and RFSU: Kafue Adolescent Reproductive Health Project (KARHP), Peer Education through Family Life Education Clubs

PART A: DESCRIPTION OF THE PROGRAM

Program Rationale and History

In 1995, the Zambian government, with assistance and funding from the Swedish International Development Authority (SIDA), developed the Kafue Adolescent Reproductive Health Project (KARHP). Kafue district was selected by the Zambian Central Board of Health (CBoH)[1] because it includes both urban and rural settings lacking sexual and reproductive health (SRH) education programs, and is a high-risk area for HIV/AIDS and other sexually transmitted infections (STIs) because it is situated along the highway to Zimbabwe and South Africa.

In 1996, The Planned Parenthood Association of Zambia (PPAZ), Family Life Movement of Zambia (FLMZ), Young Women's Christian Association (YWCA), and Swedish Association for Sexuality Education (RFSU) carried out a needs assessment. The main aim was to find out about adolescents' attitudes and behaviors regarding SRH and what factors influence these behaviors in

> Peer education is seen as having the potential to influence social norms and enhance positive attitudes as well as being a way to teach skills needed for prevention and risk reduction for HIV/AIDS, STIs, teenage pregnancies, and drug abuse.
>
> *Program coordinator*

---

1. The Central Board of Health is a national technical administrative body responsible for overall provision and development of health services.

Kafue district. It also looked at the health and educational facilities available to adolescents. Based on the results of the needs assessment, the project structure and materials were developed, and a project coordinator was appointed to manage the day-to-day running of the project.

The project began in 1997 in seven communities and nine schools (two primary, five basic, and two secondary) and targeted 10,700 in-school adolescents. The main focus of the program was the Family Life Education (FLE) Clubs in schools. In these clubs, peer educators were responsible for conveying messages to the adolescents about their SRH in a variety of ways. Toward the end of 1998, two youth-friendly clinics were also established, and two more were operational by the end of 1999.

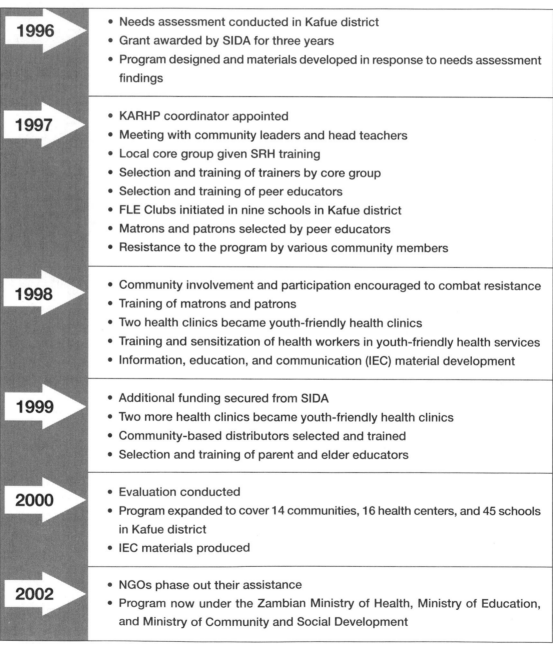

1996
- Needs assessment conducted in Kafue district
- Grant awarded by SIDA for three years
- Program designed and materials developed in response to needs assessment findings

1997
- KARHP coordinator appointed
- Meeting with community leaders and head teachers
- Local core group given SRH training
- Selection and training of trainers by core group
- Selection and training of peer educators
- FLE Clubs initiated in nine schools in Kafue district
- Matrons and patrons selected by peer educators
- Resistance to the program by various community members

1998
- Community involvement and participation encouraged to combat resistance
- Training of matrons and patrons
- Two health clinics became youth-friendly health clinics
- Training and sensitization of health workers in youth-friendly health services
- Information, education, and communication (IEC) material development

1999
- Additional funding secured from SIDA
- Two more health clinics became youth-friendly health clinics
- Community-based distributors selected and trained
- Selection and training of parent and elder educators

2000
- Evaluation conducted
- Program expanded to cover 14 communities, 16 health centers, and 45 schools in Kafue district
- IEC materials produced

2002
- NGOs phase out their assistance
- Program now under the Zambian Ministry of Health, Ministry of Education, and Ministry of Community and Social Development

Figure 1. Time Line of Major Program Events

Despite holding advocacy meetings with leaders of the community and the head teachers, the program met with some resistance from members of the community. Their main complaint was that they felt young people should not talk about sex. In response, community members were encouraged to become integrated into KARHP, and they are now actively involved and happy to support the clubs and help organize community events.

Drama and counseling are important because they reflect real-life situations. Lectures and talks are less effective because the adolescents find them boring.

Peer educator

In 2000, the University of Zambia and the Institute of Economic and Social Research conducted an evaluation. As a consequence, more funding was secured from SIDA, and the program was expanded to cover 45 (75 percent) of the government schools, 16 health clinics, and 14 communities.

In April 2002, the program was integrated into the district offices of the Ministry of Health, Ministry of Education, and the Ministry of Community and Social Development, and the assistance of the founding NGOs and the SIDA funding was phased out.

Program Overview

Aim
To deliver information and services concerning SRH to 10- to 24-year–old, in-school youth in Kafue district through strengthening the collaborations between the institutions involved (PPAZ, FLMZ, and RFSU).

Objectives
The program objectives are to

Girls and boys have some activities separately. It is good that there are some separate activities, as they help girls to build self-confidence and awareness.

Program coordinator

- promote young people's access to SRH information and services,
- increase the involvement of parents and elders in empowering adolescents to adopt healthy sexual and reproductive behavior,
- foster positive behavioral change,
- equip in-school adolescents with the necessary knowledge and skills to negotiate and practice safer sexual behaviors,
- reduce the risks of negative peer pressure, and
- help youth to develop positive attitudes about each individual's — and especially her or his own — worth.

Target Groups

Primary Target Group
Initially, the primary target group was 10,700 10- to 24-year-old adolescents and youth in nine schools (two primary, five basic, and two secondary) in Kafue district. Since 2000, the project has been scaled up to 45 schools (19 primary, 25 basic, and 4 secondary), but the numbers of youth targeted are now unknown. Any young person 10 to 24 years old can participate in the FLE Clubs as long as they are attending school.

Secondary Target Group
The program also directly targets parents and health providers, who are trained to help improve information access and services related to SRH.

Site

The program was started and is mainly based in schools in the district. It later began working in the clinics and the community.

Kafue district is situated approximately 45 km south of the capital, Lusaka. It is geographically diverse, but predominantly rural. The town is located on the transit corridor formed by the Great North Road and the railway line, which are channeled between the Kafue River and the hills to the east.

> Some of the problems the adolescents face can be complex. A strong support structure is important so that peer educators can ask for assistance.
>
> *Program coordinator*

Program Length

The average length of attendance at an FLE Club is two and a half years, and the maximum is eight years. The school-based FLE Clubs operate continuously, once a week during the school year. The club meetings do not take place during the school holidays. During the school holidays, different activities are organized, such as educational picnics and training. The clinic-based activities (youth-friendly health services) are available for young people throughout the year. The community-based activities also operate continuously throughout the year.

Program Goals

The program coordinator ranked the program goals as shown in figure 2. Behavior change was thought to be one of the most important because it is through behavior change that the other goals can be achieved.

Approaches

The main approach that has been used by the KARHP is the peer, parent, and provider (PPP) approach: The FLE Clubs and community support goups provide peers with an opportunity to learn from one another. The Parent Elder Education Program encourages parents and children to talk to one another about SRH issues within the community, and the youth-friendly health services and condom distributors allow health providers to see to the SRH needs of the youth.

Various approaches are taken in each of the three program sites. It was impossible to rank the approaches, as all were felt to be important. However, in the school setting, peer education was mentioned as one the most effective ways of fulfilling the program goals because in-school

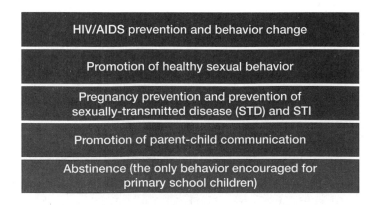

Figure 2. Program Goals Ranked in Increasing Importance by the Program Coordinator

adolescents are thought to be easily influenced by their peers and their environment. By using peer educators as positive role models, adolescents are more likely to change their attitudes, engage in safer sexual behaviors, and learn more about SRH. The main role of the clinics is to provide SRH services and information.

Activities

KARHP activities are shown in figure 4. Peer educators felt that one-to-one counseling; drama, sketches, and role play; and poems were the most effective. These were thought to be the most beneficial activities because they reflect real-life situations and because everyday, comprehensible language could be used.

> We discuss the topics that are raised by the adolescents in the clubs. We then plan to cover topics that adolescents are interested in.
>
> *Matron*

Components

The program consists of four main components:

1. FLE Clubs in schools, including peer education and counseling and matron and patron supervisors;
2. parent and elder educators to promote parent-child communication;
3. youth-friendly services in clinics; and
4. Community-based distribution of contraceptives and information on family planning.

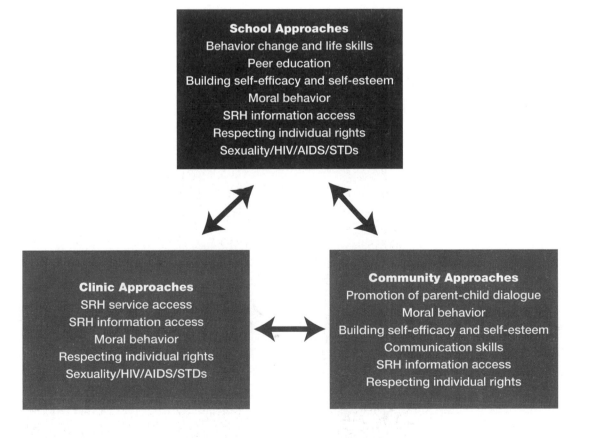

Figure 3. Program Approaches

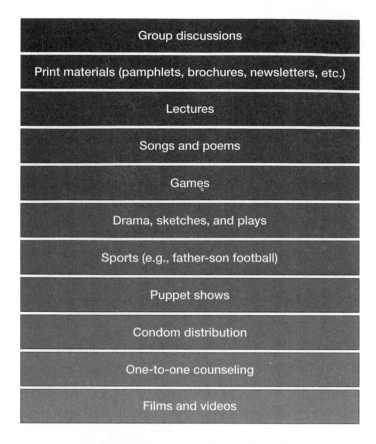

Figure 4. Program Activities Unranked

FLE Clubs

During the school term, each of the schools in the program holds an FLE Club meeting once a week after school. The clubs are organized and run by the peer educators and counselors, who are supervised by the matrons and patrons. The club meets in a classroom, and meetings last between one and two hours. Each week, a different topic related to SRH is discussed. These topics are described in the Target Group Materials section of this chapter.

> More and more members of the community are becoming aware of the purpose of the project. One mother said that nowadays she wants her child to be seen in a condom not a coffin.
>
> *Matron*

Each week, various activities are used to promote the program approaches (e.g., a discussion on respecting individual rights and moral behavior). The youth are also encouraged to suggest topics to be included in future club meetings.

Students who want individual counseling can approach trained peer educators, who will take them into another classroom, a nearby clinic, or anywhere where privacy can be found to discuss their problems. When needed, the peer educators can refer young people to the clinics for medical attention. They have referral forms to fill in that explain the problem. In cases of sexual abuse, the case is referred to the matron or patron if the adolescent concerned agrees. Then it will be taken to the KARHP, YWCA, or the victim support unit of the police service.

FLE Clubs Case Study

David is 12 years old and has been attending the FLE Club in his school for the past three months. He has just moved to Kafue from another district and did not attend an FLE Club there.

Today, he attended the FLE Club after school. The meeting's theme was dating and relationships. The peer educator began by giving a short talk. He said that even if two people in a relationship love each other, they should wait until they are married before having sex. He said that if you have sex before you are married, you may get pregnant or even catch HIV or an STD. At the end of the talk, the adolescents were encouraged to ask questions.

The peer educator then asked the adolescents to split into groups. He told them to think of a short role play about a dating couple. He said the role play should be about what to do if the boy wants to have sex and the girl does not. The groups were given time to prepare their role plays, which they then acted out for the rest of the club. The peer educator then led a short final discussion about the issues that had been raised by the role plays.

Peer educators and counselors. There are between 5 and 15 peer educators in each school. Their main task is to run the FLE Clubs. However, they also partake in community outreach activities (e.g., door-to-door campaigns, drama), youth-friendly clinic activities, organization of community events (e.g., World AIDS Day), presentations for the whole school, one-to-one talks with students who are not club members, and activities held outside the school term (e.g., picnics, sports events).

> The integration of the PEEP program into KARHP activities has increased community acceptance of the concept of sexual and reproductive health education.
>
> **Program coordinator**

Matron and patron supervisors. In each school, two matrons or patrons are appointed to help with running the FLE Club. The matrons and/or patrons meet with the school peer educators and counselors every week after school, in a classroom. They work together to plan the agenda for the next club meeting and share new ideas and information. These sessions with their supervisors also provide a feedback mechanism whereby the peer educators and counselors can discuss any new developments in the club and how to handle them.

Although the main role of the matrons and patrons is to offer the peer educators help and support, their other roles include:

- Preparation of quarterly reports on the activities of the club.
- Finding any extra materials and information needed to help run the clubs from the KARHP office, PPAZ, FLMZ, and the District Education Officer's (DEO) office. They also have an HIV/AIDS focal point in each zone[2] in the district, whom they can ask for up-to-date HIV/AIDS information.
- Raising awareness among parents and the community about the FLE Clubs. One of the ways the matrons and patrons do this is through holding short talks at parent-teacher meetings. By talking about the program, and its aims, objectives, and activities, the community is made more aware of what their children are learning and why the program is important.
- Training future matrons and patrons (some of the matrons and patrons are selected and trained to become trainer of trainers).
- Training peer educators and counselors.

2. Each district is split into several zones.

The matrons and patrons also meet with other matrons and patrons in the district and the KARHP coordinator at KARHP headquarters. They discuss any problems they are having and share their experiences. When the program was first established, the meetings took place every month. Once the program was firmly established and running smoothly, the meetings were held on a quarterly basis.

Parent and Elder Educators

The Parent Elder Education Program (PEEP) equips parents, elders, and community and religious leaders with knowledge and skills on issues of SRH to facilitate positive parent-child communication. This component is vital in the KARHP because it helps parents to examine their values and attitudes on issues of sexuality, STIs, and HIV/AIDS and make them comfortable in discussing these issues with their children. PEEP supports and complements the FLE/SRH information given to the youth through the other components of the project.

> At first, community taboos about sex meant that parents were not very willing to discuss sexual issues openly with their children. After community advocacy, awareness of the program increased and the stigma surrounding HIV was reduced.
>
> **Program coordinator**

Parent and elder educators organize community meetings, weekly door-to-door campaigns, religious meetings, and monthly Parent-Teacher Association (PTA) meetings, where they talk about the program, SRH topics, and the importance of parent-child communication. They also give written referrals to the health clinics for people requiring medical attention. The parent and elder educators explain to parents and the community that the aim of the program is to help youth learn important skills that will help protect them from HIV/AIDS, STIs, and unwanted pregnancy.

Youth-Friendly Services

An important component of the program is the establishment of youth-friendly services in the district's health clinics. One of the main roles of the clinics are to provide access to condoms and other contraceptives. In addition to such family planning services as pregnancy testing, the clinics also provide STD and HIV screening.

Certain clinic staff are specially trained in how to serve adolescents. These staff are also trained on how to give talks on SRH issues (e.g., contraception).

When the youth attend the clinics, they are first directed to "Youth-Friendly Corners," where the peer educators and counselors can discuss issues with and counsel them. Then, the young person and the peer counselor usually go together to see the nurse or other health worker. The peer educators and counselors usually offer their services three times a week in these clinics.

> Shortages of condoms and inadequate numbers of trained community distributors in rural areas means that some youth might not get the services they require.
>
> **Program coordinator**

Community-Based Distributors

The community-based distributors (CBDs) are young people trained in the delivery of SRH messages, family planning, and contraceptive methods. The main aim of this component of the program is to reduce the incidence of unwanted pregnancies, HIV infection, STIs, early marriage, and risky sexual behaviors.

The CBDs offer services to all youth (in-school and out-of school) in the communities. They work hand in hand with the local clinics that supply the materials needed (i.e., condoms, contraceptives). The CBDs also refer clients that need medical attention to the nearest clinic.

This approach to service delivery has been advocated to address the limitations of the clinic-based service delivery network: lack of trained personnel, shortages of contraceptives, inadequate coverage of rural populations, and a bias against serving adolescent sexual and reproductive health (ASRH) needs.

PART B: IMPLEMENTING THE PROGRAM

Needs Assessment

In 1996, a needs assessment was conducted in Kafue district to gather information on the sexual behavior of the young people and the factors affecting and influencing their behavior. The needs assessment also aimed at evaluating the educational, recreational, health, and other social facilities available to youth in their communities. The needs assessment took place as follows:

- It was carried out over a period of three weeks (October 29 to November 19, 1996) by a team of professionals from the PPAZ, FLMZ, RFSU, and YWCA who were familiar with Kafue district and its communities.
- Information was collected on knowledge related to HIV/AIDS and STDs/STIs, attitudes toward relationships and sex, sexual behaviors and practices, and health-seeking behavior.
- The information was collected through individual interviews, focus groups, and observations in places where young people gather.
- In total, 70 people (including young people, teachers, health staff, and community leaders) participated.

> Reaching out to young people in Kafue, and sharing and learning how young people perceive issues related to sex, has been interesting. I realized that there are a lot of rumors, myths, and misconceptions in the minds of young people, and these, unless addressed, will continue misleading them.
>
> *Youth participating in needs assessment*

The main results revealed that poverty was one of the major risk factors, leading young women and girls to engage in sexual activities in exchange for gifts and money that they use to survive and pay school fees. One of the main problems affecting boys and young men was the use of alcohol and marijuana. It was also found that early marriages, STIs (including HIV), and unwanted pregnancies were common problems.

The findings from the needs assessment and information collected from the district health officer gave a good understanding of the SRH needs in Kafue district. The results enabled the design, planning, and implementation of the project:

- establishment and implementation of FLE Clubs, community support groups, PEEP, and youth-friendly services;
- development of curriculum and training programs;
- training and sensitization of different of stakeholders; and
- youth-based community services and distribution of contraceptives and family planning information.

Program Materials

The program materials have been developed over the course of the project. Most of the initial materials were developed using the results of the needs assessment to adapt materials available from the Ministry of Health, the United Nations Population Fund (UNFPA), the Society for Family Health, PPAZ, FLMZ, and RFSU. Other materials have been produced as the program has evolved.

Most of the materials are produced in English rather than local languages. Yet local languages were particularly encouraged in the training workshops.

Target Group Materials

Family Life Education Curriculum

Family Life Education: A Curriculum for Teachers and Trainers was developed for use by trainers, peer educators, matrons and patrons, parent and elder educators, and CBDs for use in the FLE Clubs and various community meetings and trainings of all program workers. The curriculum was developed by a consortium of youth service professionals and young people themselves, with assistance from the Margaret Sanger Centre International and UNFPA. Seven agency members, namely PPAZ, FLMZ, Young Africans Welfare Association, Girl Child Adolescent Reproductive Health Project, YWCA, Community Youth Concern, and the Department of Youth Development make up this consortium, called the Adolescent Reproductive Health Project.

> I learned that in Kafue, sex is taken as a major source of income among many young people due to poverty and unemployment.
>
> *Youth participating in needs assessment*

The curriculum does not have to be followed in a strict order, but it is important that the clubs cover a range of issues to ensure that young people gain knowledge and skills on a wide range of topics. The same curriculum is covered each year in the FLE Clubs. However, the emphasis in primary schools is on abstinence, whereas in secondary schools, information on condom use is also provided.

The club curriculum is as follows:

Unit One: The Family
- Family Structures
- Family Relationships
- Family Roles

Unit Two: Self-Awareness
- Who Am I?
- Human Development
- Adolescence
- Decision-Making

Unit Three: Gender and Sexual Expression
- Gender Identity Formation
- Sexual Orientation
- Sexual Expression

Unit Four: Family Planning and Contraception
- Traditional Family Planning Practices
- Reversible Methods of Birth Control. Permanent Methods of Birth Control
- Emergency Contraception
- Abortion
- Contraceptive Use in Special Situations

Unit Five: Relationships
- Friendship
- Dating
- Love
- Marriage and Other Life Partnerships
- When Relationships Sour

Unit Six: Responsible Parenthood
- On Parenting
- Demands of Parenting
- Pregnancy and Childbirth
- Breast Feeding

Unit Seven: Personal and Sexual Health
- Zambia's Health Goals
- Critical Health Concerns
- Basic First Aid
- Preventive Health and Hygiene
- Sexually Transmitted Infections
- HIV and AIDS
- How to Use a Condom

Unit Eight: Abuse and Violence
- Child Abuse
- The Touch Continuum
- Sexual Abuse
- Domestic Violence
- Employer Abuse

Unit Nine: Drugs and Mood Altering Substances
- Drugs
- Alcohol

Unit Ten: Youth Rights
- Bill of Rights
- The Juveniles Act
- Youth and Reproductive Health Care
  This curriculum is available. Please see Available Materials in part D of this chapter.

> Using nonlocal languages can enable people to discuss issues that they would be too embarrassed to talk about in their own language. For example, adolescents were willing to name the sexual parts of the body in English but were reluctant to do so in their own language.
>
> **Program coordinator**

> One of the major problems is the high turnover rate of peer educators due to lack of motivation, changing schools, and leaving school to start work..
>
> **Program coordinator**

Brochures

Peer educators, with the assistance of resource persons from PPAZ, FLMZ, and RFSU, designed and developed IEC brochures. Five brochures on different topics addressing young people's concerns and problems were produced and pretested using structured questionnaires and focus group discussions. These brochures provide additional information to supplement the FLE activities. The five brochures are:

- *Sexually Transmitted Infections*
- *What's Up on Drugs and Alcohol?*
- *Early Marriage: Know the Facts*
- *Avoiding Many Sexual Partners: What You Should Know*
- *Facts About Growing Up*

A total of 50,000 copies (10,000 copies of each brochure) were produced. Copies of the new brochures were distributed to the peer educators, matrons and patrons, CBDs, parent and elder educators, health service providers, all schools in Kafue district, football teams under the Kafue sports advisory committee, and members of the communities.

These materials are available. Please see Available Materials in part D of this chapter.

Staff Training Materials

Family Life Education Manual

Family Life Education: A Manual for Parent Educators was designed to train and guide parent and elder educators in leading community-based education sessions with community members. The manual provides details on the kind of techniques needed when conducting community meetings and one-to-one sessions. The manual also outlines several activities that can be used to promote interest in the program among the community. It explains the purpose of each activity, gives step-by-step instructions, estimates time and materials needed for each activity, and gives fact sheets, questionnaires, case studies, and role plays. There is also advice on how each section of the manual can be adapted to suit the needs of the group and the time available for the session.

> It is recommended that the matrons and patrons receive "refresher" courses to keep them motivated and to provide more skills and information.
>
> **Program coordinator**

The manual was not specifically developed for peer educators to use in FLE Clubs. However, some of the sections have been used after revision to guide and help conduct FLE Club activities.

This manual is available. Please see Available Materials in part D of this chapter.

Staff Selection and Training

Staff selection methods may change over time. All staff go through training with the following activities:

- Question boxes: During the training, participants are encouraged to anonymously write questions they are concerned about. Every morning questions are discussed and answered.
- Steps to condom use: Different stages of condom use are written on strips of paper, and participants are asked to put the stages in order.
- "Teach back": Participants are encouraged to teach other participants what they have learned during their training.
- Pretest and posttest training: Participants are tested before and after training to assess their level of knowledge and specifically what they have learned during training.

Trainers of Trainers

- A core group, formed by representatives from PPAZ, FLMZ, and the CBoH, selected the first trainers of trainers (TOTs). The trainees were teachers, police officers, and government officials. Peer educators, matrons and patrons, and parent and elder educators have since been trained as trainers of trainers.
- Training lasts between one and two weeks and is conducted by the master trainers from PPAZ, FLMZ, RFSU, and KARHP.
- At the end of training, the TOTs should be able to plan, organize, and conduct training workshops in FLE/SRH. The training objectives include strengthening participants' knowledge on FLE/SRH, making participants understand their own attitudes toward ASRH matters, imparting skills on how to conduct FLE/SRH training, and making participants feel comfortable in their roles as trainers in FLE/SRH.
- The TOTs receive refresher courses after their initial training.
- Some of the TOTs were later trained as master trainers.

Peer Educators and Counselors

- The TOTs and the matrons and patrons select the peer educators and counselors from the members of the FLE Clubs. Peer educators and counselors should be accepted and respected by the other youth and the members of the wider community (parents, teachers, etc.). They should be willing and motivated to be trained and work as peer educators and counselors, and be committed to the goals and objectives of the program.

- The TOTs, master trainers, and/or matrons and patrons train the peer educators and counselors for 5 to 10 days, depending on the budget and availability of trainers.
- The training content is adopted from the FLE curriculum. The training also includes an introduction to the program's goals and objectives, the concept of peer education, and facilitation and communication skills.
- Refresher courses have been offered to peer educators to keep them motivated and help them learn more about SRH issues.

Matrons and patrons

- Two matrons or patrons are selected in each school by the peer educators and counselors and school heads.
- The TOTs, master trainers, and/or experienced matrons and patrons train the new matrons and patrons. The training lasts between 5 and 10 days, depending on the availability of trainers and the budget.
- The training covers human sexuality, values, facilitating skills, gender and sexuality, behavior change, equal rights, adolescence, relationships, fertility awareness, setting up FLE Clubs, condom use, abuse and violence, STDs and HIV/AIDS, roles of matrons and patrons, and work plans.
- The matrons and patrons receive refresher courses to keep them motivated and provide them with more skills and information.

Health Service Providers

- In each of the youth-friendly health clinics, the district health management team (DHMT) selects two staff members to be trained as youth-friendly health care providers. They are trained for seven days by the master trainers.

> Without community support and political will and commitment, the efforts to prevent HIV/AIDS transmission will not succeed.
>
> ***Program coordinator***

- The objectives of the training workshops are to
  - create awareness among health care providers on ASRH needs,
  - help health care providers foster positive attitudes to young people's SRH,
  - help health care providers develop communication skills, and
  - create a youth-friendly environment in all health care facilities in the district.

Parent and Elder Educators

- Initially, members of the neighborhood health committees, PTAs, PPAZ, and FLMZ nominate two or three parents per community to be trained as parent and elder educators. Later, the KARHP advertised in marketplaces, clinics, and shops. (Applicants had to fill in a form concerning their previous experiences of volunteer work with people, especially in the area of SRH and youth.) The final selection is made by KARHP assistants and the coordinator after interviews.
- The parent and elder educators are trained by the TOTs, master trainers, and/or other experienced parent and elder educators for 5 to 10 days.
- The topics include remembering your youth, sources of values, facilitation skills, nuts and bolts of parent and elder education (components of PEEP), human sexuality, fertility awareness, traditional modes of education, STIs and HIV/AIDS, family planning, responsible parenting, what hinders communication, behavior change, gender and sexuality, abstinence, victim

support unit (police), relationships and sex and love, abuse, linking prevention with care, community involvement in PEEP, community mobilization, and target groups.

- After initial training, refresher training is provided to parent and elder educators.

CBDs

- The community members selected young people from their communities to be trained as CBDs.
- The CBDs are trained by trainers from PPAZ for 14 days.
- The objective of the training is to equip the CBDs with skills and knowledge in providing family planning and SRH services in the communities to reach out to fellow youth.

Setting Up the Program

Before the program was set up, the Ministry of Health and the Ministry of Education were fully involved in the its development. Community leaders, head teachers, and other key members of the community were also consulted at all stages of its establishment.

How to Set Up an FLE Club

- Seven schools (six rural and one periurban) were selected by the CBoH, PPAZ, and FLMZ.
- Consensus meetings and sensitization workshops concerning the program (goals, activities, strategies, etc.) were held with all head teachers and teachers.
- Staff (peer educators and counselors, matrons and patrons) were selected and trained, and the first clubs were established.
- Matron and patrons meet with the peer educators and KARHP coordinator to discuss club curriculum and activities.
- The clubs are publicized in the school through school assemblies and posters on the notice board.

Youth-Friendly Services

- Health clinics are selected to become youth-friendly centers by the DHMT.
- Two staff members per health clinic are selected to be trained as youth-friendly health care providers.
- All health clinic staff are sensitized on how to create a youth-friendly environment.
- Youth-friendly services are publicized in radio programs, newspapers, and their own brochures, and in door-to-door campaigns and public places, such as bus stops.

Program Resources

The KARHP has two offices with photocopying facilities and a meeting place that project implementers can use. The coordinator has a computer (with Internet access), brochures, some videos, the FLE manual, and curriculum and other materials in his office to which implementers have access.

Advocacy

The KARHP promotes the program's aims in the community by holding workshops, picnics, and other events with all members of the community. To gain the community's acceptance, there was a concentration of these events when the program was established and during program expansion.

The Ministry of Sport, Youth and Child Development; the Ministry of Health; and the Ministry of Education have all supported the KARHP by directly ensuring partnership at regional and district levels. The overall role of these partners was to provide legitimization of the program and advocate support in the community. In addition, they allow school facilities and various community venues, such as community centers, to be used for holding club meetings, talks, and program events.

In 1999, the KARHP held a meeting with key political figures to raise awareness of the importance of HIV/AIDS prevention in the community. The workshop concluded by asking for political commitment and support to expand the program to the whole of Kafue district. The KARHP also helped form the HIV/AIDS Network Co-ordinating Committee, established in Kafue district in 1999. The committee tries to join together the efforts of all the people in the community fighting against HIV/AIDS.

Program Finances

The yearly budgets (total expenditure) were:

1997: US$148,219,
1998: US$137,842,
1999: US$123,902,
2000: US$197,316, and
2001: US$120,000 (until March 2002).

A breakdown of spending for the KARHP program is not available. It is estimated that 53,000 youth have benefited from the program at an estimated cost of US$2.26 per youth per year. However, it should be noted that 101,400 adults have also been targeted by this program since 2001.

PART C: ASSESMENT, CHALLENGES AND LESSONS LEARNED

Challenges and Solutions

Program Coordinator

- It is important that the needs assessment include both qualitative and quantitative techniques. This will aid monitoring and evaluating the program because it will be possible to see trends and changes over time.
- Certain community members, along with the religious organizations, were unhappy about the program running in their community. Hence, it is crucial to rally their support for and involvement in the program before implementation begins.

- At first, training was not long enough, and it needed to be extended so that staff would be equipped with the necessary skills and information to do their jobs. Continuous training is needed to maintain the necessary numbers of staff.

> Adolescents that participate in the clubs are the ones that are motivated to attend. It might be that those adolescents who don't attend the clubs frequently are the most at risk of contracting HIV.
>
> *Program coordinator*

- The initial aim was to work with very young children, to allow them to grow and develop with the program. However, the core group did not want a program to work for children younger than 10 years of age. In the future, the program coordinator would like to target a younger age group. This is a problem that is still being faced.
- It is important to be innovative and try out new ideas, such as educational picnics.
- One major challenge was how to scale up the program. The logistics of running the program on a large scale are far more complicated, and these need to be thought through carefully if the program is to work on a larger scale.
- There is a high drop-out rate of volunteers because of the lack of (monetary) incentives.
- Sometimes it took longer than anticipated to receive the needed funds from SIDA. These delays can cause problems.
- Sufficient quantities of materials are not always available.
- Lack of staff at senior levels has led to a backlog of work that still remains.

Evaluation

In 2000, an evaluation was carried out to assess knowledge, attitudes, and practices (KAP) in relation to SRH/FLE by Institute of Economic and Social Research at the University of Zambia. The general aim of this study was to document and evaluate the KARHP to determine its achievements and/or limitations based on process, outcome, and impact measures.

A cross-sectional survey of 10- to 24-year-old youth in households was undertaken in the project sites (371 youths) and in out-of-project sites (87 youths). In addition, focus group discussions and individual, in-depth interviews were conducted with project staff, peer educators and counselors, trainers, CBDs, parents, and teachers (altogether, 70 people). A semistructured questionnaire was used to collect information from the 458 youths.

The results showed that the problems identified in the needs assessment (prostitution, unwanted pregnancy, drug abuse, STIs, poverty, and unemployment) were still problems faced by young people, but the focus groups were unanimous that these problems were worse before the KARHP program. They felt that KARHP activities were directly responsible for these changes.

A copy of the evaluation is available. Please see Available Materials in part D.

UNAIDS Benchmarks

	Benchmark	Attainment	Comments
1	Recognizes the child/youth as a learner who already knows, feels, and can do in relation to healthy development and HIV/AIDS-related prevention.	✓	The youth have been involved in various stages of the design, planning, and implementation of the KARHP activities since the beginning of the project. The targeted youth are encouraged to express their SRH needs and find their own solutions to problems and risky sexual behaviors.

	Benchmark	Attainment	Comments
2	Focuses on risks that are most common to the learning group and that responses are appropriate and targeted to the age group.	Partially fulfilled	A needs assessment was carried out before the implementation of the program. The findings were used to develop the program. The peer educators being from the same age group as the members of the clubs ensures that the risks most common to this age group ae addressed. There is no age-specific targeting of messages. Although the messages are built upon during the course of the year, ideally different types of messages need to be imparted to different age groups. The wide age range of young people targeted could mean that some may be too young or too old to relate to their peer educator/counselor.
3	Includes not only knowledge but also attitudes and skills needed for prevention.	✓	The program tries to increase people's knowledge, and also to equip them with new skills and new attitudes. This multi-dimensional approach is more likely to result in behavioral changes than any one approach.
4	Understands the impact of relationships on behavior change and reinforces positive social values.	✓	The KAAHP actively promotes and tries to reinforce positive social values. The main principle behind the program is its focus on behavior change through peer education.
5	Is based on analysis of learners' needs and a broader situation assessment.	✓	The program design is based on an analysis of the needs of the target group and the program materials directly establish and tackle the risks the youth face. For example, even though the program advocates abstinence, it recognizes that some adolescents are sexually active, and they show their respect for this decision through the distribution of contraceptives.
6	Has training and continuous support of teachers and other service providers.	✓	Training, refresher training, and workshops are offered for all staff and members of the community who wish to be involved in the program. A support network exists so that all members of staff have someone they can refer to.

	Benchmark	Attainment	Comments
7	Uses multiple and participatory learning activities and strategies.	✓	A wide variety of activities and strategies is used to convey the program's messages, making it more likely for messages to be listened to and understood. Participatory and innovative activities include drama, sports, educational picnics, and puppet shows.
8	Involves the wider community.	✓	The program realizes that confronting HIV/AIDS requires the involvement, education, and collaboration of the entire community. It has achieved this through advocacy and collaboration between different sections and institutions within the society.
9	Ensures sequence, progression, and continuity of messages.	Partially fulfilled	The program follows a curriculum on SRH. However, because the same curriculum is covered each year, it may be hard to tackle any issues in depth or to build on existing knowledge and messages. Because the materials are not age specific, there is doubt as to whether the messages do increase in complexity as the youth grow.
10	Is placed in an appropriate context in the school curriculum.	Not applicable	The school curriculum at present does not educate youth on issues related to HIV/AIDS. Therefore, KARHP is the only medium through which they receive HIV/AIDS education.
11	Lasts a sufficient time to meet program goals and objectives.	Partially fulfilled	There is some concern that because the same curriculum is used for all age groups, some children may not attend the clubs regularly and forget the skills and knowledge they have been taught. The evaluation shows that there have been noticeable changes in the sexual behavior among those youth who have been reached by the program. The program activities have been integrated in the government offices, and thus the programs have continuity, even though the NGOs have phased out their assistance.

	Benchmark	Attainment	Comments
12	Is coordinated with a wider school health promotion program.	Not applicable	There is no school health program for the KARHP to coordinate with at present.
13	Contains factually correct and consistent messages.	✓	Young persons, with the assistance of resource persons from PPAZ, FLMZ, and RFSU, designed and developed IEC brochures for the KARHP. Five brochures on different topics addressing young peoples' concerns and problems were produced and pretested. All the materials developed by KARHP (the brochures) have gone to the IEC Committee/Zambia Information Services for approval. The other materials used by KARHP can be said to be factually correct and accurate because the main sources of information have been based on the materials developed by Ministry of Health, CBoH, UNFPA, Society for Family Health, PPAZ, FLMZ, and RFSU. Some new materials have recently been developed in response to the needs of the target groups.
14	Has established political support through intense advocacy to overcome barriers and go to scale.	✓	Advocacy has been an important element of this program. Government and the community have been involved throughout the course of development, enabling it to evolve and expand.
15	Portrays human sexuality as a healthy and normal part of life, and is not derogatory against gender, race, ethnicity, or sexual orientation.	✓	Sexuality has been portrayed as a normal part of human life that starts from a very tender age and goes on throughout one's life. The program targets youth irrespective of their gender and ethnic background. The curriculum of the training and FLE Clubs deals with and discusses issues of different sexual orientations, such as homosexuality.
16	Includes monitoring and evaluation.	✓	An effective program needs to monitor the changing needs and risks of its target group and alter the program accordingly. The program achieved this by holding meetings to discuss problems and come up with solutions. KARHP lacked continuous evaluation. It was only evaluated once by exernal evaluators, and there was no evaluation at the end of the project.

PART D: ADDITIONAL INFORMATION

Organizations and Contacts

Kafue Adolescent Reproductive Health Project (KARHP)
Francis Joseph Phiri, project coordinator
P.O. Box 360254,
Kafue, Zambia
Cell phone: +260 97 78 36 13
E-mail: kafyth@zamnet.zm

Family Life Movement of Zambia (FLMZ)
FLMZ is a voluntary NGO without religious or political affiliations that was founded in 1981. It has four provincial officers that operate in Choma, Copperbelt, Monze, and Lusaka. FLMZ also has affiliate offices in all provinces of the country.

The main objective of FLMZ is to promote a healthy and happy family life through the services offered to the communities.

Mr. Raymond Muchindo, acting executive director
P.O. Box 37644,
Lusaka, Zambia
Telephone: +260 1 221898
Fax: +260 1 221898
E-mail: flmz@zamnet.zm

Planned Parenthood Association of Zambia (PPAZ)
PPAZ is a voluntary, nonprofit, nondiscriminatory, nonpolitical NGO that is a pioneer family planning organization in Zambia, formed and registered in 1972. It receives most of its funding for program activities from the International Planned Parenthood Federation (IPPF). PPAZ operates in all nine provinces of Zambia, and it is the largest NGO providing family planning and SRH services in both the urban and rural areas of the country.

PPAZ implements projects to address SRH concerns in Zambia, including the Family Health Promotion Project, women's empowerment, the FLE Project, the Community-Based Distribution Project, the Family Planning Centers/Family Health Project, male involvement in family planning, the Integrated Project, and KARHP.

Mr. Godfrey Musonda, executive director
P.O. Box 32221
Lusaka, Zambia
Telephone: +260 1 228178; +260 1 228198
Fax: +260 1 228165
E-mail: ppaz@zamnet.zm
Website: www.ppaz.zm

Contributors to the Report

This report was prepared by Anne Salmi, M.A., Education and International Development: Health Promotion. Anne is an independent consultant living and working in Zambia (e-mail: annesalmi@yahoo.com).

It was guided by Michael J. Kelly, M.A., Ph.D., Educational Psychology. Michael has worked extensively on HIV/AIDS prevention in Zambia and is currently based at the University of Zambia (e-mail: mjkelly@zamnet.zm).

Edited by Katie Tripp and Helen Baños Smith.

We appreciate the help of the following members of Kafue district in providing much of the information in this report:

Godfrey Musonda — executive director, PPAZ
R. D. Muchindu — acting executive director, FLMZ
Francis Phiri — project coordinator
Nine peer educators and counselors from Naboye Secondary School, Kafue
Twelve matrons and patrons of the FLE Clubs from several schools in Kafue (Nakatete Basic School [2], Mutendere Basic School [3], Nangongwe Basic School [1], Kasenje Basic School [3], Soloboni School [2], and Kafue Day Secondary School [1])
Paul K. Chinyama — parent and elder educator and trainer (for organizing the focus group discussions and the visit to the Kafue Day Secondary School)
Kafue Day Secondary School headmaster, matron, peer educators and counselors, and other students

Available Materials

To obtain these materials, please contact ibeaids@ibe.unesco.org or Education for HIV/AIDS Prevention, International Bureau of Education, C.P. 199, 1211 Geneva 20, Switzerland.

"What's Up Kafue? An Assessment of the Livelihood, Sexual Health and Needs of Young People in Kafue District"
(order number: KARHP01)

Family Life Education: A Manual for Parent Educators
(order number: KARHP02)

Family Life Education: A Curriculum for Teachers and Trainers
(order number: KARHP03)

"In School Training for Peer Education Programme (PEP) 2002"
(order number: KARHP04)

"Training of Trainers Workshop 1999"
(order number: KARHP05)

Facilitator's Guide to Participatory Practice in HIV/AIDS Work: Gender and Sexuality in Young Men's Lives
(order number: KARHP06)

"National Workshop: Youth Empowerment"
(order number: KARHP07)

"Documentation and Evaluation of the Kafue Adolescent Reproductive Health Project, August 2000"
(order number: KARHP08)

Annual Report 2000
(order number: KARHP09)

"Report on the Training of Teachers in Family Life Education and Sexual Reproductive Health"
(order number: KARHP10)

"Report on the Parliamentarians' Advocacy Workshop, November 1999"
(order number: KARHP11)

"Report on the Sensitisation Workshops of Health Providers, September 2000"
(order number: KARHP12)

Brochures:
Sexually Transmitted Infections
What's Up on Drugs and Alcohol?
Early Marriage: Know the Facts
Avoiding Many Sexual Partners: What You Should Know
Facts About Growing Up
(order number: KARHP13)

APPENDIX 1. STAFF ROLES

Main Program Staff Roles

Executive Directors of PPAZ and FLMZ
The directors are in charge of the project, the allocation of funds, and approval of changes to project activities

The Core Group
The core group at central level is composed of representatives from the two local NGOs (PPAZ, FLMZ) and from the CBoH. The functions of the core group are development of annual plans, implementation, coordination, reporting, training, monitoring accounts, providing technical support to the project coordinator, and evaluation.

The local core group consists of representatives from local institutions, namely the PPAZ local branch, FLMZ local branch, Department of Social Welfare, Department of Community Development, DEO, Kafue District Council, DHMT, peer educators, and local community leaders. It provides support to project activities and aims to strengthen local collaboration. It also focuses on facilitating the integration of FLE/SRH activities into the district public health, community and social, and educational systems.

KARHP Project Coordinator
The coordinator has had previous experience in SRH and FLE and is responsible for overseeing the selection and training of staff, coordinating meetings between various program staff, and organizing community and FLE Club events.

KARHP Program Assistants
The assistants have had previous experience in SRH and FLE. They assist the project coordinator in the day-to-day running of the project.

Master Trainers
Master trainers are actively involved at the beginning of the program, and are responsible for training all staff and the TOTs.

TOTs
The TOTs are teachers, police officers, members of local government, parent and elder educators, and peer educators who have been trained to train members of staff. They are responsible for organizing all staff training, workshops, and refresher courses, and organizing outside trainers to aid training workshops.

Peer Educators and Counselors
They are the main point of contact with the youth and are responsible for the day-to-day running of the FLE Clubs and other activities.

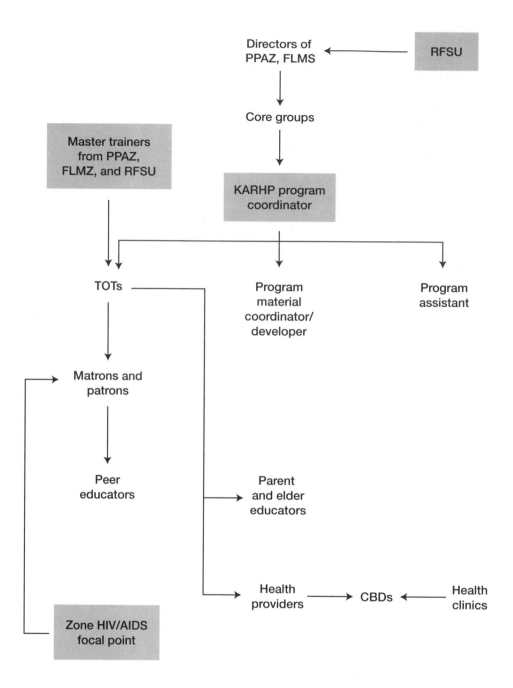

Note: All staff in boxes are collaborators but are not part of the main staff structure.

Figure A1. Staff Structure.

Matrons and Patrons

These are teachers who are trained as matrons and patrons and who are responsible for helping with the organization of the FLE Clubs and providing guidance to the peer educators.

Parent and Elder Educators

They are responsible for working among the community and mobilizing community support for the program.

Youth-Friendly Health Providers

These providers work in the clinics and provide advice to young people seeking advice about contraceptives, HIV/AIDS and STDs, pregnancy, and other issues related to SRH.

CBDs

CBDs are young people trained in the delivery of SRH messages, including other family planning and contraceptive methods (such as condoms) to youth in the communities. They help to bridge the gap between the clinic and the youth.

APPENDIX 2. STAFF DATA

	Number of staff	Position/title	Gender
Full-time and paid	1	Program coordinator	Male
	2	Program assistants	1 male, 1 female
Volunteer staff, other than peer educators (not receiving allowances/ incentives)	80 (estimated)	Matrons and patrons	Male and female
	200 (estimated)	Parent elder educators	Male and female
	13	Community-based distributors	Male and female
	20	Master trainers	Male and female
	50 (estimated)	Trainers of trainers	Male and female
	28 (300 sensitized)	Youth-friendly health providers	Male and female
Volunteer peer educators (not receiving allowances/ incentives)	500 (some 50 are counselors)	Peer educators and counselors	Male and female

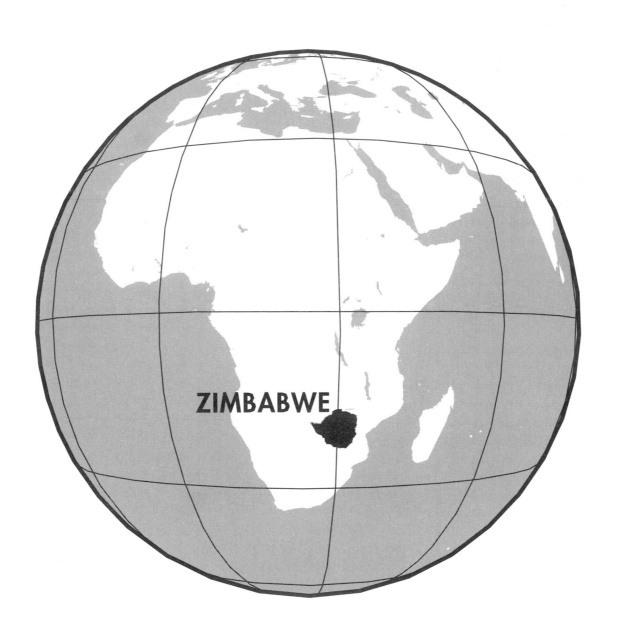

ZIMBABWE

Africare: Adolescent Reproductive Health Project; AIDS Action Clubs in Schools

PART A: THE PROGRAM

Program Rationale and History

The Zimbabwean Ministry of Education, Sport and Culture called for the participation of other sectors involved in youth AIDS education to help confront the HIV/AIDS problem. Africare, a Zimbabwean nongovernmental organization (NGO), was already conducting adolescent sexual and reproductive health (ASRH) programs in Bindura and Mount Darwin districts. Africare decided to respond to the government plea by expanding its programs to include HIV/AIDS education.

In June 2000, Africare carried out a needs assessment to examine the factors influencing youth's sexual behavior and their attitudes toward sex. Based on the findings of the needs assessment, school-based AIDS Action Clubs and income-generating programs were established in 2000. They were established in 26 schools (17 primary and 9 secondary schools) and targeted more than 20,000 in-school children and adolescents. In the AIDS Action Clubs, peer educators were responsible for establishing a variety of ways of conveying messages to young people about their sexual health. Toward the end of 2000, a further 34 clubs were established.

> Because of the major gaps between knowledge and behavior change even among the adult population in Zimbabwe, the program is making efforts to focus on teaching skills that will encourage behavior change, such as skills to negotiate, assertiveness, and the provision of role models.
>
> *Program officer*

Income generating activities were implemented to help children develop practical skills and encourage them to become self-reliant in the future. To take part in income-generating activities, a child or adolescent has to become a member of an AIDS Action

Club. Most children were very interested in income-generating activities, so this was a good way of encouraging them to join the clubs and learn about AIDS.

To ensure community support for the clubs and income-generating activities, sensitization meetings were held with community leaders such as chiefs, counselors, and youth leaders. The leaders agreed to endorse the clubs, giving them legitimacy within the community. Furthermore, the youth community development groups (YCDGs; community-based groups formed by youths and/or traditional leaders for social or economic reasons) agreed to help in the maintenance of the income-generating activities.

An evaluation was carried out by an independent consultant at the end of 2000. The evaluation showed a decrease in risky behaviors and vulnerability to HIV/AIDS among the targeted youth. As a consequence of these findings, the program is hoping to expand to other districts but is awaiting further funding.

Please see figure 1 for a time line of major program events.

> To illustrate "real life situations," educational stories of how people indulge in high-risk sexual behavior, get infected, and end up sick are taught to the club members to ensure that the youths understand the history of the disease from infection to death.
>
> *Program coordinator*

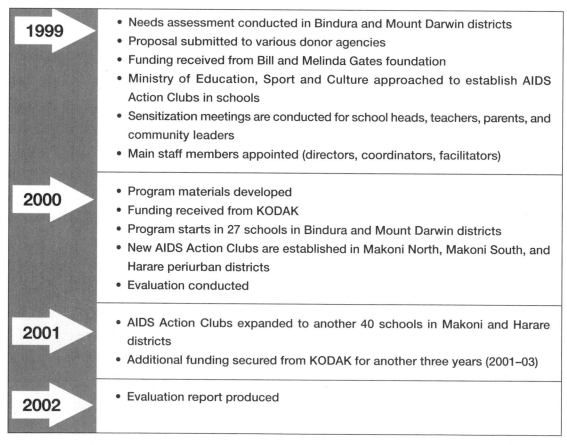

Figure 1. Time Line of Major Program Events

- **1999**
  - Needs assessment conducted in Bindura and Mount Darwin districts
  - Proposal submitted to various donor agencies
  - Funding received from Bill and Melinda Gates foundation
  - Ministry of Education, Sport and Culture approached to establish AIDS Action Clubs in schools
  - Sensitization meetings are conducted for school heads, teachers, parents, and community leaders
  - Main staff members appointed (directors, coordinators, facilitators)

- **2000**
  - Program materials developed
  - Funding received from KODAK
  - Program starts in 27 schools in Bindura and Mount Darwin districts
  - New AIDS Action Clubs are established in Makoni North, Makoni South, and Harare periurban districts
  - Evaluation conducted

- **2001**
  - AIDS Action Clubs expanded to another 40 schools in Makoni and Harare districts
  - Additional funding secured from KODAK for another three years (2001–03)

- **2002**
  - Evaluation report produced

Program Overview

Aim

The aims of the program are to effectively reach 10- to 24-year-old youths in Bindura, Mount Darwin, Makoni, and Harare districts with sexual and reproductive health (SRH) information and promote positive attitudes and behaviors toward sex. The program also aims to teach youth practical skills to generate income and become self-sufficient.

Objectives

According to the program manager, the program objectives are to

Collaboration occurs among schools through activities that are often coordinated through the District Education Offices, such as quizzes and other interschool competitions.

Program coordinator

- instill in-depth knowledge and promote positive attitudes about HIV/AIDS and sexually transmitted diseases (STDs) among youth,
- equip youth with life skills to enable them to make informed choices on SRH,
- facilitate young people's access to SRHservices,
- empower youth with self-reliant skills through business development skills training and income-generating activities,
- enhance leadership qualities and interpersonal communication skills among the youth, and
- establish and strengthen links with relevant organizations, ministries, and other key stake-holders.

Target Groups

Primary Target Group

The primary target group is 10,500 in-school and out-of-school youth aged between 10 and 24 years in Bindura and Mount Darwin districts of Mashonaland Central province, Makoni North and South districts in Manicaland province, and urban Harare.

Secondary Target Groups

The secondary target groups are

- teachers, who are trained to work as supervisors (patrons and matrons) of the AIDS Action Clubs;
- parents, who are encouraged to improve parent-child communication, especially on issues concerning SRH; and
- children in difficult circumstances — for example, orphans and other vulnerable children, who are offered support and assistance with school fees, food, and clothing from funds raised from income-generating projects.

Site

For in-school youth, the AIDS Action Clubs and the income-generating activities take place in schools. For out-of-school youth, the club activities take place in community halls and other venues available to them. The income-generating projects take place at growth points (a business center in a district designated by the government for further development) and other business centers.

The program also maintains links between the community and health centers.

Program Length

Club membership is open to any person younger than 24 years. The youth are free to continue in the program as long as they wish. Because the program has been running only for two years, the average length of stay is difficult to determine. However, no youth has yet dropped out of the program voluntarily. If a club member transfers to another school, he or she is encouraged to join a club if the new school has one.

Program Goals

According to the program coordinator, all of these goals are actually equally important because they are complementary — one cannot work without the other. However, the main focus of the program is behavior change; motivation for abstinence and delaying the age of first sexual experience are also emphasized. Behavior change is perceived as the cornerstone that will result in the achievement of all other goals. Through behavior change, the youth will be able to avoid contracting STDs and will also respect their rights and the rights of other young people.

Approaches

Club Approaches
- Behavior change,
- peer education,
- sexuality and HIV/AIDS education,
- moral behavior and social values,
- respecting individual rights,
- building self-esteem and self-efficacy,
- life enhancement skills,
- HIV/AIDS counseling,
- SRH, and
- communication skills.

Community Approaches
- Communication skills,
- moral behavior,
- HIV/AIDS counseling, and
- income-generating projects.

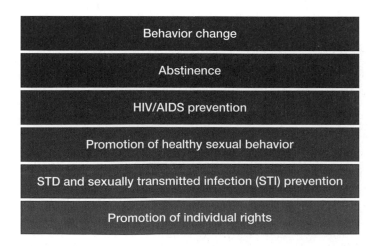

Figure 2. Program Goals Ranked in Increasing Importance by the Program Coordinator

The program emphasizes peer education and life skills training. Peer education is a critical approach because young people are thought to be the most effective mediators in influencing group norms in relation to HIV/AIDS in their own community. Life skills training equips youth with useful skills, such as communication, decisionmaking, managing emotions, assertiveness, and self-esteem building. They are also taught how to manage peer pressure, as well as relationship skills and creating awareness on HIV/AIDS, not only within the school but also in the community.

Educating patrons, matrons and school heads in parent-child communication and counseling skills is seen as important in making children's and adolescents' environment more youth-friendly.

Income-generating projects not only empower youth economically, but also enable them to distribute HIV/AIDS information. For example, when a person comes for a service, the youth use this opportunity to distribute leaflets on HIV/AIDS.

> Using peers has helped to sanction behavior among the children. For example, girls now avoid situations where they will be at risk of abuse by elders or teachers by only running errands to teachers' houses in pairs or small groups. As role models, the peers have helped instill a sense of responsibility, and this has resulted in behavior change.
>
> *Program coordinator*

Activities

The major activities carried out in the program are listed in figure 3.

It is crucial in all activities that the youth work out what their own problems are, why they have them, and come up with their own solutions. Group discussions are the primary means of considering topical issues that emerge from drama and role plays.

The program coordinator said that drama and role plays were very popular, and research has shown them to be effective tools. In addition, music was found to be very effective because song and dance are used in African culture to mobilize and inform people. Lectures were the least effective and least popular method of disseminating information because young people found them boring. It was unclear, however, which of these activities are actually most effective in promoting positive behavior change.

Components

The program consists of two main components:
1. AIDS Action Clubs and
2. income-generating activities.

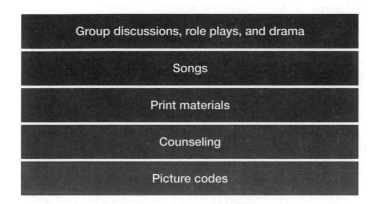

Figure 3. Activities Ranked in Increasing Frequency of Use

AIDS Action Clubs

Each club has approximately 30 members who meet once a week, either at school (for the in-school youth) or at the income-generating site or community hall (for the out-of-school youth). The club sessions last one to two hours for in-school youth, and as long as it takes to fully discuss a topic (usually a whole morning or afternoon) for out-of-school youth.

When a boy comes to collect his shoes, we put a message in the shoe. He has no choice but to notice and read it. By so doing, we reach many youth who do not want to attend our peer education sessions.

Peer educator

The clubs are organized by patrons and matrons, but it is the peer educators who decide which topics to discuss and what activities to use.

Any youth who is suffering from sexual abuse can receive one-to-one counseling from the trained patrons and matrons or from the trained program officer. With the young person's permission, he or she can also be referred to youth-friendly centers and get help with legal procedures.

Peer educators. The peer educators are members of the club. During the weekly meetings, drama, songs, and poems are performed. Practice in how to approach a person to discuss HIV/AIDS issues and child abuse, and how to use the different materials and role plays, occupies a lot of program time. The rest of the time is spent learning about HIV/AIDS, planning income-generating activities, and discussing experiences from recent peer education sessions with other students or community members.

Peer educators are responsible for club activities, as well as

- conducting one-to-one and group peer education sessions with both members and nonmembers (other youth in the school) of the clubs;
- distributing educational materials to their peers;
- developing messages for use during drama and role plays that they conduct for non–club members and the community; and
- conducting community outreach, such as door-to-door visits. (This involves visiting sick people and conducting prayers for them; offering financial support, such as paying school fees, to orphans; and encouraging other youth to join the club.)

Group sessions with girls only are also conducted as a way of building assertiveness skills and as preparation for mixed group discussions.

Case Study

Lilian, aged 13, is a member of the Chiweshe Primary School AIDS Action Club. Today the club is going to meet and discuss child abuse. Lilian has been chosen to take the role of the abused child. She is going to act with Molly, who will take the role of the mother, and Sando, who will play the uncle who abused Lilian.

In the play, Lilian appears unusually quiet to her mother, and when her mother asks what the problem is, she begins to cry. Her Uncle Sando, after hearing this, comes near so that Lilian will be afraid to say anything. Molly, however, takes her daughter to her bedroom, where, after some probing, Lilian tells her what has happened.

After the play, the children analyze the story with the help of the patron or matron.

Lizy, who is also a member of the club, says that the story helped her to identify the behavior of an abused child and what should be done to persuade her to talk. She also said that she is going to share the story with her friends and parents so that they are able to identify child abuse victims.

Patrons and matrons. There are usually two or three patrons or matrons per club (depending on the size of the school). Their major roles are to supervise the AIDS Action Club activities and support the members in their work. It is also the patrons' and matrons' job to look out for and identify signs of possible abuse and offer help in this situation. The patrons and matrons also encourage other teachers to join the clubs.

Once every quarter, patrons and matrons from different schools meet with each other and the Africare staff to share ideas and discuss problems.

AIDS action committee. The AIDS action committee, which comprises parents, peer educators, patrons, and matrons is responsible for planning the club's activities, coordinating these activities, and reviewing the progress of income-generating projects.

Income-Generating Activities

There are 21 income-generating projects in schools and 8 projects for out-of-school youth. Membership is open to youth aged between 10 and 24 years. The in-school youth work with patrons and matrons in the management of the income-generating projects, and the out-of-school youth work with traditional leaders involved in the project and with the Africare program officer.

The projects are used as a way of targeting community members with SRH education when they come to buy the products. For example, AIDS education leaflets are placed in repaired shoes.

The activities currently being implemented include carpentry, shoemaking and shoe repair, dressmaking, entertainment, poultry rearing, and oil pressing. Entertainment (particularly games) is a central component of the program activities, because the young people must enjoy themselves if they are to remain motivated.

Part of the profits is reinvested in income generation, and the rest is used for HIV/AIDS activities and providing support to the community through contributing toward school fees, uniforms, and food for orphans and other vulnerable children. A small percentage is given to out-of-school youth as an allowance.

PART B: IMPLEMENTING THE PROGRAM

Needs Assessment

The needs assessment consisted of three parts:
1. a baseline study to determine what youth know about SRH and examine their attitudes and behavior, as well as discover what problems they were facing at the individual and family levels;
2. identification of existing community-based initiatives that can be strengthened to educate, counsel, and support children, adolescents, and young adults in SRH; and
3. determination of youth interest in income-generating projects and their market feasibility.
   * The baseline survey was carried out by a team of professionals from Africare over one month.

- Information was collected on knowledge related to HIVAIDS and STDs/STIs, attitudes toward relationships and sex, and sexual behavior.
- Teachers and pupils were targeted in schools, and parents and community members were targeted in community halls.
- The information was collected through focus group discussions and individual questionnaires.
- In total, 230 people (teachers, youth, parents, and community members) participated.

The major findings showed that youth faced many problems, including STDs and HIV/AIDS, drug and alcohol abuse, unwanted pregnancies, sexual abuse, prostitution, and unemployment. The majority of youth had their first sexual encounter between the ages of 9 and 15. They indulged in sex as a form of experiment and often without any form of protection, even though awareness of HIV/AIDS, how to catch it, and how to avoid it was almost universal. Most youth also reported the unavailability of youth-friendly services where they could learn about family planning.

Most youths lacked the capacity for assertiveness in decision-making on issues related to health and sexuality.

Needs assessment

The breakdown in the family support system was reported to have left a gap of who should provide advice to the youth as they grow up. It was evident that the media, such as radio, television, and newspapers, had become the main source of information for the youth. Parents also reported that their children were not listening to them.

However, since the sample sizes used were small, it is difficult to draw any strong conclusions. Please see appendix 3 of this chapter for more details.

The findings from the baseline survey and the information collected from the district health officer gave a good understanding of the SRH needs of the target population(s).

Program Materials

Africare used the results of the needs assessment to produce a number of materials for use in the AIDS Action Clubs, including training manuals, leaflets, and posters. The training manuals took about four months to design, develop, and distribute. Africare consulted with a number of organizations involved in peer education and youth projects in preparing these manuals.

The youth were involved in the design and production of the other materials. Information, education, and communication officers from the Ministry of Health and Child Welfare also edited these materials before they were produced and widely disseminated.

All the materials were developed in such a way that the topics are not only relevant but have sequence, progression, and continuity of messages. They are written in English.

Staff Training Materials

All of the staff training materials are used to train both the patrons and matrons and the peer educators. The *Child Sexual Abuse Manual* is also used to train school heads and teachers how to identify a child suffering from abuse.

The HIV/AIDS Education and Communication Manual

The HIV/AIDS Education and Communication Manual gives steps and guidelines on how to conduct peer education training for adolescents. The manual covers these topics:
- What is HIV/AIDS?
- Does HIV/AIDS exist?
- Beliefs concerning HIV/AIDS.
- How is HIV transmitted?

- STDs.
- Signs and symptoms of HIV and AIDS.
- HIV testing.
- Prevention of HIV.
- Cultural aspects of sex and marriage.

The manual also looks at the impact of HIV/AIDS at the individual, family, and community levels, and teaches counseling and communication skills.

The manual also shows how different methods, such as drama, role play, and group discussions, can be used to teach about HIV/AIDS. Although it does not specifically target different age groups, it can be adapted to the target group. The program's messages have been consistent and revolve around abstinence and safer sex.

Copies of this manual are available. Please see Available Materials in part D of this chapter.

> Today, the aunties who used to teach our children are no longer. As a mother, I cannot teach my child about sex. That is taboo. Also, I do not trust the aunt anymore and therefore would not approve her teaching my child.
>
> *Parent*

The Child Sexual Abuse Manual

The Child Sexual Abuse Manual is a guide on how to deal with issues of child sexual abuse, including counseling, how to identify an abused child, how the family can respond to sexual abuse, treatment strategy, and therapy. For more information, please see appendix 4 to this chapter.

Copies of this manual are available. Please see Available Materials in part D of this chapter.

The Community Business Manual

The Community Business Manual gives a simple description of how to manage an income-generating project. It is used by both the patrons and those who participate in the income-generating projects.

The manual is divided into chapters that cover how to come up with an idea and determine its feasibility, business organization, production and operation, marketing and distribution, finances and bookkeeping, and sustaining and growing a community business.

For more details, please see appendix 4 of this chapter. Copies of this manual are available. Please see Available Materials in part D of this chapter.

Additional Materials

Posters and Leaflets

Africare has produced leaflets and posters in both English and local languages so that they can be understood by the greatest number of communities. Each poster or leaflet takes between two and three months to produce. The message is first discussed with the youth, then refined, edited, and printed.

Posters and leaflets used in clubs. Posters used in the clubs explain what is meant by the abbreviations HIV and AIDS. They also help to explain the immune system, how HIV infection damages it, and the types of illness that result from this damage.

Posters and leaflets used in the community. Posters promote HIV/AIDS awareness and also encourage adults to provide a youth-friendly environment and promote dialogue. They are posted in schools, halls, and shops. A leaflet entitled "Africare" describes the organization's activities, mission, and projects.

All of these materials are available. Please see Available Materials in part D of this chapter.

Staff Selection and Training

Peer Educators
- Young people join the clubs voluntarily. An average club will have about 30 members.
- They are trained by the patrons or matrons for one week using the same methods and materials used for training the patrons and matrons.
- Critically, they are taught the skills needed for healthy growth and development. They also learn skills to communicate with their peers and provide them with information on HIV/AIDS.
- At the end of the training session, participants are given a community work assignment for them to practice what they have learned.
- Quarterly refresher sessions are conducted by the Africare project officer with assistance from patrons and matrons.

Patrons and Matrons
- Patrons and matrons are volunteer teachers who are trained by professionals from Africare. There are one male and one female teacher in each club.
- The patrons and matrons are trained for five days in
  - peer education, which covers information on HIV/AIDS, and how to develop life skills;
  - how to run an AIDS Action Club; and
  - project management.
- Patrons and matrons are also trained by Africare professionals for a further five days in basic counseling skills so that they are able to deal with any problems that youth may face, particularly sexual abuse.
- Every three months, patrons and matrons attend refresher courses, which last for three days and are conducted by officers from Africare.

Head Teachers
- Head teachers are trained in counseling by the Africare project officer for 10 days.
- They are also trained in basic information on HIV/AIDS by the Africare project officer.

Parent Representatives
- Parent representatives are selected at School Development Association meetings, according to their interest in HIV/AIDS issues and their ability to understand the issues.
- They are trained in counseling by Africare for three days. This training includes parent-child communication.

Setting Up the Program

Setting Up an AIDS Action Club
- A needs assessment is conducted to determine the community's needs in terms of HIV/AIDS prevention. The community's knowledge, attitudes, and practices in relation to HIV/AIDS are examined. Other organizations implementing HIV/AIDS prevention programs are sourced for potential collaboration.
- The Africare team approaches the Ministry of Education, Sport and Culture officials in the district and province to explain the proposed program and gain support. They also present the results of the needs assessment to the officials.
- Sensitization meetings are conducted with school heads, teachers, community leaders, and parents.

- Schools are approached by Africare. Clubs are set up in schools wishing to participate.
- In participating schools, a committee is formed of patrons (one male and one female), children (usually two girls and two boys, selected on the basis of their understanding of HIV/AIDS issues and their leadership qualities), and a parent representative. The role of the committee is to coordinate the activities of the club, plan and implement HIV/AIDS awareness activities in both schools and the community, promote networking with the community members, and manage the income-generation projects. The committee also conducts meetings to review progress made by the club and promote participatory problem identification and solving.
- Teachers are trained as patrons, and club members are trained as peer educators (see above).
- The Africare project officer in the district keeps in close contact with the patrons and youth.

Setting Up an Income-Generating Project
- A workshop among club members is conducted to determine their interest in income-generating projects and what projects they would like to be involved in.
- A market survey is conducted to assess the potential of the projects.
- Youth select the projects they are interested in.
- Club members form a committee to oversee the running of the projects. The committee is made up of the Africare project officer and club members (who take the positions of chairperson, treasurer, secretary, deputy chairperson, and three committee members, to make them feel ownership of the program). Each project has a subcommittee that meets with the main committee once a month to report on activities.
- A constitution is drafted by the youth, with support from the Africare project officer. The constitution sets out the roles of the committee members, how the projects should be run, how the money should be used, and disciplinary procedures.
- Youth are trained in project management.
- The committee plans how the revenue from the income-generating projects is used.

Program Resources
The organization has a number of videos and posters, as well as a newsletter, which are kept by the project officer and also within Africare's offices. These are supplied to clubs on demand. Other materials come from the local government health clinic, the Ministry of Health and Child Welfare, and other organizations that produce such materials.

> The youth of today do not respect elders. They think we do not know anything.
>
> *Village elder*

Advocacy

Government
Before the start of the program in 1999, consultative meetings were conducted with government agencies that included Ministries of Education, Sport and Culture; Health and Child Welfare; and Public Service, Labour and Social Welfare. They agreed to give Africare their support, which helps to legitimize the program within the community. In addition, they allow school facilities and various community venues to be used for holding club meetings, talks, and program events, as well as allowing teachers to use some of their time for these activities. The Ministry of Health and Child Welfare also provides backup support through clinics and helps distribute materials and other supplies.

At the district level, regular meetings are held with the District AIDS Action Committee (DAAC), the District Education Office (DEO), and the District Social Welfare Office, who all collaborate with Africare. These meetings keep them informed of Africare's program.

Community

Community leaders and parents were consulted extensively in the development of the program content. Committees have also been established to represent the community, the parents, the school, and the youth to ensure that what happens in the program is in line with their thinking. Meetings are held three to four times per year, but this varies depending on availability.

It is also acknowledged that sustainability of the program depends on the support of the school leadership. Hence, regular meetings are held with school heads to discuss club activities and listen to the school heads' point of view.

Program Finances

So far, 25,200 in-school children and 10,000 out-of-school children have been targeted. Currently, an average of 1,200 pupils per school have been trained as peer educators.

The program received US$537,000 from the Bill and Melinda Gates Foundation in its first year and US$89,090 from Kodak in the second year. Out of these funds, 50,000 Zimbabwean dollars (ZD) are used for each of eight out-of-school income-generating projects (ZD400,000).

A breakdown of funds was not available, but the funds are mainly used for training, development of materials, consultancies, and salaries. The estimated cost per child is US$8.89 per year. (This was obtained by dividing the sum of US$537,000 plus US$89,090 by 35,200, the number of children reached, and then dividing this by the two years the program has been running.)

PART C: ASSESSMENT AND LESSONS LEARNED

Challenges and Solutions

Program Officer

Time

Peer educators are not given enough time to carry out their work or discuss all their problems. Because most schools in the program are in rural areas, most of the young people's time is taken up by doing chores at home, holding jobs, and traveling the long distance to and from school, so sessions are staggered over long periods.

Teachers

Teachers' interest in and support for the initiatives need to be maintained. One solution is for the Ministry of Education, Sport and Culture to make HIV/AIDS education in schools mandatory and examinable and provide resources to support teachers.

Monitoring and Evaluation

It is important to make sure the program changes with the needs of the target group. Periodic needs assessments are conducted by the Africare project officer through regular contacts with other program officers, the community at large, and the DAAC. However, the program would benefit from scientifically conducted monitoring and evaluation.

Empowering Children

Through peer education, the youth learn leaderships skills, responsibility, and interpersonal communication. However, it is crucial that the peer educators practice what they preach, yet in some cases this does not happen. Ways of getting around this problem are needed.

Condom Use

Despite the knowledge that some in-school youth are already indulging in risky sexual behavior, the decision to exclude condom promotion was reached as a matter of policy by the Ministry of Education, Sport and Culture; the schools; and the parents because it was seen as morally unacceptable and a sign of permissiveness. People's attitudes toward condom use need to be changed.

Sustainability

More lobbying for policy support, and for stakeholder and community involvement, is required if the initiatives are to be sustained. Furthermore, all these groups need to be involved in the planning and implementation stages if the program is to be sustainable.

Youth Involvement

Youth should be involved in the development of the program because they relate to, identify with, and respond better to messages they have some ownership of rather than those that are imposed on them. There should also be a special focus on skills building and empowerment because this is likely to be more effective in fostering positive attitudes and behaviors. Girls need to be targeted in a sensitive manner, and their participation in particular should be encouraged.

Targeting Young Children

Children should be targeted as early as possible because the younger children are the most enthusiastic and responsive in the clubs.

Materials

There is great demand from schools and the community for SRH materials. These could be obtained from other NGOs.

Orphans

There has been an increase in the number of orphans and child-headed households. The program needs to network with the government and NGOs that deal with orphans and refer orphaned club members to these organizations.

Poverty

The unstable political situation is leading to further poverty, which fuels the spread of HIV. The harsh economic environment the country is going through means the youth are also facing problems getting a market for their goods and services. Therefore, the income-generating projects should be strengthened.

Peer Educators

- Teachers need more counseling skills.
- Parents need training in parent-child communication to help improve their relationships.
- Clinics need training in how to be supportive and youth-friendly. This is particularly true for the clinics that treat sexually abused children seeking help and counseling.
- Condoms should be made more accessible.
- More needs to be done in terms of school, parent, and community support for and awareness of children who are being abused. For example, a help line could be set up or staff could be better trained in abuse issues.
- Better managers with business expertise are needed to make a success of the income-generating projects.

Evaluation

Toward the end of 2000, an evaluation was carried out by an independent consultant to determine whether Africare had met its objectives, whether the program has had an impact, and whether there had been an improvement in health outcomes. Africare staff, community members, school heads and teachers, and youths either participated in focus group discussions or were given questionnaires.

The evaluation found that the clubs have had a positive impact. The results showed that although the problems identified in the needs assessment (prostitution, unwanted pregnancy, drug abuse, STIs, poverty, and unemployment) were still there, they had been worse before the clubs started; and the clubs were directly responsible for this change. The clubs had also managed to bring about increased health-seeking behavior among the youth. For more information, please see appendix 5 to this chapter.

UNAIDS Benchmarks

	Benchmark	Attainment	Comments
1	Recognizes the child/youth as a learner who already knows, feels, and can do in relation to healthy development and HIV/AIDS-related prevention.	✓	Youth consultative workshops are a critical part of the program, and youth are also involved in the committee that runs the clubs. The youth participate in most aspects of the program, such as peer education, role plays, drama, and program planning.
2	Focuses on risks that are most common to the learning group and that responses are appropriate and targeted to the age group.	Partially fulfilled	Currently, messages target everyone in the age group 10 to 24 years old. There is therefore a need to produce materials for the primary school children who have different needs from secondary and out-of-school youth.

	Benchmark	Attainment	Comments
3	Includes not only knowledge but also attitudes and skills needed for prevention.	Partially fulfilled	The program teaches children new skills for prevention, such as assertiveness and communication. It also empowers them economically through income-generating projects.
4	Understands the impact of relationships on behavior change and reinforces positive social values.	✓	Community involvement in the program ensures that social values are maintained.
5	Is based on analysis of learners' needs and a broader situation assessment.	✓	A needs assessment was done before the inception of the program. Also, a workshop to come up with messages was conducted before the materials were produced.
6	Has training and continuous support of teachers and other service providers.	✓	Teachers who become patrons are trained in peer education and counseling. Refresher courses are held every three months to ensure that the teachers are kept up-to-date on the latest developments in HIV/AIDS.
7	Uses multiple and participatory learning activities and strategies.	✓	The program uses a wide variety of activities, including drama, role plays, peer education, and lectures.
8	Involves the wider community.	✓	The community has been involved in the planning and development of the program. Close contact is kept with them to ensure that the program will continue to be accepted and sustainable, even after donor assistance ends.
9	Ensures sequence, progression, and continuity of messages.	Partially fulfilled	The materials are not age specific, so the message does not increase in complexity as the youth grow up. However, the materials all emphasize abstinence, which shows a consistency of messages.
10	Is placed in an appropriate context in the school curriculum.	Not applicable	Although the clubs are not part of the school curriculum, they have been set up to reach as many youth as possible in an appropriate context.
11	Lasts a sufficient time to meet program goals and objectives.	✓	The program has been running for three years and is going to be extended for another two years. This is probably sufficient time for the program to show results.

	Benchmark	Attainment	Comments
12	Is coordinated with a wider school health promotion program.	Not applicable	The AIDS Action Clubs use the life skills program implemented by the Ministry of Education, Sport and Culture.
13	Contains factually correct and consistent messages.	✓	Before any materials were produced by Africare, they were circulated to experts in the Ministry of Education, Sport and Culture and in the Ministry of Health to ensure that the messages are correct, appropriate, and consistent.
14	Has established political support through intense advocacy to overcome barriers and go to scale.	✓	Africa had held a number of workshops with government, political, and community leaders to ensure that they understand and approve of the program. Advocacy activities are continuing with quarterly meetings being held with community leaders.
15	Portrays human sexuality as a healthy and normal part of life, and is not derogatory against gender, race, ethnicity, or sexual orientation.	Partially fulfilled	The program attempts to include everyone.
16	Includes monitoring and evaluation.	Partially fulfilled	Monitoring activities are carried out every month. An evaluation of the program was conducted in February 2002.

PART D: ADDITIONAL INFORMATION

Organizations and Contacts

Africare is a private, nonprofit organization dedicated to improving the quality of life in rural Africa through the development of water resources, increased food production and processing, delivery of health services, and sustainable small-enterprise development.

Further information on Africare can be obtained from

Mrs. Ruth Mufute
Country representative
Africare
P.O. Box 308
4A Hugh Fraser Drive
Harare, Zimbabwe
Telephone/fax: (263-4)-481093 or 498108 or 496453
E-mail: Africare@mweb.co.zw

Contributors to the Report

This report was prepared by Ms. Evelyn Serima, consultant to the report, and Mr. Sunday Manyenya, research assistant.

It was guided by Mr. Ebrahim Jassat, World Bank local office, and Mr. Jumbe, program director, Ministry of Education, Sport and Culture.

Edited by Helen Baños Smith.

We appreciate the help of the following members of Africare in providing much of the information in this report:

Mrs. Ruth Mufute — Country representative, Africare
Ms. C. D. Chipere — HIV/AIDS program coordinator

Available Materials

To obtain these materials, please contact ibeaids@ibe.unesco.org or Education for HIV/AIDS Prevention, International Bureau of Education, C.P. 199, 1211 Geneva 20, Switzerland.

Child Sexual Abuse Manual
(order number: Africare01)

Community Business Manual
(order number: Africare02)

"Baseline Survey"
(order number: Africare03)

"Final Evaluation Report"
(order number: Africare04)

Africare Zimbabwe pamphlet
(order number: Africare05)

Adolescent reproductive health project newsletter
(order number: Africare06)

Poster: "Empowering Youth to Celebrate Life"
(order number: Africare07)

Poster: "Equal Opportunities"
(order number: Africare08)

APPENDIX 1. AFRICARE PROGRAM ROLES

Main Program Staff Roles

HIV/AIDS Program Coordinator
Coordinates the program at the national level and provides technical support to the project officer, school heads, patrons and matrons.

Project Officer
- Coordinates the program at the district level,
- provides technical support to patrons and matrons in running the AIDS Action Clubs,
- trains schools heads, patrons and matrons in counseling,
- trains patrons and matrons as trainers of peer educators,
- conducts refresher courses for patrons and matrons,
- provides support to the out-of-school youth in running income-generating projects, and
- initiates networking activities with other NGOs.

School Heads
- Act as advisers to the AIDS Action Clubs
- promotes AIDS Action Clubs at community outreach activities.

Patrons and Matrons
- Train AIDS Action Club members as peer educators,
- ensure that club members meet weekly,
- ensure that income-generating projects are run smoothly, and
- participate in the parent, youth, patron and matron committee activities.

Peer Educators
- Are responsible for the day-to-day running of the clubs,
- provide peer education sessions to other youth, and
- function as role models for peers.

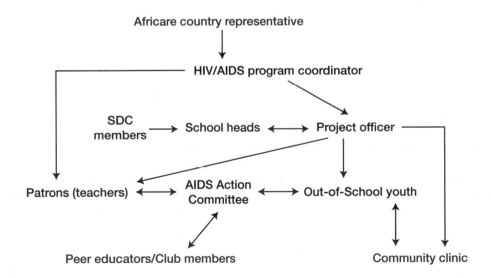

Figure A.1. NGOs: Regional and District Education Offices

APPENDIX 2. STAFF DATA

	Number of staff	Position/title	Gender
Full-time and paid	1	Program coordinator	Female
	1	Program officer	Female
Volunteer staff, other than peer educators (receiving allowances/incentives)	52	Patrons	26 Males and 26 Females

APPENDIX 3. NEEDS ASSESSMENT

Please note that because the sample sizes are very small, it is difficult to draw any strong conclusions.

Table 1. Youth Activity During Free Time

Activity	Secondary school		Out of school	
	Number	%	Number	%
At youth center	9	10.1	5	6.8
Reading novels	47	52.2	—	—
Socializing with friends	19	22.1	6	—
Growth points	—	—	15	20.3
Nothing	—	—	24	32.4
Working	—	—	14	18.9
Others	14	15.6	190	13.5
Total	89	100	254	100

Table 2. Sexual Experience

Have you ever had sex?	Secondary school		Out of school	
	Number	%	Number	%
Yes	11	12.4	47	63.5
No	78	87.6	27	36.5
Total	89	100	74	100

Table 3. Age at First Sexual Intercourse

	Adolescent category			
	Secondary school		Out-of-school	
Age group (years)	Number	%	Number	%
Younger than 10	5	50	0	0
11–15	3	30	5	11
16–19	2	20	25	54
20 and older	—	—	16	35
Total	10	100	46	100

Table 4. Whether or Not You Discuss Sex Before the Act

	Adolescent category			
	Secondary school		Out-of-school	
	Number	%	Number	%
Yes	4	40	30	63.8
No	3	30	5	10.6
It just happened	3	30	12	25.5
Total	10	100	47	100

Table 5. Reasons for Having Sexual Relations

	Adolescent category			
	Secondary school		Out of school	
Reason	Number	%	Number	%
Forced	1	10	—	—
Experimenting	7	70	10	21.3
It just happened	1	10	10	21.3
Pleasure	1	10	4	8.5
Show love	—	—	11	23.4
Wanted a baby	—	—	12	25.5
Total	10	100	47	100

Table 6. Ever Heard of HIV/AIDS (%)

	Primary school	Secondary school	Out-of-school
Yes	97.8	100	100
No	2.2	—	—
Total	100	100	100

Table 7. Respondents' Preferred Persons for Discussion of Sexuality

| | Adolescent category | | | | | |
| | Primary school | | Secondary school | | Out-of-school | |
Reason	Number	%	Number	%	Number	%
Friends	24	52.2	41	46	39	54.2
Grandparent/uncle/aunt	9	19.6	—	—	6	8.3
Parent	2	4.3	5	6	3	4.2
Teacher	—	—	16	18	8	11.1
Peer educator	—	—	14	16	—	—
Health worker	—	—	12	14	7	9.7
Partner	—	—	—	—	6	8.3
Other	11	23.9	1	1	3	4.2
Total	46	100	89	100	72	100

Table 8. Secondary School Students' Opinion on Who Should Provide Young People with Advice

	Percentage distribution (rank)
Teacher	33.0
Aunt/uncle	27.0
Parent	20.2
Grandparent	18.0

Table 9. Ways of Addressing Youth Problems

| | Percentage distribution | |
	Secondary school	Out-of-school
Sex education	41.3	32.4
Counseling	15.0	—
Projects	31.3	62.2
Recreational facilities	6.3	6.8
Workshops	—	12.2
Other	6.3	8.1

APPENDIX 4. PROGRAM MATERIALS

Child Sexual Abuse Manual

Chapter 1. Background Information
- Definitions of sexual abuse
- The extent of child abuse
- Factors associated with child abuse
- Indicators of sexual abuse
- Mediators in the effects of sexual abuse
- The family's response to sexual abuse
- The context in which the child lives
- A multisectoral approach to child abuse

Chapter 2. Counseling Skills and Treatment Strategies
- How children communicate
- How children communicate about sexual abuse
- Structuring the counseling environment
- Interviewing skills
- Obstacles in interviewing children
- Counseling skills
- A model of counseling
- Play therapy
- Use of the playroom
- Use of questions
- Assessment versus counseling
- Working with the family
- Working with groups
- Preventing revictimization of the child

Chapter 3. Issues for the Therapist
- Burnout
- Listening to stories of abuse
- The effects of your attitudes and values

The Community Business Manual

Chapter 1. Introduction

Chapter 2. Business Idea Formation
- Idea generation
- Idea evaluation
- Market research

- Resource inventory
- Choosing your business
- Applying for assistance from Africare

Chapter 3. Organizational Structure

- Organizational structure definitions

Chapter 4. Production and Operations

- Steps to create an operational plan
- Improving production and operations

Chapter 5. Marketing

- Examine the market
- Define the market
- The 4 Ps: product, price, placement, promotion
- Customers
- Competition
- Distribution/sales plan
- Advertising: word of mouth, print, events/shows

Chapter 6. Finances and Bookkeeping

- Finances
- Planning and bookkeeping
- Books: receipt book, order book, cash book, purchases book, sales book, debtors book, creditors book, stock book, asset book

Chapter 7. Sustaining and Growing Your Community Business

- Making business decisions using your books
- Understanding fixed and variable costs for your product
- Important concepts for managing your growing business
- Deciding on the uses of your profits
- Paying back the Africare loan
- Growing your business
- Reinvesting money in your local community and AIDS Action Clubs

Chapter 8. Contacting Africare

APPENDIX 5. PROGRAM EVALUATION

The main changes were

- Less denial and increasing discussion about the issues of HIV/AIDS, with high community turnout at club events.
- Increasing number of youth seeking information from the members of the AIDS Action Clubs.
- Increased number of youth referred to other service providers, including the youth-friendly services.
- Reduction in number of sexual partners among both males and females.
- Self-reported abstention and delay of onset of sexual activity.
- Fewer secondary school boy–primary school girl couples are occurring.
- Teachers have noticed a declining rate of early marriage, previously prevalent among high school girls.
- Decline in teenage pregnancy.
- One secondary school reported its highest retention rate of girls after the first two years of secondary schooling, which they solely attributed to AIDS Action Club activities.
- At the individual level, the young involved in AIDS Action Clubs have become more confident and assertive as their knowledge of SRH and interaction with the community have increased.
- Increased support from parents and leaders in the form of praise, donations (e.g., of land), and endorsement of AIDS Action Clubs–related activities.
- More compassionate treatment of people living with HIV/AIDS.
- Stronger community solidarity: Social pressure may eventually help to create new norms by discouraging behavior that is perceived as increasing risk of HIV infection.

Midlands AIDS Service Organisation (MASO): Youth Alive Initiatives Project

PART A: DESCRIPTION OF THE PROGRAM

Program Rationale and History

An HIV prevalence survey conducted in 2000 by the Zimbabwean Ministry of Health and Child Welfare showed that 27.8 percent of the youth in the 15- to 19-year-old age group were HIV positive. These high figures convinced the Midlands AIDS Service Organisation (MASO) that a program to combat the spread of HIV among youth needed to be set up.

In developing the program, two main sources of information were used. First, the findings from a needs assessments conducted by UNICEF in 1996 were used (see Needs Assessment section of this chapter for details). Second, MASO borrowed ideas from an initiative that had been established by its sister organization, the Matebeleland AIDS Council in Bulawayo district.

> The program has chosen this focus because it believes that life skills enhancement allows the youth to develop skills necessary for them to avoid high-risk situations and also empower them with negotiating skills for safer sex.
>
> *Program officer*

Before starting the program, consultative meetings were held with officials from the Ministry of Education, Sport and Culture and the Ministry of Public Service, Labour and Social Welfare. They all agreed that such a program would be useful in curbing the HIV/AIDS epidemic in schools. Meetings were also held with parents, community members, teachers, and youth to explain the idea behind the program activities and allow discussion of them before they were set up.

The program itself began in 1996 with the setting up of clubs in 12 primary schools in Gweru district. A further 19 primary schools and 10 secondary schools were added in 1997; in

2000, the program expanded to Kwekwe district, with 20 primary schools and 11 secondary schools recruited.

Both in- and out-of-school children can attend the clubs, in which a number of activities take place — including peer education, quizzes, poems, drama, songs, dance, preparations for community outreach, and production of a newsletter. The idea is that club members will be trained as peer educators and hence disseminate knowledge about HIV/AIDS and messages of behavior change to the wider community, and, in particular, their peers.

An evaluation was held in 1997 by an external consultancy agency, and a further evaluation was conducted by MASO in 1999. The evaluations examined the relevance, efficiency, effectiveness, impact, and sustainability of the project and generally found positive results. However, because there was no baseline study, it is difficult to know how effective the program actually has been.

MASO intends to expand the clubs to other districts, subject to continued funding.

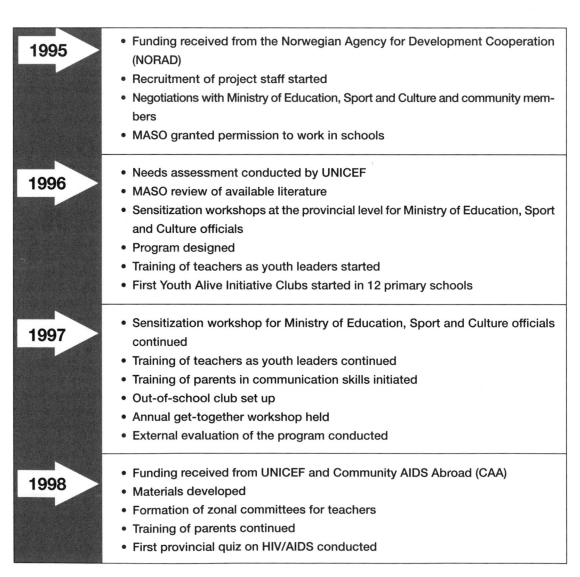

1995
- Funding received from the Norwegian Agency for Development Cooperation (NORAD)
- Recruitment of project staff started
- Negotiations with Ministry of Education, Sport and Culture and community members
- MASO granted permission to work in schools

1996
- Needs assessment conducted by UNICEF
- MASO review of available literature
- Sensitization workshops at the provincial level for Ministry of Education, Sport and Culture officials
- Program designed
- Training of teachers as youth leaders started
- First Youth Alive Initiative Clubs started in 12 primary schools

1997
- Sensitization workshop for Ministry of Education, Sport and Culture officials continued
- Training of teachers as youth leaders continued
- Training of parents in communication skills initiated
- Out-of-school club set up
- Annual get-together workshop held
- External evaluation of the program conducted

1998
- Funding received from UNICEF and Community AIDS Abroad (CAA)
- Materials developed
- Formation of zonal committees for teachers
- Training of parents continued
- First provincial quiz on HIV/AIDS conducted

Figure 1. Time Line of Major Program Events

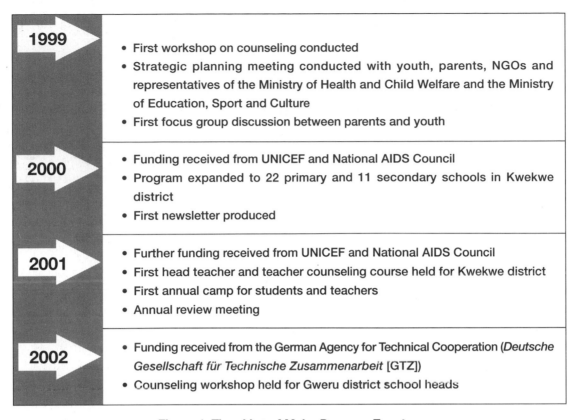

1999
- First workshop on counseling conducted
- Strategic planning meeting conducted with youth, parents, NGOs and representatives of the Ministry of Health and Child Welfare and the Ministry of Education, Sport and Culture
- First focus group discussion between parents and youth

2000
- Funding received from UNICEF and National AIDS Council
- Program expanded to 22 primary and 11 secondary schools in Kwekwe district
- First newsletter produced

2001
- Further funding received from UNICEF and National AIDS Council
- First head teacher and teacher counseling course held for Kwekwe district
- First annual camp for students and teachers
- Annual review meeting

2002
- Funding received from the German Agency for Technical Cooperation (*Deutsche Gesellschaft für Technische Zusammenarbeit* [GTZ])
- Counseling workshop held for Gweru district school heads

Figure 1. Time Line of Major Program Events

Program Overview

Aim
The main aim of the program is to equip youth between the ages of 14 and 24 years with the necessary life skills to cope with everyday life-tyle issues. This will contribute toward reducing sexually transmitted infections (STIs), HIV/AIDS, and other related problems.

Objectives
According to the program officer, the program objectives are to
- facilitate youth initiatives to prevent STIs and HIV/AIDS;
- disseminate information that is accurate, up-to-date, and clear to the target audience;
- promote a change to safer sex behaviors by target groups; and
- promote positive living among the infected and affected and ensure consistency on proven strategies of coping.

Target Groups

Primary Target Group
The primary targets are youth aged between 10 and 24 years in 74 schools (and one out-of-school club) in Kwekwe and Gweru districts who attend the Youth Alive Initiative Clubs. The program covers both rural and urban areas.

Secondary Target Group

The secondary targets are the teachers who run the clubs and those who are not members but who attend the peer educators' outreach activities (see below).

Site

The program is based in schools for in-school youth. Out-of-school youth conduct their activities in community halls, schools, or wherever they can find facilities.

Program Length

A youth can participate in the program for a maximum of 10 years and a minimum of 4 years, depending on when he or she joined the program. According to the program officer, the majority of youth who started the program in 1996 are still there. The program officer thinks youths need to attend for at least five years to gain adequate knowledge and skills to protect themselves from HIV infection and child abuse. The program itself has been operating for eight years and has the potential for continuing for at least another five years.

Program Goals

Figure 2 shows how the program officer ranked the program goals. The program focuses on behavior change and life skills enhancement through the involvement of youth and community members. The idea is that youth listen to their peers (peer educators), and by involving themselves in drama and other activities, they begin to understand issues about HIV/AIDS. Furthermore, their active participation gives them ownership of the program, and hence more incentive to maintain it.

The program emphasizes to youth that abstinence before marriage is the most effective way of preventing HIV transmission.

Approaches

According to the program officer, peer education is the best approach for considering the needs, ideas, and feelings of youth because peers understand each other better than does anyone else within the community.

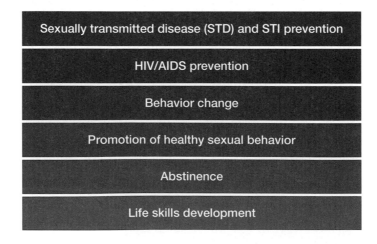

Figure 2. Program Goals Ranked in Increasing Inportance by the Program Officer

The main difference between the in-school and out-of-school youth programs is that in-school youth are not taught about contraception, including condoms.

Activities

According to the program officer, group discussions, drama, songs, and role play are the most effective methods of disseminating information to the youth and the community. This is because active involvement helps people to remember and internalize the messages, which in turn is more likely to lead to behavior change.

The program officer also felt that lectures are the least effective methods of disseminating information to the youth because they just listen and participate little. However, there was no evidence that one activity was necessarily more effective than the other.

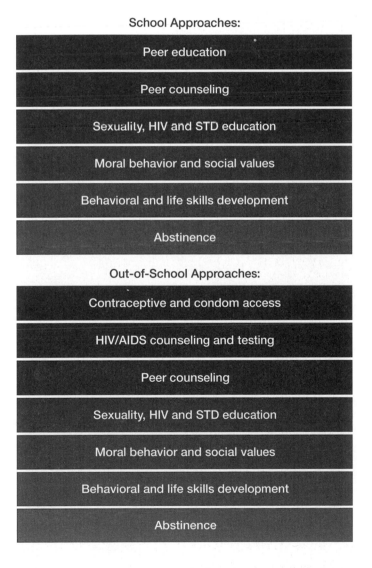

School Approaches:

- Peer education
- Peer counseling
- Sexuality, HIV and STD education
- Moral behavior and social values
- Behavioral and life skills development
- Abstinence

Out-of-School Approaches:

- Contraceptive and condom access
- HIV/AIDS counseling and testing
- Peer counseling
- Sexuality, HIV and STD education
- Moral behavior and social values
- Behavioral and life skills development
- Abstinence

Figure 3. Program Approaches Ranked in Increasing Importance

Components

The program consists of two main components:
1. Youth Alive Initiative Clubs and
2. outreach activities.

Youth Alive Initiative Clubs

The members of the Youth Alive Initiative Clubs for in-school youth meet once a week in the school during their spare time to discuss HIV/AIDS issues. This is done with supervision from youth leaders, who are teachers trained by MASO. The meetings are scheduled to take an hour, but may last longer.

> The peer approach helps youths to learn from each other and correct any misconceptions. The idea is that youth can produce their own ideas and messages.
>
> **Program officer**

In the meetings, youth are taught new topics on HIV/AIDS by youth leaders and then discuss them. They also discuss their plans for community outreach programs for the next week and review what happened in the previous week. Much time is spent practicing drama, poems, quizzes, and songs that they will perform for nonmember pupils and the community during the outreach activities. Youth also identify their fellow peers who may need assistance (for example, in the form of money for school fees or other support) and discuss how they can help.

The peer educators come up with all the ideas, but the youth leaders provide them with any information they require, and they also offer their support and guidance on how to plan the outreach activities.

Like their in-school counterparts, out-of-school youth also meet once a week with youth leaders to discuss HIV/AIDS issues and plan their community outreach schedule for the week.

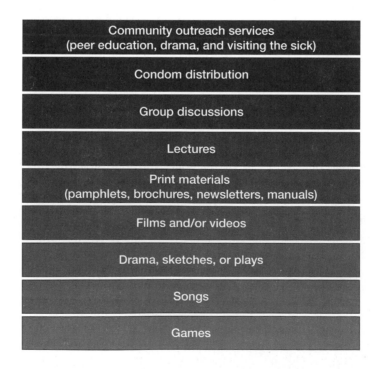

Figure 4. Program Activities Ranked in Increasing Frequency of Use

Out-of-school youth also meet every day to carry out outreach activities. As well as those activities done by in-school youth, out-of-school youth also conduct home, church, and beer hall visits; hold community meetings; and distribute literature on HIV/AIDS and condoms. They also distribute food (given to them by MASO) to people living with HIV/AIDS and sell food to those who can afford it.

Monthly feedback is given to the MASO program officer by both peer educators and youth leaders. Any plans for the month that need MASO support are discussed in these meetings.

Case Study

John is a member of the Youth Alive Initiative Club based at Midlands State University. Today the club has organized a focus group to discuss the issue of sex and peer pressure. The focus group discussion is going to be led by Chipo, a trained peer leader.

The group is made up of six male and five female students. Chipo felt that today's attendance was unusually low, possibly because students had just received their pay, so they had gone shopping.

The discussion started with the girls accusing the boys of forcing them into sex without their consent. A heated argument followed, but Chipo controlled the group by asking them to list the environments in which sex takes place. They were also asked to list the conditions that motivate them to have sex.

This list was discussed and analyzed. It was concluded that both boys and girls should try to avoid these environments because they lead young people to having sexual relations. It was also concluded that both boys and girls misunderstand each other: Boys think that if they do not have sex with their girlfriends, the girlfriend will think that they are backward; girls do not want to disappoint their boyfriends.

Youth leaders. The youth leaders are volunteer teachers who have been trained in peer education, adolescent sexual and reproductive health (ASRH), and counseling. There are usually two per school: one male and one female. They meet with the peer educators during club time, although many of them are happy to answer questions whenever they are free. The main role of the youth leaders is to run the clubs and train the peer educators. They are also responsible for conducting one-to-one counseling with youth who request it.

In addition to being responsible for the clubs, youth leaders are also responsible for referring child abuse cases to the police and youth-friendly organizations in the province, and to health clinics if the young person may have contracted an STD. Out-of-school youth leaders also do some community activities along with the out-of-school youth.

MASO organizes quarterly networking meetings for youth leaders from different schools. These are usually planning and review meetings, where progress reports from each school are given and problems are presented to MASO for discussion and consideration.

Peer educators. There are approximately 60 peer educators in each school. All peer educators are members of a Youth Alive Initiative Club. The peer educators conduct talks with their peers on different topics selected by the youth themselves. Peer education is conducted in two ways: on a one-to-one basis during a youth's spare time and in community outreach activities.

> In group discussion, youth are free to bring out their concerns and suggest solutions to deal with the problems. In drama, the youth are able to portray what happens to them in real-life situations and therefore are able to bring to the fore problems that they are facing and that the adults do not know about.
>
> *Program officer*

Outreach Activities

Peer educators conduct outreach activities as a way of reaching more youth. These might be conducted after school or in other schools and colleges (that do not have a Youth Alive Initiative Club) within the locality, as well as in community meeting areas. These activities can take a variety of forms:

- Drama and role plays are used to bring out real-life situations. The performances are followed by discussions of the problem portrayed so that the young people can learn from the stories. The audience is also encouraged to suggest possible solutions to the problem.
- Videos on various topics are used to stimulate discussions.
- Posters, leaflets, and picture codes are also used as aids to discussions.
- A newsletter for young people, *MASO Youth Alive Initiative,* is also produced. Youth contribute articles on HIV/AIDS (including poems) to this newsletter.
- Lectures and talks are presented to different youth groups and adults in the community.
- Interschool competitions are organized to integrate the community.
- Visits to give support to sick people on home-based care are made.

PART B : IMPLEMENTING THE PROGRAM

Needs Assessment

A needs assessment was carried out by UNICEF in 1996, but it was not done specifically for MASO. Rather, UNICEF wanted to conduct an analysis of the needs of youth before deciding whether to allocate funds to the region.

In-school and out-of-school, rural and urban youth aged 10 to 24 years old were asked what they knew about HIV/AIDS, where they had learned this information, and what they did in their spare time. Youth were also asked what they thought was needed in terms of sexual reproductive health (SRH) education. The major findings were:

- Young people's knowledge about HIV/AIDS was high.
- Youth were not comfortable discussing HIV/AIDS issues with their parents.
- Youth obtained most of their information from the radio and print media.
- Unemployed youth spend most of their time loitering.
- Youth are happiest with messages they have produced themselves.
- Youth would listen to peers of their age.

MASO used the idea that youth can learn from one another and that they can produce their own messages and solutions to problems when designing the program. See appendix 3 to this chapter for further details.

Program Materials

The program materials took an average of four months to develop, produce, and distribute. MASO; the Ministry of Education, Sport and Culture; the Ministry of Health and Child Welfare; and the community's youth were all involved in the materials' development. The materials were produced in English and the local language to enable every youth to understand the messages.

Materials are also obtained from the local health clinics, the Ministry of Health and Child Welfare, and other organizations working with youth.

Club Materials

MASO has produced four manuals for use by the peer leaders in the clubs. These manuals are described below in the Training Materials section.

Posters, Videos, and Leaflets

MASO has also produced leaflets, videos, and posters. The messages in these are designed to ensure continuity and consistency of messages. The youth were involved in the design of these materials.

Topics include abstinence, how to avoid drugs, and healthy eating as a way of avoiding infection or staying well if infected. The focus is on abstinence until marriage. These materials are used in both the clubs and the outreach activities. (Please see Available Materials in part D of this chapter.)

Newsletter

MASO also produces a newsletter, *MASO Youth Alive Initiative*. It is produced monthly and is compiled by MASO staff from articles submitted by youth. These articles can be poems, essays, and reports about events undertaken by the youth. In-school and out-of-school club members receive the newsletter.

> **AIDS the Killer**
>
> AIDS is not passed
> By living together
> By eating together
> Or by playing together.
>
> It is also not spread
> By shaking hands
> By kissing
> By sharing glasses or
> drinking mugs
> By swimming together
> By mosquitoes or other insects
> By giving blood at a
> blood centre or donor clinic.
>
> But AIDS is spread
> Through SEX with
> An INFECTED person.
> So be smart and say no to sex!
>
> ***By Beatrice Muvuya***
> ***Grade 6C***
> ***Mkoba 4 Primary School.***

Training Materials

As well as being used for training youth leaders, peer educators, and school heads, the manuals described below are also used in the Youth Alive Initiative Clubs.

Participatory Approaches to Community Development is primarily used by youth leaders. It informs them on how to lead the youth in the clubs in a way that ensures they are all actively participating. The manual is divided into four chapters covering these topics:
1. introduction to participatory approaches and their uses,
2. techniques and tools for collecting and analyzing data for participatory approaches,
3. how to conduct good-quality training, and
4. conducting participatory field work.

The Counseling Training Manual for Schools was designed by MASO and is used to train youth leaders, school heads, and peer educators in the counseling skills they need to talk to students, peers, and community members about HIV/AIDS. It is divided into sections that give guidance on
- the youth leader's role in counseling,
- techniques for and types of counseling,
- child abuse and how to identify it,

- how to spot a child who may have problems and what to do about it, and
- how to help children through bereavement.

Communicating About AIDS covers learning to communicate, listen, and question. Each area is dealt with in depth, and practical advice is given.

Facts About HIV/AIDS discusses HIV transmission, the course of progression from HIV infection to AIDS, signs and symptoms, and prevention. It also provides worksheets and guidelines to help work through the topics.

Copies of these manuals are available. Please see Available Materials in part D of this chapter.

Staff Selection and Training

Youth Leaders

- Youth leaders are volunteer teachers. There is one male and one female teacher in each club. When more than two teachers volunteer in a school, the youth decide which teachers they want.
- They are trained by MASO in peer education so that they are able to train the young people as peer educators. They are also trained on how to run the clubs. This involves training in planning club activities, motivating peer educators, obtaining materials, and finding contacts in the community, including other NGOs and government institutions, who can help. The training usually takes one day.
- The peer education training covers knowledge of HIV/AIDS, its transmission, signs and symptoms, and the cultural aspects of the disease.
- After the initial training, youth leaders attend three-day refresher courses everythree months.
- Youth leaders are also trained in basic counseling skills so that they are able to deal with problems that the young people may face. This training is conducted by MASO and takes one week.
- The counseling training sessions generally cover topics such as peer pressure, abstinence, facts about HIV/AIDS, supporting each other in difficult and emotional issues, and coping skills.
- Some youth leaders are also trained as trainers of trainers so that they can train more youth leaders. Their training covers presentation skills, communication skills, and participatory methodologies, and it lasts four days.

Peer Educators

- The peer educators are the only staff who are members of the Youth Alive Initiative Clubs. Each club has approximately 30 students as members.
- The peer educators are trained by the youth leaders for one week.
- The training is the same as that received by the youth leaders (see above), although less intense.
- Three-day, quarterly refresher and update sessions are conducted for peer educators by youth leaders and MASO.
- They are also trained in counseling by the youth leaders for 10 days.

School Heads

- The school heads are oriented on the importance of the Youth Alive Initiative Clubs.
- They are trained for 10 days in counseling by a MASO program officer so that they are able to deal with problems that their students might have.
- They are also trained by MASO in basic information on HIV/AIDS.

Setting Up the Program

Before MASO set up the program, the Ministry of Education, Sport and Culture and the Ministry of Public Service, Labour and Social Welfare were informed about the initiative. They all gave their consent for it to go ahead.

A three-day sensitization workshop for school heads was also conducted to inform them and encourage them to participate in the program.

How to Set Up a Youth Alive Initiative Club and Outreach Activities

The following steps are taken to set up the Youth Alive Initiative Clubs:

- A needs assessment is conducted by UNICEF to determine the knowledge and needs of the community regarding HIV/AIDS and their myths, conceptions, and attitudes toward the condition. The findings are then used to develop an appropriate program.
- MASO approaches school heads and teachers to form Youth Alive Initiative Clubs in schools.
- MASO recruits youth from within the school to join the clubs. MASO staff visit youth clubs and associations to recruit young people who are out of school.
- Committees are formed of representatives of the youth, parents, and teachers for each club. These committees meet quarterly to review program activities.
- Teachers asked to volunteer to become youth leaders. One male and one female teacher are chosen from each school to head the club.
- Volunteer teachers are trained to become youth leaders during a one-week workshop. In this workshop, they are also trained as counselors.
- Materials to be used in the program are developed by the youth, teachers, and MASO.
- Club meetings are conducted once per week to discuss issues that have arisen during the course of the week and prepare outreach activities.
- Outreach activities are organized by the youth leaders. They make arrangements with schools or community centers to be visited. Alternatively, community members approach the youth leaders and ask the club to come and give a performance.
- The MASO program officer regularly visits the project to give support and monitor progress.

> Communication between us and our parents on sexual matters is generally not encouraged within our society. Lack of communication often results in misconceptions since there is no opportunity for clarifying or dispelling them.
>
> *Youth*

Program Resources

Peer educators and youth leaders can go to the MASO offices to make photocopies and pick up any materials they need. As well as having the training manuals, posters, videos, and leaflets, MASO also has other HIV/AIDS-related materials from the Ministry of Health and Child Welfare; the Ministry of Education, Sport and Culture; and NGOs.

Advocacy

Both MASO and the community believe that community involvement is critical because youth behavior is affected by what happens in the community. If the community appreciates young people's problems, they will create an environment that is youth-friendly, which will enable youth to solve their problems. It may also encourage community members to act as role models for the youth.

Sensitization meetings in which the benefits of the program to the community were highlighted were conducted with officials from the Ministry of Education, Sport and Culture;

parents; school heads; and teachers before the start of the program. This has resulted in the program enjoying support from the community.

The club committees, composed of teachers, parents, and youth representatives, ensure that the community expectations are met in the program, and that community members have a say in the content of the program.

Program Finances

To date, US$325,245 have been received from donors to the project. The donors include NORAD, UNICEF, CAA, GTZ, and the National AIDS Council. More than 10,000 youth and 1,000 adults have benefited from the program.

During 2001, 2,000 youths and 300 adults have been involved in the program. The average cost per youth is approximately US$71 per year (that is, 2002 funding of US$143,784 divided by the current 2,000 youth beneficiaries).

See appendix 4 to this chapter for more details on program finances.

PART C: ASSESMENT, CHALLENGES, AND LESSONS LEARNED

Challenges and Solutions

MASO Director

Involvement of Youth
Involving youth in planning, implementing, monitoring, and evaluating fosters a sense of belonging and encourages commitment to the goals of the program. Working with youth as peers is more effective because they are able to relate well to each other. The importance of youth is further emphasized because there are few adult role models for youth to look up to within the community.

Lack of Technical Expertise
Training materials should be standardized so that all of the peer educators receive the same training. There is also a need for a standard monitoring and evaluation procedure.

Stigma and Cultural Taboos
AIDS still carries with it a huge stigma, and the culture does not permit open discussions on sex. Therefore, it is difficult to cover HIV/AIDS adequately in the schools because its controversial nature means it is given little time or importance.

Socioeconomics

There is a lack of human and material resources, and the current unstable political and economic situation just makes matters worse.

Continuity

The out-of-school youth and the teachers are very mobile, looking for jobs and better opportunities. Therefore, there is a high turnover rate of both youth leaders and peer educators.

> I don't like to use condoms because I think they might reduce my manhood.
>
> **Youth**

Sustainability

Use of the existing school structure ensures that the human resources, and many of the material resources, necessary to carry out a program are automatically available. This also provides easy access to a large number of youth. The use of local peer educators and other local and government structures ensured that the program would continue to go on even if MASO were to pull out. These factors help secure sustainability.

Evaluation

Two evaluations of the program have been conducted, one in 1997 and one in 1999.

1997

An evaluation of the in-school and out-of-school programs was conducted by an independent private consultancy in 1997. Interviews were held with youth, school heads, and teachers, and focus group discussions were held with parents and youth. The main aims of the evaluation were to determine the relevance, efficiency, effectiveness, impact, and sustainability of the program.

There were three main findings of the evaluation:

> The program has had a positive impact on the youth and the community they live in. Participating schools mentioned that the program had benefited them as there were signs of more responsible behavior from the children who had joined the clubs.
>
> **Head teacher**

- The youth who participated in the MASO Youth Alive Initiative Clubs had more techniques available to them to help them avoid risky behavior. This was largely due to the participatory nature of the activities used in the clubs, such as anthems, poems, drama, plays, and competitions. Club youth were also less likely to be found loitering and doing nothing productive.
- Peer education has been effective, not only in reaching the youth, but also in reaching the community leaders and parents.
- There were too many objectives and activities to be undertaken in the program for it to be effective. However, it was very difficult to measure whether the program was having a positive impact.

It is not clear what changes have been made to the program as a consequence of these findings.

1999

MASO undertook an evaluation in 1999 in collaboration with the Gweru multisectoral AIDS team, with support from UNICEF. The study looked at two main things:

- youths' impressions of the program and of sex education generally, and
- the impact of the program on youths' knowledge, attitudes, and behavior toward sex, including what they did in their spare time and where they went for information about sex.

The study covered both rural and urban areas and took the form of focus group discussions and self-administered questionnaires. A total of 241 female and 234 male youths participated.

The study found that many factors that put youth at risk were still there. For example, there was high unemployment in both rural and urban areas. The majority of the young people had a boyfriend or girlfriend: Even though they said they did not believe in sex before marriage, there was an indication that many of them were practicing unsafe sex and that condoms were not promoted within the society. A general lack of communication, particularly between different generations, probably added to the many misconceptions the youth still had. However, because no baseline data were available from before the program implementation, it is difficult to judge whether the program has improved the situation.

As a result of this evaluation, the program was enhanced further to serve the needs of the youth and community. See appendix 5 to this chapter for more details.

UNAIDS Benchmarks

	Benchmark	Attainment	Comments
1	Recognizes the child/youth as a learner who already knows, feels, and can do in relation to healthy development and HIV/AIDS-related prevention.	✓	The youth are involved in most program activities, from planning to material development, and in performances such as drama and songs.
2	Focuses on risks that are most common to the learning group and that responses are appropriate and targeted to the age group.	✓	UNICEF undertook a needs assessment that MASO took into account when designing the program. The materials produced in the program are not age specific.
3	Includes not only knowledge but also attitudes and skills needed for prevention.	✓	Besides teaching youth about HIV/AIDS, the program also involves them in income-generating activities that can empower them economically and reduce their risk of infection. The youth are encouraged to discuss what changes are necessary if they are to avoid risky behavior.
4	Understands the impact of relationships on behavior change and reinforces positive social values.	✓	The program takes into consideration the issue of peer pressure and uses peer education to promote behavior change.
5	Is based on analysis of learners' needs and a broader situation assessment.	Partially fulfilled	An evaluation was conducted soon after the program was initiated to examine the extent to which the needs of youth are taken into consideration. The program takes into account that poverty is often the cause of vulnerability. The income-generating activities are set up to prevent this.

	Benchmark	Attainment	Comments
6	Has training and continuous support of teachers and other service providers.	✓	All staff involved in the program are trained in managing clubs, peer education, and counseling. Refresher courses are held quarterly. MASO staff visit the project sites and schools from time to time to offer support.
7	Uses multiple and participatory learning activities and strategies.	✓	Participatory learning techniques — such as drama, songs, dance, poems, and role of plays — are used in the program.
8	Involves the wider community.	✓	The program involves the wider community in planning and implementation. This has been done through sensitization and planning workshops.
9	Ensures sequence, progression, and continuity of messages.	Partially fulfilled	The way the training manuals are designed ensures that there is continuity of messages. There is no age-specific targeting of materials.
10	Is placed in an appropriate context in the school curriculum.	Not applicable	There is a link between the school curriculum and what is taught in the Youth Alive Initiative Clubs, although more topics are covered in the clubs.
11	Lasts a sufficient time to meet program goals and objectives.	✓	The program runs for 10 years, which may be sufficient time to meet program objectives. However, because of youth mobility, some may leave the area before acquiring the necessary skills for behavior change.
12	Is coordinated with a wider school health promotion program.	Not applicable	The program is school based. However, besides lessons on life skills and HIV/AIDS, there are no lessons that focus on health. The program does not regularly involve itself with local clinics or other health-related institutions, but youth both in and out of school collect some leaflets from clinics on HIV/AIDS and STDs.
13	Contains factually correct and consistent messages.	✓	The materials that have been produced by MASO have been edited by experts from the Ministry of Health and Child Welfare and the Ministry of Education, Sport and Culture to ensure that they contain correct messages.

	Benchmark	Attainment	Comments
14	Has established political support through intense advocacy to overcome barriers and go to scale.	✓	Advocacy meetings are continually being held with political leaders. The government is supporting the program through the National AIDS Trust Fund from the National AIDS Council.
15	Portrays human sexuality as a healthy and normal part of life, and is not derogatory against gender, race, ethnicity, or sexual orientation.	Partially fulfilled	The program acknowledges that sexuality is a normal way of life.
16	Includes monitoring and evaluation.	✓	The program places importance on monitoring and evaluation. Monthly and quarterly meetings are held to review the progress of the program.

PART D: ADDITIONAL INFORMATION

Organizations and Contacts

MASO was formed as a volunteer organization in 1991 by citizens of the city of Gweru in the Midlands province of Zimbabwe who were concerned about the growing HIV/AIDS crisis. The organization seeks to provide emotional, physical, and spiritual support for persons living with AIDS (PWAs) and their families and friends. To prevent the spread of HIV infection, it also provides support and guidance for those who feel they are at risk.

More information on MASO and its activities can be obtained from

Director
MASO
30B 7th St.
P.O. Box 880
Gweru, Zimbabwe
Telephone: 263-54-21029 or 263-54-21937
Fax: 263-54-25237
E-mail: maso@adtech.co.zw

Contributors to the Report

This report was prepared by Ms. Evelyn Serima, consultant to the report, and Mr. Sunday Manyenya, research assistant.

It was guided by Ebrahim Jassat, World Bank local office.

Edited by Helen Baños Smith.

We appreciate the help of the following people in providing much of the information in this report:

Mr. Ticharwa Masimira — Director, MASO
Mr. Michael Matimura — Program officer, MASO
Sr. Bhebhe — Youth leader, Midlands State University
Victor Mundara — Peer educator
Beatrice Mwale — Peer educator
Fortunate Chinanga — Peer educator
Tobias Gushura — Peer educator

Available Materials

To obtain these materials, please contact ibeaids@ibe.unesco.org or Education for HIV/AIDS Prevention, International Bureau of Education, C.P. 199, 1211 Geneva 20, Switzerland.

The Counselling Training Manual for Schools
(order number: MASO01)

Participatory Approaches to Community Development: A Trainer's User Guide
(order number: MASO02)

"Peer Education Training: Timetable"
(order number: MASO03)

"Module 1A: Communication"
(order number: MASO04)

"Module 1B: Effective Communication"
(order number: MASO05)

"Module 3: Facts About HIV/AIDS"
(order number: MASO06)

"Module 4: Facts About STDs:
(order number: MASO07)

"Evaluation Report"
(order number: MASO08)

"Orphans Sensitization Workshop; Program Timetable"
(order number: MASO09)

"School Heads Sensitization Workshop; Program Timetable"
(order number: MASO10)

"Annual Report 1998"
(order number: MASO11)

"AIDS Is Our Problem"
(order number: MASO12)

"Orphan Care Program"
(order number: MASO13)

"Enrolment Certificate"
(order number: MASO14)

Poster: "Healthy Eating in the Midst of HIV/AIDS, and Some Suggestions"
(order number: MASO15)

Poster: "Smart Girls"
(order number: MASO16)

Poster: "Smart Boys"
(order number: MASO17)

Poster: "Girls and Boys and AIDS"
(order number: MASO18)

The following videos are also available directly from MASO (see contact details in part D):

More Time: Feature film produced by Media for Development (MFD) Trust, Harare, about a teenager whose life spins out of control: Thandi has to learn that playing with love may mean playing with her life. For copies, contact Media for Development, mfdadmin@mango.zw or www.samara.co.zw/mfd.

Everyone's Child: The message is that "everyone can do something to support orphaned or stressed children, and can do it well. We have the resources. The problems people experience can be overcome — in particular, the physical and emotional needs of children." (MFD, Harare)

Neria: A young woman loses her husband, and her brother-in-law invokes tradition to inherit all of her possessions yet makes no attempt to care for his late brother's family. When he tries to take the children as well, Neria fights back and seeks justice. (MFD, Harare)

The Silent Epidemic: STI/AIDS documentary produced in Uganda.

Time to Care: The Dilemma: (Uganda: Ministry of Health/USAID). Television drama, produced by the Ugandan Ministry of Health and the United States Agency for International Development (USAID), about the consequences of a married man bringing an STD into his family after a fling with an old girlfriend.

Time to Care: Face It: In the sequel to *Time to Care: The Dilemma,* the characters present mixed reactions to a newly introduced counseling and testing service in the community.

Side-by-Side: Women and AIDS in Zimbabwe: (Vision Films/Harvey McKinnon. English and Ndebele Versions). This short film, produced by Vision Films/Harvey McKinnon in both English and Ndebele versions, follows two women — a social worker and a theater director — as each uses her skills in mobilizing the community to overcome the effects of AIDS.

Karate Kids: A cartoon aimed at city kids, especially those living on the streets. Karare says, "Anyone can get AIDS. So we must protect ourselves and protect our friends." Produced by the National Film Board of Canada and Street Kids International, it can be ordered from nfbkids@nfb.ca.

APPENDIX 1. MASA PROGRAM: STAFF ROLES

Main Program Staff Roles

Program Officer
- Coordinates the program at district level;
- provides technical support to youth leaders in running the Youth Alive Initiative Clubs;
- trains school heads, youth leaders, and Youth Alive Initiative Club members in counseling;
- trains Youth Alive Initiative Club members as peer educators;
- conducts refresher courses for youth leaders and club members;
- provides support to the out-of-school youth program projects; and
- initiates networking activities with other NGOs.

Youth Leaders
- Train Youth Alive Initiative Club members as peer educators,
- ensure that club members meet weekly,
- provide counseling to club members and other youth, and
- participate in the parent, youth, and youth leader committee activities.

Peer Educators

- Are responsible for the day-to-day running of the clubs,
- provide peer education sessions to other youth,
- function as role models for peers, and
- carry out outreach activities.

NGOs: Regional and District Education Offices

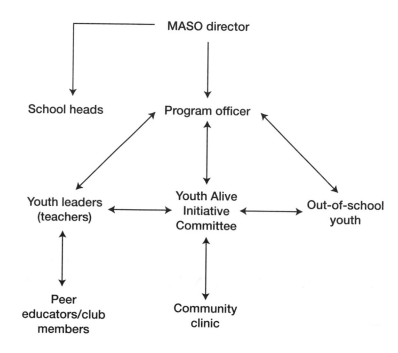

Figure A.1. Staff Structure

APPENDIX 2. STAFF DATA

	Number of Staff	Position/title	Gender
Full-time and paid	1	Project officer	Male
Volunteer staff, other than peer educators (not receiving allowances/incentives	200 teachers 140 parents	Youth leaders	50% female and 50% male
Volunteer peer educators (not receiving allowances/ incentives)	30	Peer educators	20 male and 10 female

APPENDIX 3. NEEDS ASSESSMENT

	Urban youth (%)	Rural youth (%)
Unemployed	62	78
Have a boyfriend/girlfriend	63	63
Do not believe in sex before marriage	74	69
Believe in sex on mutual agreement	16	16
Have felt peer pressure to have sex	44	21
Cannot identify someone who is HIV+	56	73
Have seen someone with AIDS	67	54
Can list three safe sex choices	65	65

APPENDIX 4. PROGRAM FINANCES

A breakdown of expenditures for 2001 shows that of the US$143,784 given to the program (NORAD, US$90.500, National AIDS Council, US$9,985.50; UNICEF, US$10,533.71; and the rest from MASO program funds), the money was spent as follows:

Spent on	Amount (US$)	Total (%)
AIDS literature and publications	49,212.67	34
Training expenses	23,954.18	17
Salaries	32,969.96	23
Vehicles	13,260.73	9
Other expenses	24,386.55	17

APPENDIX 5. EVALUATION RESULTS

Out-of-School Program

- *Relevance:* The youth program was found to be relevant because the youth targeted would otherwise be idle if there were no income-generating projects and therefore would be at a very high risk of HIV infection. Also, the rapid change in culture, loss of cultural values, experiments in drugs and alcohol, and peer pressure make fertile ground for the MASO program.
- *Efficiency:* The training of trainers approach, targeting peer educators, community leaders, and parents, used in the program has given leverage and mileage to the resources. More people are reached. The program also uses existing political and social structures, such as nursing officers, councillors, chiefs, church leaders, village community workers, and other government structure.
- Effectiveness: It was found that there was consistency between objectives, strategies, inputs, and outputs. The program design has been formulated from the identified needs. It was found, however, that there were too many objectives and activities of the program. From focus discussions with parents and youth, it was evident that the program had a positive impact. However, the evaluation noted that impact was not easily measurable.
- *Sustainability:* The evaluation concluded that the program had laid some foundation for future sustainability through the effective use of community mobilization, participation, and community ownership strategies. The use of local peer educators and other local and government structures has helped the program to anchor firmer roots within the community. Financially, the program was not sound, because most costs were funded by donors.

In-school program

- *Relevance:* The prime objective of "catching the youth before they catch AIDS" was found to be relevant in reducing HIV/AIDS among school-going youth. Students become sexually active as early as 10 years old. The MASO program was found to be more dynamic than the ministry's sex education curriculum. This was largely due to the participatory nature of the strategies through such activities as anthems, poems, drama, plays, and competitions.
- *Efficiency:* This program has managed to tap the existing school structure and requires minimal resources, motivation, and supervision.
- *Effectiveness:* The program began well and has gathered momentum. The teachers and parents at participating schools mentioned that they had benefited because there were signs of more responsible behavior from the youth who had joined the clubs.
- *Sustainability:* The program activities tapped into an existing school structure and were satisfactorily run with minimal supervision from MASO. Ownership of the program was rooted in the beneficiaries, and indications were that they were involved in planning the program activities.

Section 4: Appendix

Lessons from School-Based Approaches
to Reducing HIV/AIDS-Related Risk

Appendix.
Lessons from School-Based Approaches to Reducing HIV/AIDS-Related Risk

Please note that these reviews are derived from experience in both developing and more developed nations. "Quality" programming is essential to realizing the potential of HIV/AIDS prevention education.

The following principles are central to maximizing program outcomes.

Quality of Learner

Recognizing the Child

Recognize what the learner already knows, feels, and can do in relation to healthy development and HIV/AIDS-related risk prevention. Individuals and communities often have established mechanisms and practices for supporting children and young people to learn and develop, and these should be embraced. Encouraging learning from each other — peer to peer, teacher, family, and community — can integrate the unique and valuable knowledge and experience of learners that can make school programs more relevant and effective. Some learners will be more affected by HIV/AIDS than others — they may be orphans themselves, or they may be already caring for others who are sick, or caring for siblings. The starting point for effective teaching and learning is working toward ensuring that all learners are healthy, well nourished, ready to learn, and supported by their family and community in gaining access to education.

Relevance

Focus on the risks most likely to occur among the learners, as well as those that cause the most harm to the individual and society. Some issues attract media attention and public concern, but these may not be the most prevalent or most harmful. The program objectives, teaching methods, and materials need to be appropriate to the age, sexual experience, and culture of children and young people and the communities in which they live. Both direct and indirect factors need to be considered, for example, understanding gender and power relations and preventing violence should be integrated into programs, along with other factors where they are evident in the lives of learners. Well-targeted research, including listening to what young people believe and already know, can help to address motivation for behavior and ensure an acceptable and appropriate program.

Quality of Content

Theoretical Underpinnings

Use social learning theories as the foundation of the program.[1] Some common elements exist across these theories, including the importance of personalizing information and risk, increasing motivation for change and action, understanding and influencing social norms, enhancing personal ability to act, and developing enabling environments.[2]

More Than Information

Make decisions about the information, attitudes, and skills to include in the program content on the basis of relevance to preventing HIV/AIDS risk, developing protective behaviors, and related attitudes. Programs that address a balance of knowledge, attitudes, and skills, such as communication, negotiation, and refusal skills, have been most successful in changing behavior. Examples of risk factors for HIV/AIDS include ignorance, discriminatory attitudes toward those affected by HIV/AIDS, or lack of access to or use of condoms. Examples of protective factors include obtaining accurate information, developing positive personal values and peer groups that support safe behavior, identifying a trusted adult for support, using health services, and using condoms if sexually active.

Interrelationship

Ensure an understanding of HIV/AIDS, characteristics of individuals, the social context, and the interrelationship of these factors within program content. Programs that address just one of these components may neglect other significant influences, which can limit success. Information is necessary, but not sufficient, to prevent HIV/AIDS. The values, attitudes, and behaviors of the community, as well as of the individual, need to be addressed along with the basic facts. Responsible decisions by learners are more likely when peer and community groups demonstrate responsible attitudes and safe behavior.[3] Therefore, reinforcing clear values against risky behavior and strengthening individual values and group norms are central to HIV/AIDS prevention programs.[4]

Quality of Processes

Evidence

Build programs based on research, effective teaching and learning practice, and identified learner needs. Unilateral or single-strategy approaches — such as testimonials alone, or information alone — have failed in many cases because they ignore local needs and tend to be based on unevaluated assumptions. Analysis of learner needs and broader situation assessment should be an important source of information for shaping programs.

1. Bandura 1986; McGuire 1972; Kirby et al. 1991; Schinke et al. 1981.
2. McKee 2000.
3. Ballard, R., A. Gillespie and R. Irwin 1994. *Principles for Drug Education in Schools.* University of Canberra, Faculty of Education.
4. Kirby, D. 1997. *School-Based Programs to Reduce Sexual Risk Behaviors: A Review of Effectiveness.*

Preparation and Training

Deliver programs through trained and supported personnel within or attached to the school. The classroom teacher is in some cases the optimal person to deliver the program. In other cases, other trained facilitators or peer educators are needed. However, in cases where teachers do not deliver the program, they should be involved and activities should be reinforced in the broader school environment. Training and support at both preservice and in-service levels are required.

Teaching and Learning Methods

Use a range of teaching and learning methods with proven effects on relevant knowledge, attitudes, and risk behavior. Although there is a place for teacher-centered delivery of information or lecture, interactive or participatory methods have been proven more effective in changing key HIV/AIDS-related risk behaviors, such as delaying sex, increasing confidence or using condoms, and reducing number of sexual partners.[5] Programs with a heavy emphasis on (biological) information can improve some knowledge, but are generally not effective[6] in enhancing attitudes and skills or changing actual risk behavior.

Participation

Develop mechanisms to allow involvement of students, parents, and the wider community in all stages of the program. A collaborative approach can reinforce desired behavior through providing a supportive environment for school programs. The participation of learners and others in HIV/AIDS prevention education can help to ensure their specific needs and concerns are being met in a culturally and socially appropriate way. It can also foster commitment to or ownership of the program, which can enhance sustainability.[7]

Timing and Duration

Ensure sequence, progression, and continuity in programs over time, throughout schooling.[8] Messages about HIV/AIDS need to start early, be regular and timely, and come from a credible source. The age and stage of the learner needs to be taken into account, moving from simple to complex concepts, with later lessons reinforcing and building on earlier learning.

Placement in the Curriculum

Place HIV/AIDS prevention education in the context of other related health and social issues, such as sexual and reproductive health and population, that are relevant to children, young people, and the community in which they live. For example, "carrier subjects" such as health education or civic education can accommodate the necessary balance of knowledge, attitudes, and skills together. Over time, programs that are "integrated" or "infused" thinly throughout a curriculum without a discrete, intensive module have been generally disappointing.[9] Programs that are part of the national curricula and officially timetabled can have the advantage of greater coverage as well as greater likelihood of training, support, and actual delivery. Where nonformal approaches are utilized, they should be clearly linked to other school-based activities. Whether formal or nonformal approaches are employed, isolated or one-off programs should be avoided, as they tend to be unable to address the complexity and interrelationship of the full range of relevant issues.

---

5. Kirby and DiClemente 1994.
6. Wilson et al. 1992.
7. UNICEF. 1996. *Education: A Force for Change. World Congress Against Commercial Sexual Exploitation of Children.* Stockholm.
8. Kirby and DiClemente 1994; Botvin 2001.
9. CDC 1995; *Journal of School Health.* Gachuhi, 2000 for UNICEF, East and Southern Africa Region.

Going to Scale

For a vision of national program coverage of high quality, establish early partnerships with key ministries. Without such a vision and political commitment, activities will not move beyond pilot program status. Political investment of ministries of education and health are often central to establishing large-scale school-based programs. Encouraging links with other ministries particular to the setting, nonformal mechanisms, and the community will augment scope and capacity to reach all learners

Quality of Environments

Garnering Commitment

To influence key national leadership and mobilize the community to overcome the key barriers, use intense advocacy from the earliest planning stages. In too many cases, policymakers are not aware of key information such as the extent of HIV infection, sexually transmitted infections, teen pregnancies, and other sexual health problems among young people. Advocating with accurate and timely data can convince both communities and national leaders of the importance of prevention from an early age. It can also help ensure that programs focus on the real health needs, experience, motivation, and strengths of the target population, rather than on problems as perceived by others.[10] Communicating the evidence, listening and responding to community concerns, and valuing community opinions can help garner commitment, and effective resource mobilization will underscore the effectiveness of such efforts.

More than Education Alone

Over time, coordinate education programs with other consistent strategies, such as policies, health services, condom promotion, community development, and media approaches. Education programs work best in the context of other consistent strategies over time. Because the determinants of behavior are varied and complex, and the reach of any one program (e.g., schools) will be limited, a narrow focus on prevention education alone is unlikely to yield sustained behavior change in the long term.

Consistency

Ensure that HIV/AIDS prevention messages are consistent and coherent across the school environment. Finding ways to encourage open communication among learners, teachers, families, and the broader community is essential to recognizing and clarifying the many myths and misunderstandings that exist in relation to HIV/AIDS. School policies and practices that reinforce the program objectives maximize the potential for success.

Quality of Outcomes

The Goal

Focus on prevention and reduction of HIV/AIDS-related risks as the overall goal. Program objectives should concentrate on key behaviors that are linked to achieving the goal, such as avoiding unprotected sex and unsafe drug use, including abstinence and avoidance of intravenous drugs.

---

10. Baldo 1994.

Realizing Outcomes

Consider the full range of available strategies known to contribute to the program objectives. Some strategies are marginalized because of lack of understanding or political, religious, or cultural issues (e.g., condom use or needle exchange programs). Gathering all the available evidence from credible sources is important to choosing the most effective and acceptable strategies, and to adapting them wherever possible. Some strategies are used because they are popular, fun, or interesting, but unless they are also linked to the achievement of the objectives, the value of such approaches for achieving the intended outcome is questionable.

Long-Term View

Select programs, activities, materials, and resources on the basis of an ability to contribute to long-term positive outcomes among learners and in the school environment. Some approaches may attract media and public attention in the short term, but these may not be the most effective, especially where they are not coordinated with existing strategies. A coordinated series of short-term programs linked with longer-term outcomes should be given priority over superficially attractive stand alone, one-off, or quick-fix alternatives.

Research, Monitoring, and Evaluation

Evaluate program objectives, processes, and outcomes using realistic indicators, and allow enough time for results to be observed.

At the outset, an evaluation plan and monitoring mechanisms should set the stage for measuring the degree to which progress is made toward the objectives over time. Setting objectives that are too ambitious, and indicators that are too difficult to collect or do not accurately reflect what the program is attempting to change, are common problems. In general, much more process evaluation than outcome evaluation information is collected, and probably only a fraction of that is reported.[11] Accurately assessing and reporting the extent to which the program was implemented as planned is equally important as the ultimate outcome — changes among learners.

Address comments and suggestions to A. Valerio (avalerio@worldbank.org) and D. Bundy (dbundy@worldbank.org).

---

11. Kinsman et al. 2001.